Promoting Abstinence, Being Faithful, and Condom Use with Young Africans

Promoting Abstinence, Being Faithful, and Condom Use with Young Africans

Qualitative Findings from an Intervention Trial in Rural Tanzania

Mary Louisa Plummer

LEXINGTON BOOKS
Lanham • Boulder • New York • Toronto • Plymouth, UK

Published by Lexington Books
A wholly owned subsidary of The Rowman & Littlefield Publishing Group, Inc.
4501 Forbes Boulevard, Suite 200, Lanham, Maryland 20706
www.rowman.com

10 Thornbury Road, Plymouth PL6 7PP, United Kingdom

British Library Cataloguing in Publication Information Available

Library of Congress Cataloging-in-Publication Data

Plummer, Mary Louisa.
  Promoting abstinence, being faithful, and condom use with young Africans : qualitative
findings from an intervention trial in rural Tanzania / Mary Louisa Plummer.
     p. cm.
  Includes bibliographical references and index.
  ISBN 978-0-7391-6844-8 (cloth : alk. paper)—ISBN 978-0-7391-6845-5 (electronic)
  1. Youth—Sexual behavior—Tanzania. 2. HIV infections—Tanzania—Prevention.
  3. Safe sex in AIDS prevention—Tanzania. I. Title.
  HQ18.T34P58 2012
  362.196792009678—dc23   2012031713

Printed in the United States of America

Contents

Tables

Figures

Case Studies

Boxes

Acknowledgments

Figa moja haliinjiki chungu
One stone cannot support a cooking pot (over a fire).
[More than one person is needed to achieve a goal.]

—Swahili proverb

This book and its companion volume would not have been possible without the dedicated efforts of many people. First and foremost, I thank the villagers in Mwanza, Tanzania, who participated in this study. I am especially grateful to the families that hosted participant observation researchers, to the young people who researchers accompanied in their daily activities, and to those who participated in formal and informal interviews.

I am also indebted to the extraordinary qualitative researchers in the Health and Lifestyles Research (HALIRA) Project, who collected almost all of the data presented in this book: Halima Abdallah, Neema Busali, Gerry Mshana, Kija Nyalali, Zachayo Salamba Shigongo, and Joyce Wamoyi. Each of these individuals demonstrated remarkable fortitude and adaptability in collecting sensitive data in often trying field conditions. All of them also contributed to data coding, data summarizing, and report writing post-fieldwork. I am grateful to each of them for their many unique contributions, in particular Joyce's prolific, discerning documentation; Zachayo's invaluable critical reflections; Kija's enthusiastic and astute questioning; Gerry's articulate analytical skills; Neema's thoughtful diligence; and Halima's cheerful adaptability. It was a pleasure and an honor to work with such good-natured, hard-working, and insightful individuals.

Angela Obasi, the *MEMA kwa Vijana* intervention coordinator, also played a crucial role in the creation of this book. Critically, she developed and led the carefully designed, large-scale, and sustainable sexual health program

xv

that is examined closely here. She and her team also conducted extensive monitoring and evaluation of the intervention, and those findings provide an important complement to the HALIRA data presented in this book.

I am also very grateful to the principal investigators of the HALIRA study and the *MEMA kwa Vijana* intervention trial whose work was vital to this book and its companion volume. Daniel Wight, the lead principal investigator for the HALIRA project, developed the initial study design and helped supervise fieldwork, analyze data, and draft publications, including chapter 11 of this book, and this book's companion volume (*Young People's Lives and Sexual Relationships in Rural Africa*, Plummer and Wight, 2011). David Ross, the *MEMA kwa Vijana* trial director, led the quantitative evaluation of intervention impact while also supporting and contributing to the design, management, and write-up of both the intervention and the HALIRA study. Richard Hayes, a principal investigator for both the *MEMA kwa Vijana* trial and the HALIRA study, was generous in his time and critical input throughout the research process.

I also thank other *MEMA kwa Vijana* intervention and research staff who provided me with important logistical assistance and discerning advice during data collection and beyond, including Alessandra Anemona, John Changalucha, Kenneth Chima, Bernadette Cleophas-Mazige, Aoife Doyle, Heiner Grosskurth, Maende Makokha, Pieter Remes, Jenny Renju, Jim Todd, Deborah Watson-Jones, and Helen Weiss. Throughout the study I benefited from the support of many other administrative intervention and trial staff at the Tanzanian National Institute for Medical Research, the African Medical and Research Foundation, and the London School of Hygiene and Tropical Medicine. Of particular note are the trilingual translators, Stanslaus Shitindi, Samuel Gogomoka, Eustadius Kabika, William Kasubi, Deogratius Mazula, Daudi Ngosha, and Henry Nyalali, who brought great skill and patience to their work, as did the bilingual transcribers, Mbango Mhamba, Happiness Ng'habi, Mwanahawa Maporo, and Fatma Bakshi. Nicola Desmond, Caroline Ingall, and Tom Ingall provided indispensable assistance in coding the data analyzed in this book. Preliminary analysis of specific topics in this book was helpfully provided by Bernadette Cleophas-Mazige (youth-friendly health services) and Tom Ingall (condom use, and *MEMA kwa Vijana* school program process evaluation).

Several people generously volunteered their time and expertise to read and comment on chapters in this book. I am particularly indebted to Janet Seeley and Mustafa Kudrati, both of whom reviewed the manuscript in its entirety prior to submission. I also am grateful to others for their review of specific chapters, namely: Angela Obasi (chapters 4–6); Karen Flynn (chapters 8–10);

and Aoife Doyle, Richard Hayes, David Ross, and Daniel Wight (chapters 7 and/or 11).

At Lexington Books I thank this book's acquisition editors, Justin Race and Sabah Ghulamali, production editor Stephanie Brooks, proofreader Annette Van Deusen, and typesetter Rhonda Baker, for their patience, advice, and assistance in bringing this book to press.

Many of the people mentioned above are my friends as well as colleagues and gave me invaluable personal support during the decade of work that culminated in this book and its companion volume. In addition, I am very grateful for the humor, care, and assistance of other dear friends throughout this time, including Alexandra Terninko, Ann Ireland, Anna Sassi, Ben Steinberg, Graham Anderson, Jennifer Schoenstadt, Kathy White, Kelsey Heeringa, Kulindwa Kasubi, Lida Junghans, Ma-nee Chacaby, and Susan Cook. Members of my family—Amina, Munir, and Yasmin Kudrati-Plummer, Bascom and Nancy M. Plummer, Bob and Nancy D. Plummer, Kaye Carmichael Plummer, Gulamabbas Kudrati, and Shirin, Azher, Ammar, and Mariya Karimjee were also sources of great love and support during this work. My deepest thanks go to my husband, Mustafa Kudrati, who was patient and enthusiastic during every day, week, month, and year of this project. My final stretch of work on these books included over two years of long hours, no pay, and many sacrifices by our family, but Mustafa's loving support never wavered. Neither book would have happened without it.

The HALIRA project fieldwork and preliminary data analysis were funded by a UK Medical Research Council grant. Subsequent data analysis and publication writing were partially funded by a British Academy Post-Doctoral Fellowship and the Medical Research Council Social and Public Health Sciences Unit.

Part I

BACKGROUND

Chapter One

Introduction

Shija is a young woman who completed Year 7 of primary school when she was sixteen years old. Unlike most of her classmates, she abstained from sex while schooling because her parents were very strict and would have punished her severely if it were discovered. She also had participated in a sexual health intervention and felt supported by its message about a girl's right to refuse sex. In her last month of school, Shija meets a young farmer who she likes and who gives her monetary gifts. After three weeks they have sex for the first time, and one week later she elopes with him, because she believes a man is unlikely to marry a woman if they have an extended premarital sexual relationship. One year later Shija gives birth to a child and begins to use oral contraceptives. One year after that, she tells an interviewer she does not feel at risk of contracting HIV, because her husband is the only sexual partner she has ever had. Nonetheless she tests positive for two other sexually transmitted infections, herpes and trichomonas.

—Case Study 2.1

Makoye is a young man who was fourteen years old and in Year 4 the first time he had sex. Over the next several years he occasionally has sex with the same school girl again, and twice has onetime sexual encounters with other school girls he meets at special events. When he is seventeen years old, Makoye experiences painful genital symptoms and is diagnosed and treated for syphilis. At the age of eighteen he explains that this experience—combined with his participation in a sexual health intervention—led him to decide to abstain from sex. However, over the subsequent two years he finds it too difficult to abstain. Instead, he tries to be monogamous with a low-risk partner, but he occasionally still has onetime, unprotected sexual encounters with women he has just met. Seven

3

years later, at the age of twenty-seven, Makoye is married and working in a fishing village. At that time he explains that, unlike many male acquaintances, he actively tries to reduce his sexual health risk by avoiding sex with bar maids and other women who he considers to be high risk, or by using condoms with them. In contrast, he has unprotected intercourse with women who he considers to be low risk and who he believes will be faithful to him, such as school girls, or his wife. At this age, Makoye tests negative for HIV and other sexually transmitted infections.

—*Case Study 3.3*

Since the onset of the AIDS epidemic, the three "ABC" behaviors—abstinence, being faithful, and condom use—have been widely promoted as ways to reduce sexual health risk. At first glance these behaviors seem simple and straightforward. As Shija's and Makoye's experiences illustrate, however, each behavior can be challenging and complicated to practice safely and consistently long-term. For example, in settings where young people experience multiple pressures to have sex, long-term abstinence can require extraordinary discipline and assertiveness, and few people wish to abstain completely once they reach adulthood. Like Shija, some decide to practice long-term fidelity with one partner, but nonetheless become infected if that partner enters the relationship infected, or contracts an infection from a concurrent relationship. Like Makoye, some try to reduce their risk by only having unprotected sex with partners who they perceive to be low risk and trustworthy, while using condoms if they have sex with others. However, one's ability to assess a partner's relative risk based on appearance, observed behavior, or livelihood is inevitably limited.

Three decades into the AIDS epidemic the challenge of practicing low-risk sexual behaviors and avoiding HIV and other sexually transmitted infections remains great for young people in sub-Saharan Africa. In 2009, thirty-three million people were estimated to be infected with HIV globally, of whom 68 percent live in sub-Saharan Africa, although that region only holds 10 percent of the world's population (UNAIDS, 2010). In total, 5 percent of fifteen- to forty-nine-year-olds in sub-Saharan Africa are believed to be infected with HIV (UNAIDS, 2010).

There is some evidence that ABC promotion can increase age at sexual debut, reduce partner number, and/or increase condom use. Nonetheless, this impact has been limited, and in recent years there has been substantial debate about the relative appropriateness, feasibility, and effectiveness of each of the ABC behaviors in reducing HIV transmission. Despite this controversy, few studies have closely scrutinized how adolescent sexual health programs in Africa target each of these behaviors, examining program potential and challenges in each area in depth. Few also have studied the backgrounds and experiences of young Africans who try to practice one or more of the ABC behaviors, to better understand their motivations, strategies, and the protective and supportive factors in their lives.

This book draws on an extraordinarily large and representative qualitative study to examine both of these issues in depth. First, it evaluates a large-scale, sustainable adolescent sexual health intervention that was implemented in rural Tanzania, focusing on the program's strengths and limitations in promoting abstinence, low partner number, fidelity, and condom use. Second, it closely examines the lives, relationships, and decision-making of young people in the study area who plausibly and consistently reported those behaviors, regardless of whether they had participated in a sexual health intervention. In examining these issues, the book builds upon the findings of a companion volume (Plummer and Wight, 2011), which provided an in-depth description of the lives and sexual relationships of typical young rural Tanzanians in the absence of intervention.

This introductory chapter is divided into several sections. It begins with a description of socioeconomic conditions and the AIDS epidemic in sub-Saharan Africa at the start of the twenty-first century. This will be followed by a review of HIV prevention in the region with focus on the ABC behavioral goals, intervention approaches, and methods of program evaluation. The chapter concludes with an overview of the study that is the basis for this book, and a brief description of each of the chapters to come.

SUB-SAHARAN AFRICA AT THE START OF THE TWENTY-FIRST CENTURY

Africa south of the Sahara desert is very diverse, with forty-eight countries and over a thousand ethnic groups and languages (National Research Council, 2002), so any general overview risks gross simplification. Nevertheless, it is indisputable that most sub-Saharan countries are among the poorest in the world at the start of the new millennium. Socioeconomic circumstances vary within and between countries, but most Africans have extremely limited financial and material resources, and very poor access to health, education, water, and sanitation services (World Bank, 2006).

An estimated 63 percent of Africans and 72 percent of Tanzanians live in rural areas, which have particularly poor infrastructures and services (IFAD, 2001; Mamdani and Bangser, 2004; National Bureau of Statistics and ORC Macro, 2005). Rural residents have lower quality health, higher rates of infant mortality, and more stunted growth than urban residents (World Bank, 2005a). Most rural households cope with poverty by diversifying their sources of income, for example, raising small livestock or fishing while also cultivating cash crops and food staples, such as maize, millet, sorghum, yams, or cassava (IFAD, 2001). However, even in relatively productive seasons most rural families' diets are based almost exclusively on a few staples. In less productive seasons, consumption of even those staples can reduce substantially, causing malnourishment (IFAD, 2001).

The majority of people in both urban and rural Africa are young, largely due to high fertility and the impact of AIDS on older populations (United Nations, 2007). In 2005, 41 percent of Africans were fourteen years old or younger. By 2030, the global population of youth aged fifteen to twenty-four years is expected to increase by 17 percent, but in Africa it is expected to increase by 84 percent (United Nations, 2004).

Sexual and Reproductive Behavior and Health

Before considering sexual risk reduction in sub-Saharan Africa, it is important to review sexual and reproductive health beliefs and practices in general. Historically, it has not been unusual for young people to be sexually active by their mid-teens, whether or not they were married formally (Caldwell, Caldwell, and Quiggin, 1989). Fertility has been highly valued, almost all women have married at an early age, and couples have prioritized conceiving a pregnancy very soon after marriage (Caldwell and Caldwell, 1987; Cohen, 1998). Efficient contraception has been extremely low, including condom use. This has resulted in women giving birth to an average of six or seven children in their lifetimes. However, in recent decades fertility has declined in rural and especially urban areas, primarily due to greater use of modern contraception (Kirk and Pillet, 1998), and to a lesser extent, older age at first marriage (Cohen, 1998; Harwood-Lejeune, 2000) and the AIDS epidemic (Hinde and Mturi, 2000; Terceira et al., 2003). Contraceptive use has increased overall, because unmarried women seek to delay childbearing (Gage-Brandon and Meekers, 1993), while married women wish to increase the intervals between their children, to protect their children's health and their own future reproductive capacity (Cohen, 1998). Extramarital relationships have been common in many African societies, particularly for men (e.g., Cory, 1953; Caldwell, Caldwell, and Quiggin, 1989; Omorodian, 1993; Ferguson et al., 2004; Parikh, 2007; Jana, Nkambule, and Tumbo, 2008; Smith, 2009).

More recent research on young people's sexual behavior in sub-Saharan Africa suggests that many of these general patterns continue. For example, a review of national surveys found that in seven of nine East African countries, 11 to 23 percent of fifteen- to nineteen-year-old girls reported sex before the age of fifteen years, while 8 to 27 percent of boys reported this (Doyle et al.,

2012). More broadly, when considering national survey data for fifteen- to twenty-four-year-olds in twenty-four African countries, the review found that rural youth (particularly females) were more likely than urban youth to report early sex and childbearing, and less likely to report multiple sexual partnerships or condom use.

Relatively little is known about the history of sexually transmitted infections in sub-Saharan Africa, because there were few studies historically and they were of highly variable and questionable quality (Setel, 1999a). During the colonial period, for example, venereal syphilis was often confused with yaws, a non-sexually transmitted illness caused by a similar bacterium to the one that causes syphilis (Setel, 1999a). Similarly, in Africa there have been few historical studies of Herpes Simplex Virus 2 (hereafter simply referred to as "herpes"). Blood samples collected in the early 1980s provide some of the earliest data, revealing that herpes was very prevalent among adults in urban areas such as Brazzaville, Congo (71 percent in 1982) and Kinshasa, Zaire (41 percent in 1985) (O'Farrell et al., 1999). In general, sexually transmitted infections are prone to being underestimated because they may not have obvious symptoms, and even when they do, people may be reluctant to seek treatment because of potential stigma and cost (Gerbase et al., 1998; O'Farrell et al., 1999; Chalamilla et al., 2006). Poor health services and inconsistent collection of medical data in most African countries only exacerbate such problems (Caldwell, Caldwell, and Quiggin, 1989; Setel, 1999a). Based on the available studies, the World Health Organization estimated that in 1999 12 percent of adults in sub-Saharan Africa had a curable sexually transmitted infection (chlamydia, gonorrhea, syphilis, or trichomonas), which was a far higher rate than found in any other region in the world (WHO, 2001). The proportions of people infected with incurable sexually transmitted infections such as HIV, herpes, or Human Papilloma Virus are often higher, because once people become infected they remain infected for life.

The AIDS Epidemic

The first cases of what came to be known as the Acquired Immunodeficiency Syndrome (AIDS) were identified in North America around 1980, and shortly afterward also in central and eastern Africa (Caraël, 2006). However, the virus that causes AIDS—the Human Immunodeficiency Virus (HIV)—originated in non-human primates in Africa, and probably was transmitted to humans who hunted them or handled their meat. Genetic and molecular studies suggest that some people in west-central Africa were already infected with HIV by the early twentieth century (Etienne, Delaporte, and Peeters, 2011). Indeed, the earliest known specimens of HIV were found retrospectively in stored blood from 1959 and a stored biopsy from 1960, both of which had been collected in what is today the Democratic Republic of Congo.

Today, most countries in the world have *low level* HIV epidemics in which the HIV prevalence does not exceed 5 percent in any major subpopulation, or *concentrated* epidemics in which it exceeds 5 percent in at least one subpopulation, such as injecting drug users, men who have sex with men, or sex workers (UNAIDS, 2007; Inter-Agency Task Team on HIV and Young People, 2009; Mavedzenge et al., 2011). Several African countries, however, have *generalized* epidemics in which HIV has spread to the general adult population and can be found in more than 1 percent of pregnant women. In eastern Africa, for example, most countries have an HIV prevalence of 6 to 7 percent amongst fifteen- to forty-nine-year-olds, including the three largest countries, Kenya (6 percent), Tanzania (6 percent), and Uganda (7 percent), which together represent approximately 100 million people (UNAIDS, 2010). HIV prevalences are by far the highest in most southern African countries, where the epidemic is highly generalized or *hyperendemic*, having a prevalence exceeding 15 percent in the general adult population.

The AIDS epidemic has had a great impact on health, education, and economic growth in sub-Saharan Africa, contributing to an increase in already high infant mortality rates, and a reduction in already low average life expectancies (World Bank, 2006; UNAIDS and WHO, 2009; Beegle et al., 2010). In Swaziland, for example, which has been severely affected by the epidemic, the average life expectancy halved between 1990 and 2007, dropping to only thirty-seven years (UNAIDS and WHO, 2009).

Many factors are believed to have contributed to the particularly severe course the AIDS epidemic has taken in sub-Saharan Africa. Biological factors such as the high prevalence of urinary schistosomiasis, malaria, and sexually transmitted infections are clearly important, because they can facilitate HIV transmission and acquisition (Aral and Over, 2006; Modjarrad and Vermund, 2010; Sawers and Stillwaggon, 2010a; Smith et al., 2010). Social factors also play an important role, such as very limited services to diagnose and treat infections, and low rates of male circumcision (i.e., the surgical removal of the foreskin which covers the tip of the penis), as this can be protective against HIV transmission and acquisition (Schomogyi, Wald, and Corey, 1998; Buvé, Bishikwabo-Nsarhaza, and Mutangadura, 2002; Weiss et al., 2010). Added to these factors are broad socioeconomic, cultural, and historical features such as poverty, labor migration, wars and conflicts, and the subordinate position of women (Setel, 1999b; Parker, Easton, and Klein, 2000; Buvé, Bishikwabo-Nsarhaza, and Mutangadura, 2002; Kim and Watts, 2005). Sexuality and sexual behavior have clearly influenced the African epidemic, but there has been substantial debate about how this has occurred (e.g., Caldwell, Caldwell, and Quiggin, 1989; Le Blanc, Meintel, and Piche, 1991; Ahlberg, 1994; Heald, 1995; Helle-Valle, 1999; Undie and Benaya, 2006; Lurie and Rosenthal, 2010; Morris, 2010; Tanser et al., 2011).

One striking pattern of HIV infection across sub-Saharan Africa is that young people are severely affected, and adolescent girls in particular have had consistently higher rates of HIV infection than boys of the same age. In Tanzania, for example, fifteen- to twenty-four-year-old women face nine times the risk of HIV infection of young men of the same age range (Hallett et al., 2010). A number of issues are believed to contribute to this phenomenon, including biological factors, such as easier genital transmission and higher rates of non-symptomatic sexually transmitted infections, and behavioral factors, such as relatively early age at first sex and older sexual partners (Laga et al., 2001; Gregson et al., 2002; Pettifor et al., 2004; Leclerc-Madlala, 2008; Mavedzenge et al., 2011; Doyle et al., 2012).

Throughout sub-Saharan Africa the epidemic has been most concentrated and severe in cities. In the 1980s and 1990s, research and interventions thus focused on urban areas and/or on highly vulnerable subpopulations, including commercial sex workers and migrant workers, such as truck drivers, soldiers, and miners (Dyson, 2003). Increasingly other high-risk subpopulations are also being identified and targeted, such as men who have sex with men and injecting drug users, two groups which are largely hidden in sub-Saharan Africa due to stigma and criminalization of their activities in many countries (Hoffmann, Boler, and Dick, 2006; UNAIDS, 2010).

As already noted, the majority of sub-Saharan Africans live in rural areas, where some people may have sexual behaviors that are equally or more risky as those of urban populations (e.g., Eaton, Flisher, and Aarø, 2003; Nzioka, 2004; Voétèn, Egesah, and Habbema, 2004; Coffee et al., 2005; Adelore, Olujide, and Popoola, 2006; Sambisa, Curtis, and Stokes, 2010). Particularly vulnerable are settlements on truck routes or near mines, and those that experience high mobility or migration rates, such as fishing villages (e.g., Campbell and Williams, 1999; Boerma et al., 2002; Cowan et al., 2005; Desmond et al., 2005; Kissling et al., 2005; Ferguson and Morris, 2007; Béné and Merten, 2008; Mojola, 2011; Seeley et al., 2012). In some countries, for example, large sections of the rural male population are migrant workers who live apart from their families for much of the year, contributing to very high rates of extramarital relationships (e.g., Campbell, 2003; Sambisa and Stokes, 2006).

Promisingly, HIV incidence fell by more than 25 percent between 2001 and 2009 in twenty-two countries in sub-Saharan Africa, including in Tanzania, where an estimated 1.4 million people were living with HIV in 2009 (UNAIDS, 2010). However, most HIV-positive people in Tanzania as elsewhere in sub-

Saharan Africa still do not know that they are infected, and may not learn this until late in their infection, if ever (UNAIDS, 2010). A study in rural Tanzania found that, in the absence of antiretroviral therapy, only half of those infected with HIV survived for twelve years or longer (Isingo et al., 2007). Similarly, a study in rural Uganda found that in the absence of antiretroviral therapy HIV-infected individuals typically lived about nine years before developing AIDS, and another nine months before dying, similar to what has been found in high income countries (Morgan et al., 2002; United Nations, 2007).

HIV Testing and Antiretroviral Therapy

At the turn of the millennium, HIV testing and counseling services were extremely limited in Africa (UNAIDS and WHO, 2003; Hardon and Dilger, 2011). In the last decade, however, the rapid scale-up of HIV testing and antiretroviral therapy services in sub-Saharan Africa has had a tremendous impact on the epidemic. Expansion of testing services and especially on-site rapid HIV tests have meant a sizable minority of the adult population has been tested and received their results at least once. Between 2005 and 2009, for example, a median of 17 percent of women and 14 percent of men in the generalized epidemics in sub-Saharan Africa had both been tested for HIV and knew their results (Padian et al., 2011). The extent of HIV testing of young people aged fifteen to twenty-four years remains highly variable between countries, but some countries have implemented intensive campaigns to promote this. For example, a recent review of national survey data in twenty-four African countries found that the proportion of sexually active young people who have had an HIV test in the last twelve months and knew their results ranged from 1 percent (Niger, 2006) to 49 percent (Lesotho, 2009) among females, and from 0 percent (Ghana, 2008) to 23 percent (Kenya, 2008–2009) among males (Doyle et al., 2012).

Within health facilities, HIV testing increasingly is initiated as a routine procedure by providers rather than clients (e.g., Ntabaye and McMahan, 2008; Hardon et al., 2011). In addition, numerous strategies are being employed to promote HIV testing on a large scale outside of health facilities, such as mobile or door-to-door free testing, which reduces barriers of cost and accessibility (e.g., Wolff et al., 2005; Angotti et al., 2009; Mindry et al., 2011; Ostermann et al., 2011). Such services are likely to contribute to early detection and treatment of HIV infection as well as a reduction in new infections.

The rapid expansion of antiretroviral therapy services in the last decade has also greatly improved the quality of life and reduced illness and death for many HIV-positive Africans. By the end of 2009, 41 percent of HIV-positive adults and children who were eligible for antiretroviral therapy in eastern and southern

Africa were receiving it (UNAIDS, 2010). In addition, antiretroviral therapy shows great promise as a way to prevent new HIV infections (Ramjee, Kamali, and McCormack, 2010; Padian et al., 2011). First, the possibility of transmitting HIV to a partner during unprotected intercourse decreases markedly if an HIV-positive person is on antiretroviral therapy (Porco et al., 2004; Attia et al., 2009). Second, HIV-negative people can reduce their chance of acquiring HIV if they are on antiretroviral therapy themselves, either topically or orally (Karim and Karim, 2011; Padian et al., 2011). Such an approach may be critical in protecting people who are not certain of an HIV-positive partner's adherence to therapy, sexual fidelity, and/or willingness to use a condom.

Despite this great progress there remain daunting challenges to the comprehensive provision of HIV testing and antiretroviral therapy services in sub-Saharan Africa. There is a need to increase the demand and provision of testing services for both individuals and couples, particularly for the large numbers of healthy people who do not attend health services routinely (e.g., Angotti, 2010; Karau et al., 2010; Matovu, 2011; Ostermann et al., 2011; Padian et al., 2011). Challenges in providing antiretroviral therapy to HIV-positive people include accommodating the millions of people who are still in need of therapy and providing quality long-term monitoring and care in areas with very poor health services (e.g., Mills et al., 2006; Heimer, 2007; Rosen, Fox, and Gill, 2007; UNAIDS and WHO, 2009; Cooper and Mills, 2010; Harries et al., 2010; Hecht et al., 2010; Menon, 2010; Hardon and Dilger, 2011; Quinn and Serwadda, 2011; Somi et al., 2012). Even in the best of circumstances, HIV-positive individuals receiving therapy must maintain a daily drug regime for the rest of their lives, and face the possibilities of side effects and viral resistance (e.g., Oyugi et al., 2007; Bratholm et al., 2010; Fox et al., 2010; Mattes, 2011). There are also many fiscal, ethical, and implementation challenges inherent to providing preventive antiretroviral therapy for HIV-negative individuals, such as how to prioritize their needs relative to those of HIV-positive individuals in areas with scarce resources (Weber, Tatoud, and Fidler, 2010; Karim and Karim, 2011).

HIV PREVENTION

All of the challenges above highlight the continuing importance of preventing new HIV infections. HIV can be transmitted in a number of ways, including through unprotected sexual intercourse; from mother to child during pregnancy, childbirth, or delivery; and through intravenous drug use, an infected blood supply, or contaminated medical equipment. Since the onset of the epidemic, a range of intervention programs have been developed to prevent each of these modes of HIV transmission (Auerbach, Hayes, and Kanda-thil, 2006; Wegbreit et al., 2006). In sub-Saharan Africa, however, the vast majority of HIV infections are transmitted through heterosexual intercourse (UNAIDS, 2010), and prevention of such infections among rural young people will be the focus of this book. Within this population certain sexual behaviors are believed to increase risk of HIV transmission, including having concurrent sexual relationships, high rates of partner change, a high number of sexual partners, and particular sexual mixing patterns, while not using condoms (Caldwell, Caldwell, and Quiggin, 1989; Halperin and Epstein, 2004; Buvé, 2006; Chen et al., 2007; Harrison and O'Sullivan, 2010). Sexual mixing patterns refer to how people with similar or distinct characteristics tend to be linked to each other sexually (Aral and Foxman, 2003).

Behavioral Prevention

In the 1980s most HIV prevention interventions in sub-Saharan Africa as elsewhere in the world followed the "Information/Education/Communication" approach, which seeks to teach people correct information about HIV and AIDS in order to empower them to make better decisions and reduce behaviors that put them at risk. This approach was moderately successful in raising awareness of HIV and AIDS in general populations, but is believed to have had only a very limited impact on sexual behavior (Hankins and Zalduondo, 2010). By the 1990s, new "Social and Behavior Change Communication" approaches were developed, which involve more interactive communication, emphasize behavioral skills development, and try to create supportive environments in which people can initiate and sustain low-risk behaviors (Hankins and Zalduondo, 2010).

The approaches described above have often been based in behavioral theories. These theories attempt to identify key behavioral determinants, that is, psychosocial cognitions and environmental factors which determine behavior. Interventions then try to target those determinants in order to change behavior, ideally resulting in fewer sexual risk practices and improved sexual health (UNAIDS, 1999a). Some researchers have argued that the most effective HIV prevention interventions are those which have an explicit basis in behavioral theories (e.g., Fishbein, 2000; Michie et al., 2005). However, some program reviews have found little or no evidence that theory-based interventions are more effective than those founded on more implicit and pragmatic processes (e.g., Gallant and Maticka-Tyndale, 2004; Maticka-Tyndale and Brouillard-Coyle, 2006; Lewin, Glenton, and Oxman, 2009).

Two of the most well elaborated and tested theories are the Social Cognitive Theory and the Theory of Reasoned Action (Bandura, 2004; Michie et al., 2005; Aarø, Schaalma, and Åstrøm, 2008). They identify largely overlapping sets of behavioral determinants, including *knowledge* of health risks and benefits of different practices; *perceived susceptibility* to negative outcomes of behaviors; *perceived self-efficacy* that one can exercise control over one's behavior; *outcome expectations* about the likely costs and benefits for different behaviors; the behavioral *intentions* or *goals* people set for themselves (and the concrete plans and strategies for realizing them); *observational learning* or *modeling* by watching the actions of others and learning the consequences of behaviors; and social, cultural and economic *facilitators* of and *impediments* to desired behavior. These theories have been developed and tested in North America and Europe since the mid-twentieth century, but they have only recently been used to develop sexual behavior interventions in sub-Saharan Africa (e.g., Klepp et al., 1994).

Most HIV-related behavior change theories consider it important to provide intervention participants with adequate knowledge about HIV and AIDS, but this step is considered relatively easy to achieve compared to other necessary steps, such as improving participants' risk perceptions, anticipated outcomes, and self-efficacy to achieve desired behaviors (e.g., Bandura, 2004). Nonetheless, basic misunderstandings about HIV and AIDS persist in sub-Saharan Africa (e.g., Bastien, Sango et al., 2008; Dixon-Mueller, 2009; Robins, 2009; Bogale, Boer, and Seydel, 2010; Mkumbo, 2010; Dimbuene and Defo, 2011). Indeed, the 2010 Global Report on the AIDS Epidemic found that less than half of young people living in fifteen of the twenty-five countries with the highest HIV prevalences could answer five basic questions about HIV correctly (UNAIDS, 2010). All of those are countries in sub-Saharan Africa, including Tanzania.

Skills development is also considered to be an important part of most behavior change theories. Programs may, for example, try to develop participants' skills in communication, negotiation, decision-making, critical thinking, assertiveness, and/or refusal. All of these may help youth to practice low-risk sexual behaviors, such as resisting peer pressure to have sex or negotiating condom use with a sexual partner. Toward that end, adolescent HIV prevention information has sometimes been integrated within broader sexual health or life skills programs which teach facts, promote values of mutuality and respect between sexual partners, and seek to develop participants' relationship and interpersonal skills (Stone and Ingham, 2006).

Efforts to promote low-risk sexual behaviors have had limited and mixed results in sub-Saharan Africa (Ferguson, Dick, and Ross, 2006; The International Group on Analysis of Trends in HIV Prevalence and Behaviours in Young People in Countries Most Affected by HIV, 2010; Michielsen et al., 2010; UNAIDS, 2010; Katsidzira and Hakim, 2011; Mavedzenge, Doyle, and

Ross, 2011). In many countries the epidemic has stalled or reversed, most notably in Uganda and Senegal in the 1990s, and Kenya, Zambia, and Zimbabwe in the first decade of the twenty-first century. Some researchers have attributed such changes to the promotion of abstinence, reduction of partner number, fidelity, and/or condom use (e.g., Cleland and Ali, 2006; Hallett et al., 2006; Pool, Kamali, and Whitworth, 2006; Sandøy et al., 2007; Gregson, Todd, and Żaba, 2009; Halperin et al., 2011). As noted earlier, however, the causal relationships and the relative roles played by the ABCs in such promising findings have been the subject of much debate (e.g., Shelton et al., 2004; Stoneburner and Low-Beer, 2004; Roehr, 2005; Murphy et al., 2006; Green, 2011). In addition, many other efforts to promote the ABCs in sub-Saharan Africa have shown little or no impact on behaviors or biological markers, such as pregnancy, HIV, and other sexually transmitted infections (Coates, Richter, and Caceres, 2008; Merson et al., 2008; Michielsen et al., 2010; Mavedzenge, Doyle, and Ross, 2011).

Finally, in many African settings sexual health interventions which specifically target adolescents have been controversial, because adults have been concerned that discussing sexual activity with adolescents might cause them to have an earlier sexual debut or otherwise increase their sexual risk-taking. Reviews of adolescent sexual health interventions have found very little evidence to support this possibility (Johnson et al., 2003; Gallant and Maticka-Tyndale, 2004; Stone and Ingham, 2006; Michielsen et al., 2010). To the contrary, many studies of young people's reported behavior suggest that such programs delay the onset of sexual activity and generally lower sexual risk-taking.

Structural Prevention

Two of the main findings of this book's companion volume are that poverty and gender inequality are important structural barriers to young people's sexual risk reduction in rural Tanzania (Plummer and Wight, 2011). The term "structure" refers to features of an environment that can influence individual risk and vulnerability to HIV infection, including physical, ecological, cultural, organizational, economic, legal, and policy factors. By definition, these features are beyond a person's control and may undermine that person's agency to protect him or herself, or others. Some authors have conceptualized this by distinguishing between risk and vulnerability, with "risk" referring to the probability that a person may acquire HIV through individual behavior, and "vulnerability" to broader factors which influence people's risk and reduce their ability to avoid infection (UNESCO, 2008; Inter-Agency Task Team on HIV and Young People, 2009).

These and other findings in sub-Saharan Africa suggest that HIV prevention programs which target individual behaviors are unlikely to succeed if they do not also work to make the broader environment safe and supportive of low-risk behaviors. Because structural factors are so broadly defined, however, their linkages to HIV are difficult for programs to target and challenging for research to evaluate, so structural HIV prevention interventions have been quite limited in sub-Saharan Africa to date. The main ones which have been implemented and evaluated are microcredit and conditional cash transfer programs which increase girls' and women's income with the goal of reducing their economic dependency on men, and related sexual risk behaviors (e.g., Gupta et al., 2008; Dworkin and Blankenship, 2009; Kim et al., 2009; Dunbar et al., 2010).

Biomedical Prevention

In addition to a range of behavioral, interpersonal, and structural interventions, and the HIV testing and antiretroviral therapy services already discussed, some other biomedical interventions currently show great potential in reducing the transmission of HIV and other sexually transmitted infections in sub-Saharan Africa today. Two of the most promising of these—male circumcision and Human Papilloma Virus vaccination—only require a few contacts with health workers and short-term behavior change (e.g., abstinence for six weeks post-circumcision) (Louie, de Sanjose, and Mayaud, 2009; Smith et al., 2010; Weiss et al., 2010). However, some other biomedical interventions require long-term, intimate sexual behavior change, and these have proven to be more difficult to promote and more difficult to adopt. For example, most female-controlled biomedical methods have shown little or no evidence of preventing HIV transmission or acquisition to date, including the female condom (a plastic or latex pouch worn inside the vagina); a diaphragm with lubricant gel (a latex barrier covering the cervix and upper genital tract); and some vaginal microbicides (antimicrobial products applied to the vagina that destroy HIV) (Vijayakumar et al., 2006; Padian et al., 2007; Ramjee, Kamali, and McCormack, 2010). To use these methods properly, women need to be consistent in inserting a product into their vaginas prior to intercourse, and their sexual partners may become aware of their use of the product and oppose it (Sahin-Hodoglugil et al., 2009). However, new female-controlled substances and methods are being explored which may be more effective and/or less dependent on routine adherence, such as implants or slow-release topical approaches (e.g., Karim et al., 2010; Padian et al., 2011).

Combination Prevention

There is increasing consensus that HIV prevention interventions are most likely to succeed if they combine promising behavioral, structural, and biomedical approaches, such as those described above (Coates, Richter, and Caceres, 2008; Piot et al., 2008; Hankins and Zalduondo, 2010; Kurth et al., 2011). To maximize effectiveness, such "combination prevention" may need to work at different levels of society, including at the individual level, the interpersonal level (e.g., within a couple, families, or with peers), the sexual or social network level (e.g., within migrant populations), and the structural level of broader community and society (UNAIDS, 1999a; Latkin and Knowlton, 2005; UNAIDS, 2007; Coates, Richter, and Caceres, 2008; Gupta et al., 2008; UNESCO, 2008; Inter-Agency Task Team on HIV and Young People, 2009; Hankins and Zalduondo, 2010; McCoy, Watts, and Padian, 2010; Mojola, 2011; Padian et al., 2011).

ABC promotion remains one important component of combination prevention today. This raises two critical questions: Why has ABC promotion had such limited effectiveness in sub-Saharan Africa to date? And how can it be improved? Three decades into the AIDS epidemic, we know that there are no simple answers to these questions. Nonetheless, they warrant renewed scrutiny and engagement. A central goal of this book is to explore both of those questions in depth.

THE ABC BEHAVIORAL GOALS

The "ABC" acronym is often used as a quick and easy way to refer to low-risk sexual behaviors. Use of the term has been criticized specifically because of that simplicity, that is, because it is not tailored to particular populations or settings, it does not include other forms of HIV prevention (e.g., needle exchange for injecting drug users), and/or it focuses on individual behavior change, which has proven difficult to promote and to practice effectively (e.g., Collins, Coates, and Curran, 2008). The acronym has also become somewhat politicized, having become associated with debates about the relative importance of each of the ABC behaviors and different types of HIV prevention in sub-Saharan Africa and elsewhere. Such controversy may distract from the fact that abstinence, fidelity, and condom use remain fundamental, complementary ways to potentially reduce sexual risk, whether for one individual at different stages of life or for many people with different priorities and desires. And for all of its limitations, the ABC acronym remains one of the most efficient and accessible ways of concisely referring to those behaviors together.

The following discussion will examine each of the ABC behaviors individually, reviewing the main ways that each has been promoted with young people in sub-Saharan Africa, some of the difficulties encountered in collecting valid data on them, and evidence of program effectiveness.

Abstinence

In many studies in sub-Saharan Africa one-third to one-half of fifteen- to nineteen-year-olds report having already had sex (e.g., Munguti et al., 1997; Singh et al., 2000; Gueye, Castle, and Konate, 2001; Dixon-Mueller, 2009). There is a good possibility that such figures are underestimates, because adult disapproval and punishment of unmarried adolescent sexual activity can contribute to underreporting of such activity and overreporting of abstinence; this will be discussed more later in the chapter. Reported early sexual debut has been associated with a higher risk of HIV and other sexually transmitted infections, possibly because it is associated with higher sexual risk behavior in general (such as high partner number), and because girls who are physically and immunologically immature may be more susceptible to injury and infection (Greenberg, Magder, and Aral, 1992; Zabin and Kiragu, 1998; Buvé, 2006; Dixon-Mueller, 2009).

The "Abstinence" goal of the ABC approach refers to delaying age at first sexual intercourse ("primary abstinence") as well as stopping sexual activity after it has already begun ("secondary abstinence"). Abstinence mainly has been promoted for never-married adolescents and young adults within programs which can be categorized as "abstinence-only," "abstinence-plus," or "comprehensive" programs. "Abstinence-only" programs present abstinence as the best and only way to prevent sexual transmission of HIV before marriage, and provide little or no information about other low-risk sexual behaviors. In the first years of the twenty-first century, such programs were strongly promoted within the United States and in many US government-funded interventions in low income countries (Stone and Ingham, 2006; Hardon and Dilger, 2011; Nixon et al., 2011). However, systematic reviews of abstinence-only programs in both developed and developing countries found they had little or no impact on sexual behavior, whether this was measured by participant self-report, or, less frequently, sexually transmitted infections or other biological markers (O'Reilly et al., 2004; Underhill, Montgomery, and Operario, 2007). A review of such programs in the United States further found they often contained false, misleading, or inaccurate information about condoms and other forms of contraception (Dworkin and Santelli, 2007).

"Abstinence-plus" programs instead present young participants with a hierarchy of risk reduction practices, promoting abstinence as the safest strategy but also providing education about other low-risk sexual practices (Dworkin and Santelli, 2007). Programs in this category have been diverse in their emphases, ranging, for example, from those which barely mention condom use to those which actively and intensively promote it for sexually active youth (Dworkin and Santelli, 2007; Nixon et al., 2011). In a systematic review of abstinence-plus intervention trials in high income countries, half

reported a protective effect on at least one sexual behavior, although sometimes this was quite modest, e.g., a delay of three to six months in sexual
initiation (Underhill, Operario, and Montgomery, 2007).

Finally, "comprehensive" programs intend to provide complete, age-
appropriate education on human sexuality—including abstinence, fidelity,
and condom use—without identifying any one as better than another (Dworkin and Santelli, 2007). Some have argued that such an approach is more
appropriate than an abstinence-only or abstinence-plus approach, because
interventions which prioritize abstinence may inadvertently discourage condom use for those young people who continue to be sexually active (Nixon et
al., 2011). However, the review of abstinence-plus programs in high income
countries mentioned above found that a primary promotion of abstinence did
not seem to detract from program messages about condom use, as several
abstinence-plus intervention trials found protective short-term and long-term
effects on reported condom use, and no trial found an adverse effect (Underhill, Operario, and Montgomery, 2007).

Evaluation of abstinence promotion with young people in Africa has been
limited. In settings where sexual activity is forbidden for unmarried youth,
one challenge is that young people may falsely report abstinence, particularly
after participating in an intervention program that promoted it. Nonetheless, a
2004 review of eleven school-based HIV prevention programs in sub-Saharan
Africa identified only two programs in which participants reported significantly later ages at first sex than non-participants (Gallant and Maticka-Tyndale, 2004). The same review found very little evidence of young people who
had already had sex choosing to become abstinent. The authors concluded
that teaching young people about low-risk behaviors prior to sexual debut is
likely to be more effective than changing high-risk behaviors once they have
become established, suggesting that interventions will be more effective if
they target younger adolescents.

Being Faithful

The "being faithful" goal of the ABC behaviors generally is interpreted to mean
having only one sexual partner. As straightforward as this goal may first seem,
it can be ambiguous and interpreted in diverse ways which have quite different
implications for sexual health risk (e.g., Painter et al., 2007; Lillie, Pulerwitz,
and Curbow, 2009; Leclerc-Madlala, 2009; Baumgartner et al., 2010; Kenyon
et al., 2010). For example, "being faithful" usually is used synonymously with
"being monogamous," but someone can reduce their partner number and their
sexual health risk without being monogamous. In addition, polygyny (i.e., a
man having multiple wives) is a widespread, legal practice in sub-Saharan

Africa, so it is also possible for a man to be faithful to multiple wives. Even individuals who consistently practice monogamy may do so in different ways that involve variable risk. One may, for example, have a series of monogamous relationships ("serial monogamy"), or a long-term monogamous relationship with a partner who may or may not also be monogamous. Sexual health risk can also vary within mutually monogamous partnerships, depending on any infections the individuals brought into the relationship when it began, and their subsequent use of condoms. During the first decades of the AIDS epidemic in sub-Saharan Africa, it was very rare for people to be tested for HIV before beginning a new relationship—or to be tested at any point in the course of that relationship—because testing services were exceedingly rare. However, the recent scale-up of testing services means that "being faithful" without condom use potentially can be a much lower risk practice today, if couples test themselves before having unprotected intercourse, and continue to test themselves at routine intervals afterward.

The 2010 UNAIDS Global Report on the AIDS Epidemic identified unprotected sex with multiple partners as the greatest risk factor for HIV in sub-Saharan Africa (UNAIDS, 2010). In recent years there has been substantial debate about the risks involved in different kinds of multiple partnerships in this region, particular the relative risks of serial monogamy or concurrency, and the implications they might have for how to best promote the "be faithful" message (e.g., UNAIDS, 2007; Research to Prevention, 2009; Lurie and Rosenthal, 2010; Harrison and O'Sullivan, 2010; Morris, 2010; Tanser et al., 2011). Concurrent relationships are those in which one or both partners have other sexual partners while continuing to have sexual encounters with an original partner.

Research suggests it is common for men to have concurrent sexual relationships in many parts of sub-Saharan Africa (e.g., Caldwell, Caldwell, and Quiggin, 1989; Jana, Nkambule, and Tumbo, 2008; Research to Prevention, 2009; Mbago and Sichona, 2010; Kenyon et al., 2010). Increasingly studies suggest that, in some areas, it is also fairly common for women to have concurrent partnerships, although their secondary relationships may involve fewer partners, longer relationship durations, and greater secrecy than men's (e.g., Nnko et al., 2004; Tawfik and Watkins, 2007; Hattori and Dodoo, 2007; Jana, Nkambule, and Tumbo, 2008; Harrison and O'Sullivan, 2010; Kenyon et al., 2010). Some researchers have suggested that the overall rates of long-term, concurrent relationships are higher in sub-Saharan Africa than in many other parts of the world, while numbers of lifetime partners are similar or lower (Halperin and Epstein, 2004).

When compared to other kinds of multiple partnerships, concurrency may involve relatively high risk of HIV transmission because the virus can pass between any partners who are linked to each other directly or indirectly, for as long as the relationships overlap. HIV can also be transmitted indirectly through a series of monogamous relationships, but this is generally a slower process and, critically, it only goes in one direction, so that earlier uninfected partners remain uninfected (Doherty et al., 2006). Several researchers have argued that the non-linear nature of network connectivity means that small differences in concurrency potentially can contribute to large differences in a sexually transmitted infection epidemic (e.g., Potterat et al., 1999; Morris, 2010). Others have argued that, if concurrent sexual partnerships are very common within a population, it can allow rapid transmission of an infection from person to person to person even if relatively few individuals have many contacts, such as sex workers and frequent clients of sex workers (UNAIDS, 2007). Concurrent partnerships may also involve relatively high risk because people who are newly infected with HIV have high amounts of it in their blood and semen, so if a person has more than one partner during that period there is more chance of the virus being transmitted further (Pilcher et al., 2004; Wawer et al., 2005). This is less likely to happen in a series of mo-nogamous relationships, unless they involve very short relationships and fast partner change (Morris and Kretzschmar, 1997; Buvé, 2006).

The level of risk for individuals in concurrent relationships is believed to depend on many factors, including the number of partners (and part-ners' partners), the timing and duration of partnerships, the frequency of sexual encounters, knowledge of whether a partner has concurrent partners, consistency of condom use, and the duration of the specific infection and its prevalence in the population (Morris and Kretzschmar, 1997; Man-hart et al., 2002; Moody, 2002; Drumright, Gorbach, and Holmes, 2004). All of these factors—and the sensitive nature of many concurrent sexual partnerships—make accurate measurement of concurrency very challeng-ing. Indeed, research on concurrency and its possible association with HIV transmission has been very limited, and some researchers question the hy-pothesis that concurrent relationships involve substantially higher risk than serial monogamy with the same number of partners and the same frequency of encounters. Some authors have argued that high partner number overall is more important in determining risk than whether those partnerships are serial or concurrent (Sawers and Stillwaggon, 2010b; Tanser et al., 2011). They believe that a special focus on concurrency complicates and confuses the main intervention message to have few partners.

Despite the potential importance of the "be faithful" message, to date it has not received as much focus within HIV prevention work in sub-Saharan Af-rica as messages related to abstinence and condom use (Gallant and Maticka-Tyndale, 2004; Shelton et al., 2004; Grills, 2006; UNAIDS, 2007; Wilson and Halperin, 2008; Leclerc-Madlala, 2009; Lurie and Rosenthal, 2010; Green, 2011). Generally HIV prevention programs have produced simple messages, such as "have few partners" or "be faithful," but they have not addressed the challenging and sometimes complex issues involved in practicing those behaviors safely. To truly be low risk, for example, fidelity must involve a long-term, closed network of mutually faithful, uninfected partners—or infected partners who use condoms consistently. This suggests that, to be maximally effective, interventions may need to go beyond the individual to engage with couples about their relationships. To date, intervention programs which have focused on reducing sexual partner number and promoting fidelity in sub-Saharan Africa mainly have tried to reduce men's extramarital relationships (e.g., Parikh, 2007). The extent to which such interventions are effective is unclear, because so few have been developed and implemented, let alone evaluated rigorously. Interventions for unmarried youth have been even less likely to address fidelity with any depth, because this would require acknowledgement of unmarried young people's sexual relationships. Fidelity promotion for unmarried youth may also be challenging if many participants are not at a stage of their lives when they feel prepared for a long-term or exclusive sexual commitment.

Condom Use

A male condom consists of a disposable sheath of thin rubber or latex that is rolled on to an erect penis prior to intercourse, providing a snug barrier that prevents the exchange of body fluids. A different form of condom has been developed for women but is far less common in sub-Saharan Africa, so in this book the term "condom" will only be used to describe male condoms, unless otherwise specified. Consistent and correct condom use is one of the most effective ways to prevent the transmission of HIV during sexual intercourse (Holmes, Levine, and Weaver, 2004). As such, it has been strongly promoted in most African HIV prevention programs, including some of the work that has been carried out with young people (Hearst and Chen, 2004; Foss et al., 2007). Some evidence of success can be seen in such efforts (e.g., Wegbreit et al., 2006; Bankole et al., 2009; UNAIDS and WHO, 2009). From 1993 to 2001, for example, there was a median annual increase of 1.4 percent in young women's reported condom use in eighteen African countries (Cleland and Ali, 2006). Similarly, there was a two to three fold increase in condom sales in some countries in the 1990s (Hearst and Chen, 2004). However, a review of condom sales statistics in four countries found sales were poor indicators of actual condom use (Meekers and Van Rossem, 2005). Specifically, the authors found that drastic fluctuations in annual sales in each country reflected wholesaler and distributor inventories and stock-ups, not consumer use.

Like abstinence and fidelity, it can be difficult to collect accurate and meaningful data on condom use for a number of reasons. While it is possible to ask survey respondents fairly simple questions, such as whether they have ever used condoms, or if they used a condom at last sex, such data may not reflect how well individuals protect themselves with condoms over time. In addition, as with other low-risk behaviors, people who have participated in condom promotion interventions may overreport their condom use because they believe it to be a desirable behavior; this will be discussed more later in the chapter.

Different data sources suggest that condom use is generally low in sub-Saharan Africa, even in casual relationships and even after condom promotion interventions (e.g., Lagarde et al., 2001; Cleland and Ali, 2006; Foss et al., 2007; Rutherford, 2008; UNAIDS, 2010; Papo et al., 2011). A review of condom promotion efforts in the developing world noted that high HIV transmission rates generally have continued even when reports of condom use were relatively high (Hearst and Chen, 2004). The authors concluded that the impact of condoms in sub-Saharan Africa has been limited by low and inconsistent use among those at highest risk. A number of other factors may have limited the success of condom promotion efforts in Africa. Condom distribution and access have been problematic in many countries, particularly in rural areas (e.g., Lamptey and Goodridge, 1991; Meekers, Ahmed, and Molathegi, 2001; Shelton and Johnston, 2001; Myer, Mathews, and Little, 2002; Bosmans et al., 2006; Papo et al., 2011). For example, a 2007 study in Kenya found that the distance from respondents' households to the nearest outlet with free condoms was eighteen times farther in rural areas than urban areas (4.45 versus 0.25 kilometers, respectively) (Papo et al. 2011).

However, the main reason for low condom use is not believed to be limited supply as much as little demand, as negative beliefs and attitudes toward condoms have been powerful deterrents of use in sub-Saharan Africa, even when condoms have been readily available (e.g., Taylor, 1990; Karim et al., 1992; Lamptey and Goodridge, 1991; Bond and Dover, 1997; Hart et al., 1999; Campbell, 2003; Thomsen, Stalker, and Toroitich-Ruto, 2004; Maticka-Tyndale and Kyeremeh, 2010; Stadler and Saethre, 2011; Nixon et al., 2011). Commonly reported negative beliefs include that condoms: reduce sexual pleasure; indicate infidelity or a lack of trust in a partner; are inherently dangerous; and/or are associated with sexually transmitted infections, casual sex, or prostitution. Other factors which may discourage condom use include embarrassment and shyness; a lack of perceived personal risk; male control of sexual decision-making; and the importance of male potency, male and female fertility, or the exchange of body fluids during sexual intercourse.

Condom promotion for unmarried sexually active adolescents has also been controversial in sub-Saharan Africa, as adults have often been concerned it would lead to increased sexual activity (e.g., Fuglesang, 1997; Mkumbo, 2009). For example, a review of school-based HIV prevention programs for African youth found that all but two of the programs that attempted to address condom use encountered resistance from communities and teachers (Gallant and Maticka-Tyndale, 2004). That review found that, in several programs, teachers entirely omitted the recommended material on condom use, regardless of whether it was identified as standard or optional (e.g., Kinsman et al., 2001; Klepp et al., 1994; Visser, 1996; Klepp et al., 1997).

PROGRAM APPROACH AND STRUCTURE

Sub-Saharan African countries are diverse in their political, historical, economic, and sociocultural characteristics, and national and local responses to the AIDS epidemic have been similarly diverse. Within and between countries, HIV prevention interventions have varied in their content, structure, intensity, and scale. They range, for example, from national radio programs providing basic information about HIV and AIDS; to targeted condom social marketing campaigns; to in-depth, multi-component interventions based at schools, health facilities, or religious institutions. Some communities which have experienced high HIV prevalences have demonstrated great initiative and engaged in intensive indigenous HIV prevention efforts, as seen, for example, at a national level in Uganda and the regional level in Kagera, Tanzania (Green and Witte, 2006; Thornton, 2008; Frumence et al., 2010). However, three decades into the AIDS epidemic there are still many parts of sub-Saharan Africa where populations have received only superficial and inconsistent HIV prevention information, particularly in rural areas (e.g., Singh, Bankole, and Woog, 2005).

Young people have been targeted for HIV prevention in sub-Saharan Africa in five main ways: through the mass media, schools, health facilities, initiatives within geographically defined communities, and initiatives targeting young people who are most at risk (Ferguson, Dick, and Ross, 2006; Stone and Ingham, 2006). In the course of evaluating the *MEMA kwa Vijana* adolescent sexual health intervention, this book will closely examine the potential of three of these approaches, namely, those through schools, health facilities, and initiatives within geographically defined communities.

To maximize potential impact, HIV prevention interventions should be designed to be sustainable, feasible to scale-up, and replicable (Bell et al., 2007; UNAIDS, 2007; Bertozzi et al., 2008; Altman, 2009; Galárraga et al., 2009; Padian et al., 2011). A *sustainable* intervention is one that continues to be implemented and to benefit the community even after major assistance from intervention developers and donors ends. This is especially important in HIV prevention interventions for young people, because new generations of children continually enter adolescence and eventually becoming sexually active. An intervention that is *feasible to scale-up* is one that can be substantially increased in size or extent in real-world scenarios. It is not sufficient to develop effective programs which are small in scale and require great expense or resources, as it is unlikely they can be scaled-up to have an impact on a broader population and epidemic. Finally, a *replicable* intervention is one that can be independently and effectively adapted and reproduced elsewhere.

INTERVENTION EVALUATION METHODS

HIV prevention programs in sub-Saharan Africa frequently are undertaken with good intentions, limited resources, and dedicated, hard work. Unfortunately, such efforts do not insure that a program is effective in reducing risk behaviors or new infections with HIV and other sexually transmitted diseases. Some interventions are not implemented as planned, which can substantially affect their impact (e.g., Kinsman et al., 2001; Visser, Schoeman, and Perold, 2004; Harrison et al., 2010). Others are implemented as intended, but still do not have the desired impact on sexual health (e.g., Pronyk et al., 2006; Jewkes et al., 2008; Cowan et al., 2010). It is thus critical to carefully evaluate both the process and the impact of an intervention, so that effective programs can be identified, sustained, scaled-up, and replicated, while ineffective ones can be improved or discontinued.

Evaluation of a program's impact typically involves measuring participant knowledge, attitudes, and reported behaviors before and after an intervention, or in comparison to individuals in a control group that did not receive the intervention. Such an impact evaluation can be critical in determining whether a program succeeded or failed, and to what extent this was the case. Many such impact evaluations have been conducted in sub-Saharan Africa, although the quality of research has varied widely and few published studies have used strong and transparent evaluation designs (Ferguson, Dick, and Ross, 2006; Gallant and Maticka-Tyndale, 2004; Michielsen et al., 2010).

Some researchers believe a randomized controlled trial is the most rigorous way to evaluate the impact of a sexual health intervention, because it is the only study design able to control for unknown or unmeasured confounders (Bonell, Bennett, and Oakley, 2003; Lewin, Glenton, and Oxman, 2009). A randomized controlled trial is a study in which people are allocated by chance to one of two (or more) groups, one of which is a standard of comparison or control, while the other receives an intervention. After randomization the groups are followed up in the same way, with the only difference being exposure to the intervention being assessed. After receiving the intervention, outcomes are then measured and compared using statistical tests which assess the probability that differences between intervention and control groups have occurred by chance.

Few disagree that a randomized controlled trial provides a scientifically rigorous experimental design, but some argue that it is nonetheless not suitable for evaluating behavioral interventions. Their concerns are both conceptual and practical, including concerns related to randomization, generalizability, isolation of experimental and control groups, and cost (e.g., Bonell et al., 2006; Pettifor et al., 2007; Laga et al., 2012). For example, Kippax (2003, 20) argues:

> The [sexual] practices we are talking about are significant human practices, ones in which there is considerable psychological and emotional investment. This makes them difficult to change, unlike most commercial purchasing practices, where the advertiser is involved in the essentially frivolous task of persuading the buyer to choose brand X over brand Y. Sexual practice is extremely complex and its meanings dynamic, fluid, and changing. . . . What all this means is that the requirement of experimental manipulation for an exact relationship between variables, that is, relating outcomes to trial arms, cannot be met.

Indeed, a 2010 review of HIV prevention intervention trials found that thirty-three of thirty-nine trials had found no effect on HIV, including all of those evaluating behavioral interventions (Hayes et al., 2010). The five trials showing a positive effect consisted of all three trials of male circumcision for prevention of HIV acquisition, one of the nine trials of syndromic management of sexually transmitted infections, and one vaccine trial that showed a marginally significant impact. Syndromic management involves treating patients for all possible infections that could cause symptoms when laboratory tests are not available for more precise diagnoses (Grosskurth et al., 1995). In that review, the one trial showing a clear negative effect was a trial of the vaginal microbicide nonoxynol-9. Hayes and colleagues (2010) identify three main reasons why so many HIV prevention trials may have flat results, including: the basic intervention concept is flawed; the underlying concept is sound, but the specific intervention strategy is inert or too weak to have a significant effect; and the design and/or conduct of the trial precludes demonstrating an effect that, in reality, could be clinically or programmatically important (e.g., if the trial does not have sufficient statistical power, or participants do not adhere to the intervention).

In contrast to evaluations of a program's impact, a process evaluation examines its general context, the quality of its implementation, the completeness of its delivery, and the extent to which participants engaged with and were satisfied by it (Wight and Obasi, 2003; Saunders, Evans, and Joshi, 2005; Oakley et al., 2006). As such, process evaluations can be very valuable in understanding the impact of an intervention, or the lack thereof. Reed and Baxen (2010) propose that process evaluations of HIV prevention programs should examine an intervention's implicit or explicit theoretical basis, its pedagogical orientation (e.g., curriculum), and its actual process (e.g., structure, development, implementation, and delivery). Process evaluations can be based on routine data collected in the course of monitoring and supervising intervention programs, as well as specially conducted qualitative and quantitative research with program participants, implementers, and broader community members. Despite the importance of detailed process evaluation of HIV prevention interventions for young sub-Saharan Africans, very few have been published to date (e.g., Kuhn, Steinberg, and Mathews, 1994; Wolf, Tawfik, and Bond, 2000; Kinsman et al., 2001; Campbell, 2003; Visser, Schoeman, and Perold, 2004; Ahmed et al., 2006; Mukoma et al., 2009; Reed and Baxen, 2010).

The main research methods which are used in evaluating the impact and process of interventions are described below.

Surveys of HIV and Other Biological Markers

The most obvious way to assess the effectiveness of an HIV prevention program is to measure its impact on HIV prevalence (i.e., the proportion of infected people in a population at a specific time) or HIV incidence (i.e., the rate at which new infections occur in a population during a specific period of time). However, biomedical surveys are often costly and impractical because they require a high level of expertise and involve complex technology (Schachter and Chow, 1995; Fishbein and Pequegnat, 2000). Biological test performance may also be limited by a range of factors, including a test's ability to identify people who are truly positive and truly negative, the prevalence of an infection in a study population, and field conditions (e.g., the quality of specimen collection, the maintenance of appropriate cold chains, and the speed of transportation to laboratories) (Schachter and Chow, 1995; Ku et al., 1997; Cowan and Plummer, 2003). Maintaining adequate field conditions can be particularly challenging in low income countries where resources and training may be extremely limited (Sterne et al., 1993; Fishbein and Pequegnat, 2000). Finally, even when an infection is measured accurately, biological results only provide very basic information about the sexual behavior of participants who test positive. For example, they may simply indicate that a person has had sex sometime in the past, but not explain more complex issues related to risk behavior, such as partner number or frequency of sexual encounters (Catania et al., 1993; Zenilman et al., 1995; Weir and Feldblum, 1996; Fishbein and Jarvis, 2000; Aral and Peterman, 2002).

Because biomedical research is challenging to conduct in low income countries, it is rarely undertaken. A recent review of youth HIV prevention interventions in sub-Saharan Africa found only five studies had evaluated intervention impact on HIV (Mavedzenge, Doyle, and Ross, 2011). These were the *MEMA kwa Vijana* program in Tanzania, which is discussed in detail in this book (Ross et al., 2007), as well as another school-based intervention in Zimbabwe (Cowan et al., 2010), and three interventions in South Africa: the Stepping Stones program, which consisted of fifty hours of participatory, same-sex health education sessions (Jewkes et al., 2008); the Intervention with Microfinance for AIDS and Gender Equity (IMAGE), which combined HIV education and a microfinance program for adult women (Pronyk et al., 2006); and the national loveLife HIV prevention program, involving mass media, multi-purpose youth centers, and health facilities (Pettifor et al., 2005).

Each of those studies found some significant improvement in participants' HIV-related knowledge, attitudes, and/or reported sexual behaviors. However, only the national program was found to have a significant impact on HIV, in that a cross-sectional household survey found HIV was lower in those who reported intervention experience (Pettifor et al. 2005). In addition, while the fifty-hour Stepping Stones program did not have a significant impact on HIV among the program's self-selected, volunteer participants, it did have a significant impact on herpes (Jewkes et al., 2008).

Surveys of Knowledge, Attitudes, and Self-Reported Behavior

As an alternative to measuring HIV itself, many program evaluators use indirect measures and ask intervention participants about their knowledge, attitudes, and sexual risk behaviors in formally structured surveys (Gallant and Maticka-Tyndale, 2004; Michielsen et al., 2010). Surveys involve asking the exact same questions of a large number of people, and recording their responses numerically so that the data can be analyzed using statistical methods. An advantage to interviewing large numbers of people is that the results are more likely to be representative or generalizable, that is, they are more likely to reflect the total population and not specific subgroups

(Bulmer and Warwick, 2000). Importantly, participant knowledge can be assessed objectively in surveys, as unlike reported attitudes and behavior it is not falsified easily.

However, the large number of structured interviews involved in surveys means that topics usually are only addressed briefly and superficially, and there is little possibility for flexible and in-depth investigation (Smith and Morrow, 1996; Nelson et al., 2007). This is a particular concern when trying to collect accurate data on sexual behavior, given the sensitive and sometimes complex nature of sexual histories. Self-reported sexual behavior can be inaccurate due to poor recall, misunderstanding, or intentionally false statements made to avoid anticipated criticism or embarrassment (Catania et al., 1993; Huygens et al., 1996; Brewer, Garrett, and Kulasingam, 1999; Gersovitz et al., 1998; Stycos, 2000; Fenton et al., 2001; Hewett, Mensch, and Erulkar, 2004; Gersovitz, 2007; Palen et al., 2008; Beguy et al., 2009; Turner et al., 2009; Koffi et al., 2012). While biased self-reports can occur in any setting, they may be a particular problem in cultures where greater value is placed on courtesy, and—in the case of young people—on deference, than is placed on accuracy, as may sometimes be the case in sub-Saharan Africa (Bulmer and Warwick, 2000; Turner et al., 2009). The few studies which have assessed the validity of young people's reported sexual behavior in sub-Saharan Africa generally have found reports to be inconsistent at the individual level (Plummer, Ross, et al., 2004; Plummer, Wight, et al., 2004; Palen et al., 2008; Beguy et al., 2009; Cremin et al., 2009).

In addition to the issues already mentioned above, there are several other reasons why young people may provide inconsistent reports in sub-Saharan Africa. First, unmarried adolescent sexual activity typically is condemned by adults, inhibiting disclosure; second, there is very little experience of non-judgmental research, so study neutrality and confidentiality may be doubted; and third, poor education can contribute to misinterpretation of questions or inaccurate responses, such as age estimates and questions about the exact timing and duration of partnerships (Gersovitz et al., 1998; Cowan et al., 2002; Wijsen and Tanner, 2002; Mensch, Hewett, and Erulkar, 2003; Nnko et al., 2004; Helleringer and Kohler, 2007).

Young people generally are believed to underreport sexual behaviors for fear of punishment or stigma, but there are exceptions, as when boys may exaggerate their sexual experience to appear more masculine, or intervention participants falsely report a promoted activity, such as condom use (Catania et al., 1990; Agnew and Loving, 1998; Kaaya et al., 2002; Devine and Aral, 2004). The potential for intervention-related bias in reported condom use is a great concern because reported condom use is one of the most common ways to evaluate HIV prevention programs (UNAIDS, 2007). For example, in a review of sixty-two studies of intervention impact on reported condom use in Asia and Africa, forty-two studies found statistically significant increases in reported condom use after interventions, and this was interpreted as evidence of intervention effectiveness (Foss et al., 2007). However, a separate review of twelve African studies investigated associations between reported condom use and HIV infection, and only two of those studies showed significant associations: one suggested that condom use increased rates of HIV infection, and the other suggested it decreased it (Slaymaker, 2004).

There are a number of reasons why intervention experience might result in significantly higher reported condom use, but higher reported condom use might not lead to significantly reduced HIV infection (Catania et al., 1990; Catania et al., 1993; Zenilman et al., 1995; Turner and Miller, 1997; Agnew and Loving, 1998; Goodrich, Wellings, and McVey, 1998; Aral and Peterman, 2002; Geary et al., 2003; Devine and Aral, 2004; Hearst and Chen, 2004; Groes-Green, 2009a). For example, the true impact of condom use may be too small to significantly influence HIV rates. Alternatively, individual-level condom use may be too variable and complex for basic survey questions to capture well, for example, one person may only increase condom use with one of several partners after an intervention, while another may use condoms inconsistently with all partners. A third possibility is that, as noted earlier, some intervention participants may falsely report condom use because they know it is a promoted behavior.

Given the possibility of biased self-reported sexual behavior, such information should not be taken at face value in evaluating an intervention's impact. Ideally, survey reports should be scrutinized to assess their logic and consistency within and between survey questionnaires, and when possible they should be compared to several other sources of information. Returning to the example of condom use: self-reported survey data can be compared to pregnancy and sexually transmitted infection data, as well as sexual partners' reports, condom sale records, and findings from qualitative studies (Sheeran and Abraham, 1994; Goodrich, Wellings, and McVey, 1998).

Qualitative Research

Qualitative research methods such as in-depth interviews or focus group discussions offer an alternative or complement to survey self-reports in assessing intervention process and impact. Like surveys these methods often involve asking respondents about their behavior, so they can face similar self-reporting biases. However, qualitative interviews usually take longer than survey interviews, giving the respondent more time to develop rapport and trust with the interviewer, and helping to foster honesty about sensitive behaviors. In addition, qualitative interview questions typically are open-ended and semi-structured, allowing respondents to give complex responses in their own words. Topics can thus be explored in more depth and subtlety than is possible in surveys, which can be valuable in collecting information about private and sometimes complicated topics such as sexual behavior (Ankrah, 1989; Huygens et al., 1996; Agadjanian, 2005).

Simulated patient exercises and participant observation are other qualitative methods which can be used to evaluate an intervention. Neither method solely relies on the reports of intervention implementers or participants, reducing potential self-reporting biases. In simulated patient exercises, trained local community members visit health facilities in the assumed role of clients in order to assess the quality of services (Boyce and Neale, 2006). Given intervention participants may alter their behavior when they know they are being observed by a researcher (Babbie, 1986), clinical staff usually agree to participate in simulated patient exercises well in advance of such visits and are not told exactly when they will occur. In participant observation, researchers instead live and work among members of a target population for an extended period of time, carefully recording their informal conversations and observations of everyday life (Pool and Geissler, 2005). In such studies, participants also may alter what they say and do because of a researcher's presence, but this may reduce as they share activities, have empathic conversations, and develop rapport with researchers over a long period of time in their normal social environment. The strengths and weaknesses of each of these methods will be discussed more in the next chapter.

Qualitative studies can be valuable in assessing intervention impact, particularly when the subject is highly sensitive and prone to social desirability bias (Ankrah, 1989; Huygens et al., 1996). However, unlike survey research, qualitative research usually is not conducted with a large population because it is less structured and more intensive and time-consuming (Huygens et al., 1996; Bulmer and Warwick, 2000). The broader representativeness of qualitative findings may thus be quite limited. Qualitative research generally is considered most useful for intervention process evaluation, providing context and depth to better understand and interpret the more representative findings of a quantitative impact evaluation (Wight and Obasi, 2003; Oakley et al., 2006).

Lewin, Glenton, and Oxman (2009) outline several ways qualitative research can complement a randomized controlled trial. First, it can precede the trial to explore research questions within the local context, to generate hypotheses to examine in the trial, to develop and refine the intervention, and to develop and select appropriate outcome measures. Second, qualitative research during a trial can examine whether an intervention was delivered as intended, scrutinize implementation and change processes, and explore implementer and participant responses to an intervention. Third, qualitative research after a trial can be useful to understand and interpret trial results, to explain variations in effectiveness within the sample, to examine the appropriateness of the theory underlying the intervention, and to generate further questions and hypotheses.

In their review of 100 randomized controlled trials of complex health-care interventions, Lewin, Glenton, and Oxman (2009) state there is increasing consensus that qualitative studies can provide a valuable complement to such trials. However, the reviewers also found that such qualitative research is uncommon, that it usually is limited to research before a trial, and that it often has methodological shortcomings. They further note that few qualitative studies which are affiliated with intervention trials actually integrate their findings with the trial results during data analysis and interpretation, and thus few attempt to explain trial outcomes (Lewin, Glenton, and Oxman, 2009). Such an in-depth triangulation of qualitative and quantitative trial results is one of the main goals of this book. Chapters 4 to 7 will draw on multiple data sources to evaluate the process and impact of the *MEMA kwa Vijana* adolescent intervention in Mwanza, Tanzania, which is introduced below.

STUDY OVERVIEW

This book primarily is based on the findings of the Health and Lifestyles Research (HALIRA) Project, a large qualitative study that took place in four rural districts of Mwanza Region, Tanzania from 1999 to 2002 (figures 1.1 and 1.2). The HALIRA study was developed as a complement to the *MEMA kwa Vijana* adolescent sexual and reproductive health intervention trial which took place in the same districts from 1997 to 2002. HALIRA had four main objectives: to investigate the lives and sexual behavior of adolescents; to determine behaviors which put young people at risk of infection with HIV or other sexually transmitted infections; to develop and evaluate quantitative and qualitative research methodologies for use with rural African adolescents; and to contribute to the evaluation of the *MEMA kwa Vijana* intervention. The first three objectives were examined in depth in a companion volume to this book (Plummer and Wight, 2011). The fourth is one of the main topics examined in this book.

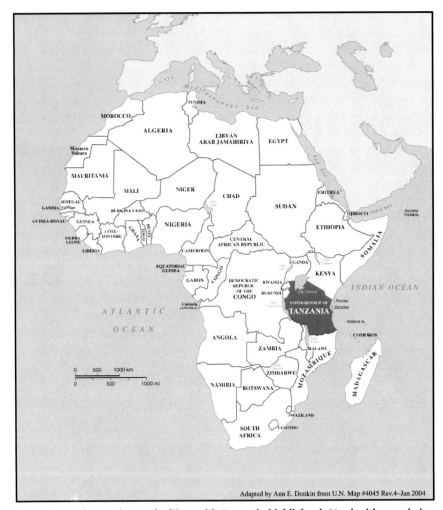

Figure 1.1.   The continent of Africa, with Tanzania highlighted. Used with permission of Karen Coen Flynn. 2005. *Food, culture, and survival in an African city*. Palgrave: NY.

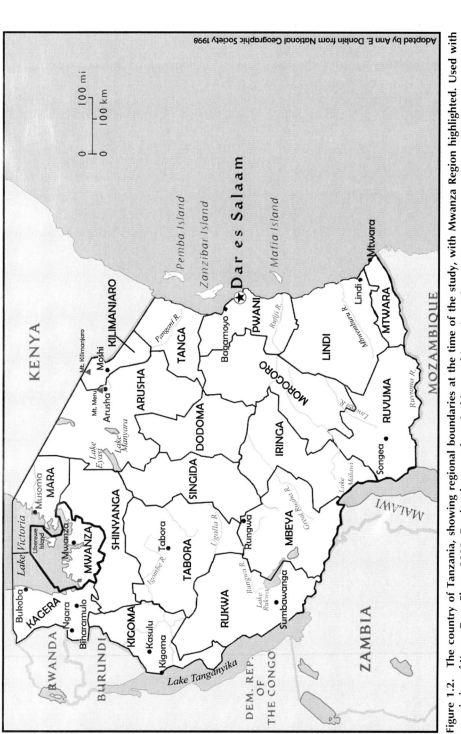

Figure 1.2.   The country of Tanzania, showing regional boundaries at the time of the study, with Mwanza Region highlighted. Used with permission of Karen Coen Flynn. 2005. *Food, culture, and survival in an African city*. Palgrave: NY.

Setting and Population

Tanzania is similar to many sub-Saharan African countries in that it gained national independence from colonial powers in the mid-twentieth century, it underwent tremendous political and economic change since then, and at the start of the twenty-first century it has a largely rural population, limited financial and material resources, and very poor health, education, water, and sanitation services (World Bank, 2006). From 1990 to 2003, for example, 60 percent of Tanzanians lived on less than $2 per day and 29 percent of children under five years of age were underweight (Palmer et al., 2007).

Important ways that Tanzania differs from most other sub-Saharan African countries include that: its primary national language (Swahili) is indigenous to Africa; it has been extraordinarily stable politically since independence; and it has one of the smallest secondary and higher education systems in the world (Cooksey and Riedmiller, 1997; Topan, 2008). At the end of the study period in 2002–2003, for example, the average number of students enrolled in secondary education as a percentage of the population of official school age was 28 percent for sub-Saharan Africa overall, but only 7 percent for Tanzania (Palmer et al., 2007).

At the time of the study, Mwanza Region was a 19,592 km^2 area just south of the equator on the southern shore of Lake Victoria. The region was home to approximately three million people, half a million of whom resided in the regional capital, Mwanza City (United Republic of Tanzania, 1997; National Bureau of Statistics and ORC Macro, 2004). The region also had six semi-urban centers with populations of approximately twenty thousand each, while the remaining 80 percent of the population lived in rural areas (Changalucha et al., 2002). At that time there was one teaching hospital, one regional hospital, and two private hospitals in Mwanza City, as well as six district hospitals and three missionary hospitals elsewhere in the region (Changalucha et al., 2002). Ninety percent of Mwanza residents were of Sukuma ethnicity, and most people in rural Mwanza spoke Sukuma[1] as a first language, with many children only learning Swahili in primary school (Bessire and Bessire, 1997). Other ethnic groups common to the area were the Zinza, Haya, Sumbwa, Nyamwezi, Luo, Kurya, Jita, and Kerewe (United Republic of Tanzania, 1997).

The people described in this book are fairly typical of rural populations throughout sub-Saharan Africa. They lived in settlements of varying remoteness, some on international thoroughfares or near economically vibrant towns, and others relatively isolated. They mainly were small farmers reliant on a combination of subsistence crops, cash crops, and cattle. The vast majority lived in mud-built houses without electricity and used traditional pit latrines. Women in most households had to walk for approximately half an hour to obtain untreated water for domestic use, and most of the population were poorly served by education and health services. Such conditions continue to be common in Tanzania today (National Bureau of Statistics and ICF Macro, 2011).

Sukumas make up the largest ethnic group in Tanzania and numbered approximately five million people at the time of the study. There are some broad similarities between the Sukuma and many other African ethnic groups. Caldwell, Caldwell, and Quiggin (1989) argue that most Africa societies share characteristics which the authors define as part of an "African system," and historically Sukuma culture shared most of those characteristics. These include: placing great importance in ancestry, descent, and fertility; believing in ancestral spirit intervention in the affairs of the living; respecting the old (particularly men) and typically valuing intergenerational links over marital bonds; payment of bridewealth to the bride's family upon marriage; marked spousal separation of economic activities and responsibilities; husbands usually being much older than wives; polygyny being more common than in the Eurasian system; and divorce also being fairly common (Cory, 1953; Tanner, 1955a; Abrahams, 1967; Varkevisser, 1973; Caldwell, Caldwell, and Quiggin, 1989).

Almost half of Mwanza Region's population was under fifteen years of age at the time of the study (National Bureau of Statistics and ORC Macro, 2004). A 1997–1998 survey of 9,445 fifteen- to nineteen-year-olds in rural Mwanza found that 1 percent of males and 2 percent of females were HIV-positive (Obasi et al., 2001). A 2007–2008 survey in Mwanza Region similarly found that 1 percent of males and 6 percent of females aged fifteen to twenty-four years tested positive for HIV (TACAIDS et al., 2008).

The *MEMA kwa Vijana* Adolescent Sexual Health Intervention Trial

The *MEMA kwa Vijana* intervention consisted of four interrelated components: a teacher-led, peer-assisted primary school program; training of health facility workers to provide youth-friendly services; the promotion and distribution of condoms by out-of-school youth; and community mobilization (Obasi et al., 2006). During the trial, intervention implementers conducted ongoing monitoring and evaluation of the program. The process of the intervention was further evaluated by external evaluators, process evaluation surveys, and ongoing qualitative research within the HALIRA project. Process evaluation findings were used to inform and improve intervention design and implementation over the three years of the trial.

The impact of the *MEMA kwa Vijana* intervention primarily was evaluated through the community randomized trial, in which twenty communities were randomly assigned to either the intervention or a control group (Hayes et al., 2005). Each community was roughly equivalent to a ward, which was a local administrative unit with its own health, education, and governance structures. Each ward consisted of five or six villages, five or six primary schools, one or two government health units, and an average total population of seventeen thousand people. To assess intervention impact, three surveys were conducted with 9,645 young people in intervention and control communities between 1998 and 2002 (table 1.1). Trial participants were fourteen years old or older at recruitment, and 94 percent were fourteen to seventeen years old in the first year of the intervention. The trial surveys collected data on participants' knowledge, attitudes, self-reported behavior, and biomedical outcomes, that is, HIV, other sexually transmitted infections, and pregnancy (Ross et al., 2007).

After the trial ended in 2002, the intervention was continued in the same schools and health facilities. From 2004 to 2008 it was also expanded ten-fold to all government primary schools and health facilities in the four project districts (Renju, Andrew, Medard et al., 2010; Renju, Andrew, Nyalali et al., 2010; Renju, Makokha et al., 2010). In 2007–2008, a cross-sectional survey was conducted with 13,804 intervention participants to evaluate long-term intervention impact (table 1.1) (Doyle et al., 2010).

The Health and Lifestyles Research (HALIRA) Project

The main research methods used within the HALIRA project were participant observation, in-depth interviews, group discussions, and simulated patient exercises. Data usually were collected by a team of two male and two female East Africans in their twenties, although staff turnover meant that six different young researchers were involved from the start to the end of the fieldwork.

Participant observation visit length, geographic range, and researcher differences were selected to maximize the representativeness of the qualitative data collected. The six fieldworkers represented different sexes, ethnicities, linguistic skills, and education levels. The nine selected villages and seventeen host households were typical of the range of sociodemographic conditions within rural Mwanza, that is, primarily agricultural or fishing, entirely Sukuma or multiethnic, and dispersed/remote or larger villages.

Participant observation took place for a total of 158 person-weeks. The four main villages were intervention-control pairs that were visited by one or two researchers for approximately seven weeks per year for three years (table 1.1). Another five villages were also visited for participant observation, either in pilot studies for the main participant observation work or as sociodemographic complements to the four main villages. During participant observation visits, each researcher lived in a village household and accompanied

Table 1.1. Timeline of the *MEMA kwa Vijana* Intervention, Surveys, and HALIRA Qualitative Research

Year	Intervention[a]	Surveys[b]	Participant Observation	In-depth Interviews	Other Qualitative Methods
1997	Development				
1998	Testing and Training	Impact Evaluation 1 (Trial Baseline)			Observation of Training Courses
1999	Trial Year 1	Process Evaluation 1	Pilot Tests and Round 1	Pilot Tests and Series 1	Pupil Group Discussions
2000	Trial Year 2	—Impact Evaluation 2 (Trial Interim) —Process Evaluation 2			—Young Adult Group Discussions —Simulated Patient Exercises
2001	Trial Year 3	Impact Evaluation 3 (Trial Final)	Round 2		
2002	Continuation		Round 3	Series 2 and 3	
2003					
2004	Ten-fold Scale-Up				
2005					
2006					
2007		Impact Evaluation 4 (Cross-sectional Follow-up)			
2008					
2009				Series 4	

[a]Obasi et al., 2006; Renju, Andrew, Medard et al., 2010; Renju, Andrew, Nyalali et al., 2010; Renju, Makokha et al., 2010.

[b]The first three impact evaluation surveys were part of the *MEMA kwa Vijana* randomized controlled trial (Todd et al., 2004; Hayes et al., 2005; Ross et al., 2007). Each of these surveys involved biomedical data collection and face-to-face questionnaire interviews with the entire trial cohort, and assisted self-completion questionnaire interviews with a sub-sample. The fourth impact evaluation survey consisted of biomedical data collection and face-to-face questionnaire interviews with a large sample of young people that overlapped with the trial cohort (Doyle et al., 2010).

young people in diverse daily activities (e.g., fetching water, preparing meals, going to market, farming, fishing, and socializing) and at special events (e.g., funerals, drumming-dancing events, video shows, and Christian and national holidays). Each day, researchers spent one to two hours writing field notes in Swahili or English.

In addition to participant observation research, 184 formal in-depth interviews were conducted with ninety-two trial participants (forty-nine intervention, forty-three control), including seventy-six who were randomly selected, thirteen who were HIV-positive, and three who were pregnant in primary school. Seventy-one of those individuals or their family members were interviewed first in 1999–2000 and again in 2002. Twenty-three of the respondents who had been intervention participants were then interviewed for a third time in 2009 (table 1.1).

A first series of eight group discussions involved *MEMA kwa Vijana* class peer educators and other pupils. Those discussions focused on pupil experiences and impressions of the in-school component of the *MEMA kwa Vijana* intervention. A second series of three or four discussions were conducted with each of six groups of out-of-school young people in trial control communities. Those twenty-one discussions and their fifty follow-up in-depth interviews explored sensitive sexual topics which had been particularly difficult to investigate through participant observation or in-depth interviews.

Finally, simulated patient exercises consisted of trained rural young people visiting nineteen *MEMA kwa Vijana* trial health facilities (ten intervention, nine control) with scripted concerns about sexually transmitted infection symptoms and/or requests for contraception or condoms.

BOOK OVERVIEW

One goal of this book is to describe young rural Africans' perspectives on sexual health intervention and effective sexual risk reduction. Toward that end, the main chapters draw heavily on interview quotes and participant observation conversations. In addition, there are three series of case studies which describe the family and school backgrounds, sociodemographic activities, and sexual relationship histories of individual young people who gave plausible accounts of trying to be abstinent, to reduce their partner number, to be faithful, and/or to use condoms.

Another goal of this book is to present the study's findings in a way that is clear and useful to people from a wide range of backgrounds. As the outcome of a rigorous, multidisciplinary research project, it is written with specialists in social sciences, public health, and areas studies in mind. Toward that end, the book's arguments are supported by detailed evidence and they are contextualized within the broader academic literature. However, it is also hoped that this material will be accessible and useful for program developers, policy makers, government officials, undergraduate students, and interested members of the general public in East Africa and elsewhere. Toward that end, academic jargon is avoided in the text, and when specialized terms are necessary, they are explained upon introduction.

The chapters in this book are divided into four broad sections: a background (chapters 1–3); a process and impact evaluation of the *MEMA kwa Vijana* intervention (chapters 4–7); an in-depth description of young people who practiced the ABC behaviors (chapters 8–10); and recommendations for more effectively promoting those behaviors with rural young people in sub-Saharan Africa (chapter 11).

More specifically, the next chapter (chapter 2) describes the study's background, design, and individual methods in detail. Chapter 3 then summarizes findings from this book's companion volume on typical young people's lives, sexual behavior, relationships, and health in the absence of an intervention (Plummer and Wight, 2011).

Chapters 4 through 7 describe and evaluate the *MEMA kwa Vijana* adolescent sexual health intervention in depth. Chapter 4 provides an overview of the intervention as well as a detailed description of community mobilization activities. Chapter 5 describes the content of the school curriculum and examines the role of teachers and peer educators within the intervention. Chapter 6 assesses the clinical and outreach services provided by health workers, as well as the work of out-of-school youth condom distributors. Finally, chapter 7 discusses qualitative and quantitative findings of intervention impact—or lack thereof—on theoretical determinants of sexual behavior, different sexual risk practices, and sexual health.

The intervention evaluation section of this book is followed by a section examining the motivations and strategies of young people who practiced low-risk sexual behaviors, regardless of intervention status. Chapter 8 considers HALIRA findings for young people who practiced primary or secondary abstinence. Chapter 9 considers findings for young people who tried to have few partners and/or to practice fidelity. Chapter 10 then examines the data collected on young people who used condoms. Case study series before each of these chapters detail the lives and sexual relationship histories of young people who tried to practice one or more of these low-risk behaviors. Finally, chapter 11 will review the book's findings and discuss broad principles to better promote low-risk sexual behaviors with young rural Africans. It will also review promising interventions which could complement and improve the effectiveness of school and health facility programs.

NOTE

1. Some contemporary writers in English refer to the Sukuma and Swahili languages and peoples by the terms that would be used within either language, e.g., **Basukuma** (the Sukuma people), **Kisukuma** (the Sukuma language), and *Kiswahili* (the Swahili language). This is not practiced for most other languages and peoples, for example, when speaking English, German people are not referred to using the German term "die Deutschen" and the German language is not referred to as "Deutsch." This book thus uses the conventional English practice of simply referring to the "Sukuma" and "Swahili" languages and peoples.

Chapter Two

Research Methods

This chapter describes the Health and Lifestyles Research (HALIRA) Project in detail. As noted in chapter 1, the HALIRA study was developed as a complement to the *MEMA kwa Vijana* adolescent sexual and reproductive health intervention trial that took place in rural Mwanza, Tanzania from 1997 to 2002 (table 1.1) (Todd et al,. 2004; Hayes et al., 2005; Obasi et al., 2006; Ross et al., 2007). The qualitative methods introduced in chapter 1 were all used within the HALIRA project, including participant observation, in-depth interviews, group discussions, and simulated patient exercises. A more in-depth description of the broader research process, such as the recruitment of the multilingual research team and challenges encountered during fieldwork, can be found in this book's companion volume (Plummer and Wight, 2011).

THE HALIRA PROJECT AND STAFF

Early in the *MEMA kwa Vijana* trial, the principal investigators recognized that it would be valuable to conduct detailed qualitative studies of trial participants' lifestyles and sexual behavior, to better evaluate the *MEMA kwa Vijana* intervention and contextualize and interpret the trial results. Ideally, such qualitative research would begin before intervention development in order to optimally inform it. However, funding for the HALIRA project was not obtained until the first year of intervention development was completed and baseline trial data had already been collected. Prior to beginning fieldwork, the HALIRA proposal was approved by the Tanzanian Medical Research Coordinating Committee and the UK London School of Hygiene and Tropical Medicine Ethics Committee.

The HALIRA project began in April 1999. From April to September, HALIRA staff were hired and trained, and research protocols and instruments were designed, pre-tested, and piloted. The main fieldwork then took place in Missungwi, Kwimba, Sengerema, and Geita Districts of Mwanza Region from September 1999 to August 2002 (table 1.1). Figure 2.1 shows the locations where different types of qualitative research were conducted relative to the *MEMA kwa Vijana* trial intervention and control communities.

The HALIRA project had three British principal investigators who were employed by the London School of Hygiene and Tropical Medicine and the UK Medical Research Council: David Ross (a clinical epidemiologist), Richard Hayes (a statistician), and Daniel Wight (a social anthropologist),

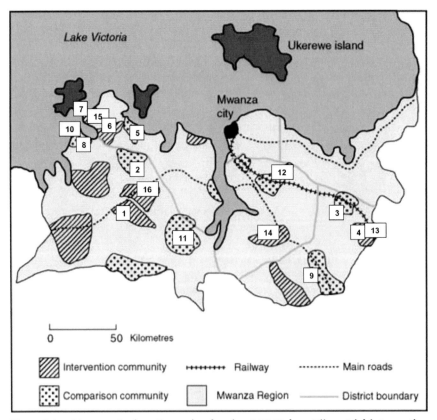

Figure 2.1.   Mwanza Region, Tanzania, showing *MEMA kwa Vijana* trial intervention and control communities, and locations of HALIRA fieldwork. In-depth interviews were conducted and simulated patient exercises attempted in all twenty trial communities. Villages numbered 1–9 = participant observation; 10–12 = young adult group discussions; 13–16 = pupil group discussions.

the last of whom led the design and supervision of the project. At the start of the project, this book's author (Mary Plummer) was a thirty-three-year-old American with a background in social sciences, biology, languages, and HIV/ AIDS education. She was employed by the London School of Hygiene and Tropical Medicine and, as the *MEMA kwa Vijana* social science coordinator, she was responsible for co-designing and co-managing quantitative and qualitative social science research within the trial, including coordination of the HALIRA project. At any given time, HALIRA fieldwork primarily was conducted by a team of four young East Africans: one male and one female Swahili-speaking university graduate, and one male and one female Sukuma-speaking secondary school graduate. Gerry Mshana was a twenty-seven-year-old Tanzanian and Joyce Wamoyi a twenty-five-year-old Kenyan when they joined HALIRA as graduate researchers. As native Swahili speakers from urban Tanzania and Kenya, they were "partial" outsiders who were fluent in the national language, and they also brought analytical skills from other disciplines to their work. The Sukuma researchers—Zachayo Salamba Shigongo, Halima Abdallah, Kija Nyalali, and Neema Busali—were Tanzanians in their early twenties when they began the research. They had quite limited training prior to being hired by the project, but they were highly intelligent and personable and brought an intimate understanding of local cultures and languages to their work. These six HALIRA researchers were all employed by the Tanzanian National Institute for Medical Research during the study.

The field researcher training included: detailed discussions of the research objectives and key methodological texts; formal and informal seminars on specific research methods; pilot field research for each method alone or with senior researchers; debriefings partway through and immediately after fieldwork; instruction and detailed feedback on writing field notes, compiling data summaries, and drafting summary reports; individualized mentorship; and collective development of a qualitative data coding frame. Over the three years of data collection the field researchers were closely supervised and their ability to analyze data and generate new research questions improved with each round of fieldwork. Three of the researchers stayed for all three years of fieldwork. This continuity was important, because the trusting relationships they built during participant observation and in-depth interviews in the first year of research allowed them to re-establish rapport easily on subsequent visits, and gave them a deeper understanding of the transitions that young people experienced in the interim. The first two female Sukuma researchers (Halima Abdallah and Kija Nyalali) left the HALIRA project for university after its first and second years, respectively, but they returned to work for it during their university vacations.

PARTICIPANT OBSERVATION

As discussed in chapter 1, participant observation typically involves a researcher living with those they are studying and/or participating in their activities for an extended period of time (Wight and Barnard, 1993; Bernard, 1995; Pool and Geissler, 2005). Historically, participant observation has usually taken the form of an individual anthropologist living in a village for one or more years. While the resultant findings may be highly valid for that particular community, they may not be typical of the broader population of interest and they will be shaped by the specific characteristics of a single researcher. This study thus attempted to maximize the representativeness of participant observation data by conducting research in many villages selected for their representativeness. In addition, during any period of fieldwork there were four field researchers of different gender and ethnicity collecting data, reducing the chance that findings were strongly influenced by one individual's characteristics. Data collected at systematic intervals over an extended period of time were also used to try to identify and monitor trends.

Prior to participant observation, HALIRA researchers received permission to conduct research from regional, district, ward, and village-level elected and appointed officials, as well as the heads of household where the field researchers were to live. Early in a village stay, field researchers usually also participated in public meetings in which they explained that they were studying the health and lifestyles of village youth. In those meetings and one-to-one conversations afterward, fieldworkers answered any questions people had about the research.

Village and Household Selection

In total, nine villages were visited for participant observation for a total of 158 person-weeks. The main participant observation villages were selected as intervention-control pairs with similar characteristics, to better compare findings from intervention and non-intervention settings. One pair of representative villages was selected in each of three districts, including a pair of large, primarily Sukuma, roadside villages near a gold mine (1 and 2); a pair of remote, dispersed, and almost entirely Sukuma villages (3 and 4); and a pair of large, multiethnic roadside fishing villages near Lake Victoria (5 and 6) (figure 2.1). Specific characteristics of these villages, the host households for participant observation, and the number and lengths of visits are detailed in table 2.1.

Table 2.1. Description of Participant Observation Villages and Households

Village No. (Intervention/ Control)	Number Annual Visits (Total Person-weeks)	Village Characteristics[a] Months Visited: Seasonal Events	Village Facilities	Head of Household Characteristics[b] (Number in Household)[c]	Number Informants in MEMA kwa Vijana Trial[d]
1 (intervention)	three (35)	• Large, roadside villages, approximately 6 km from gold mines. • Water sources mainly unprotected hand-dug ponds. • Vast majority Sukuma. Minorities included Sumbwa, Rongo, Ha, Nyamwezi, and Nyaruanda. *December–January:* —*Weeding crops, end cultivation, start of some harvesting.* —*Christmas and New Year*	One law court, 8 shops/ kiosks, two mills, two storage facilities, one bar, and two churches.	Poor farmer, monogamous couple (8) Very poor farmer, Protestant widow (8)	21
2 (control)	three (36)		One government health facility, 15 shops/ kiosks, one mill, three storage facilities, one bar, two churches and a mosque.	Kiosk owner, political leader, farmer, monogamous Protestant couple (18) Poor farmer, divorced female (9)	24
3 (control)	three (25)	• Remote villages with dispersed populations; neighboring villages were on main roads or railway line. • Cattle important to economy. • Water sources mainly 1 to 2 protected wells per sub-village, built by charities. • Almost 100% Sukuma.	Three seasonal kiosks, one storage facility, and two churches.	Poor farmer, alcohol brewer/seller, monogamous couple (14) Poor farmer, polygynous couple (9)	17

(continued)

Table 2.1. *(continued)*

Village No. (Intervention/ Control)	Number Annual Visits (Total Person-weeks)	Village Characteristics[a] Months Visited: Seasonal Events	Village Facilities	Head of Household Characteristics[b] (Number in Household)[c]	Number Informants in MEMA kwa Vijana Trial[d]
4 (intervention)	three (27)	*(continued)* June–July: —Harvesting and selling crops. —Relaxing, socializing and ngoma (drumming-dancing) celebrations —**Bulabo** (Christian Eucharist) and Saba saba (Farmer's Day)	Several kiosks, one mill, one storage facility, and two churches.	Very poor farmer, previously polygynous couple (8) Kiosk owner, alcohol brewer/seller, political leader, farmer, Nyakyusa Seventh Day Adventist widow (6); Traditional healer, farmer, polygynous Muslim husband and wives (12)	26
5 (control)	one (7)	• Large, roadside villages on or near Lake Victoria. • Many involved in fishing economy. • Water sources included the lake, deep wells, protected deep ponds, and/or unprotected seasonal shallow ponds. • Majority Sukuma ethnicity. Minorities included: Zinza, Jita and Kerewe; also some Haya, Luo, Rundi, and Nyaruanda.	Over 30 shops and kiosks, two mills, two storage facilities, 4 churches and a mosque.	Teacher, kiosk and bar owner, farmer, polygynous Sukuma/ Zinza couple (7)	
6 (intervention)	one (7)		Many shops and kiosks, one mill, two cement buildings, two storage facilities, and 4 churches.	Retired teacher, farmer, monogamous Protestant couple (4)	

Village	No. of researchers[c]	Description	Household heads[b]	No. in household[c]
7 (intervention)	one (10)	(continued) Villages 5 and 6: *July–August* Village 7: *April–May (Easter)* Village 8: *June (pilot)*	Many shops and kiosks, two mills, several bars and video halls, three guest houses, two churches and one mosque. Private church facilities (an air strip, a dispensary, schools).	Poor fisherman, farmer, monogamous couple (14) — — Poor fisherman, farmer, monogamous Kerewe couple (8) — 13
8 (control)	one (1.5)		One law court, a police post, 15 shops and kiosks, three mills, one storage facility, one bar/video hall, and one guest house.	Government employee, landlord, monogamous couple (11) —
9 (control)	three (9)	• Remote village with dispersed population. Roads impassable in rainy season. • Cattle important to economy. • Water source was seasonal river that flowed during rainy season, and in which people dug unprotected ponds in dry season. • Almost 100% Sukuma. *March, June, October, December (pilots)*	One storage facility, three seasonal kiosks.	Poor farmer, monogamous couple (6) Poor farmer, polygynous couple (10) Tailor, farmer, polygynous husband and wives (9) — 17

[a] In all villages, most villagers engaged in farming cotton, cassava, maize, sweet potatoes, peanuts, cow peas, millet, and/or sorghum. In all villages, many families also kept cattle.

[b] Heads of household were Sukuma and Catholic, unless otherwise noted. "Polygynous couple" signifies that another formally recognized wife lived in another household.

[c] Number in household was total number over 2 to 3 visits, so this could be greater than the number present at any one point in time.

[d] Villages 5, 6, and 8 were only visited in 1999 by one researcher each. At that time, information was not collected on whether informants were also *MEMA kwa Vijana* trial participants.

Villages 1–4 each were visited for approximately two months per year for three years (tables 1.1 and 2.1). Villages 5 and 6 were each only visited once for approximately two months due to researcher time constraints, although another intervention village (7) with similar characteristics was visited by other researchers for approximately two months later in the study period. The remaining two villages (8 and 9) were in control communities and were used for one-week participant observation pilot and training visits. After the onset of the study, village 9 was visited by each new researcher during training, while accompanied by an experienced researcher.

Upon first arriving at a village, participant observation researchers enlisted the support of village authorities to identify households of *MEMA kwa Vijana* trial participants where they might live. Each researcher requested to stay with a typical family, that is, one that was not unusually wealthy, educated, religious, or otherwise distinct. They also took into consideration the characteristics of the other participant observation host families in order to achieve a demographically representative range of households. Researchers usually visited three or four households before selecting one. Pairs of researchers lived in different households within the same village, and they almost always returned to live in those same households on subsequent visits to the village.

Researcher Integration in Villages

The researchers were generally welcomed as guests by their hosts. However, they contributed to households by paying for some basic staples, helping in chores, and writing or reading as requested by semi-literate or illiterate hosts. The researchers did not pretend to be villagers, but they sometimes altered their appearance and habits to avoid stark differences. For example, female researchers did not wear trousers during fieldwork, because this was very uncommon in rural areas.

During the first days of a first visit to a participant observation village, fieldworkers found that local people were often cautious with them, treating them politely but with some reserve. The levels of curiosity and wariness about researchers varied within and between villages. Within a few days of familiarity, however, villagers usually seemed to become comfortable with fieldworkers and to take their presence for granted. The Sukuma researchers were particularly successful in quickly and effectively integrating into households and villages. They could easily follow and participate in informal discussions and exchanges, which were often in Sukuma, and this was very important in quickly building rapport with villagers. Being in their early twenties, they were also several years younger than the graduate researchers and sometimes were perceived to be even younger.

Most village households consisted of an immediate family and one or more extended family members who came from within and beyond the village, including young people who might join a household for some months or years. The Sukuma researchers' backgrounds were so similar to other villagers that they were treated very similarly to such young people and others in the household of their age and gender. Of all of the researchers, the young Sukuma women seemed the least likely to be perceived as guests within households and villages, and they were readily expected to participate in the routine menial tasks expected of other girls and young women.

The graduate researchers were not absorbed into households and villages in the same way as Sukuma researchers. Neither graduate researcher was a member of a local ethnic group nor spoke a local language other than Swahili, and the female graduate researcher spoke a Kenyan dialect of Swahili. These attributes, combined with the graduate researchers' somewhat older, urban identities, always indicated that they were visitors to the area, even after they built rapport with many villagers and learned basic Sukuma terminology. Graduate researchers assisted in some daily chores within households and farms—particularly the female researcher, since domestic work was largely done by women—but this was less frequent and was not taken for granted in the same way that it was for Sukuma researchers, particularly the females. Nonetheless, there were times when the graduate researchers' identities as urban, professional "outsiders" seemed advantageous. Villagers could be particularly patient and detailed with them when explaining beliefs and practices which they might have felt were self-evident to others of a similar background.

Participant observation researchers began and continued their fieldwork by accompanying the young people in their households in their normal daily activities outside of school. These activities included work, such as cultivating or harvesting crops, cattle herding, running errands (for example, grinding flour at a mill, or buying fish at Lake Victoria), and, for women only, domestic chores such as peeling and pounding cassava, cooking, and collecting water and firewood (figure 2.2). Researchers also accompanied young people during their leisure time, such as when they strolled and mingled in the village center in the evening, talked with their family over meals, attended choir practice, or, usually for boys and men only, played soccer, netball, or traditional board games. Over time, young people in the host household and others that researchers met in the course of daily activities were befriended, informally interviewed, and accompanied to social settings, such as markets, weekly church services, weddings, funerals, video shows and *ngoma* (traditional drumming-dancing) events, as well as celebrations related to Christian holidays such as Christmas and Easter, and national holidays such as *Saba saba* (the July 7th national holiday).

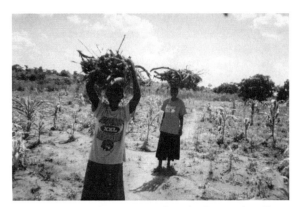

Figure 2.2. A Sukuma researcher (background) collecting firewood with a seventeen-year-old.

Informants

During the three years of fieldwork, the participant observation researchers identified a total of 927 informants of various ages. The term "informant" is used here to mean anyone for whom information was documented; the amount of information varied from very brief (for example, someone was seen playing cards) to detailed and lengthy. In the villages which were only visited by one researcher in 1999, information was not collected on whether informants were also *MEMA kwa Vijana* trial participants. In the remaining six villages, 118 of the informants were trial participants (table 2.1).

Most informants were aged between fourteen and twenty-five years. Fieldworkers tried to engage with as wide a range of young people in each village as possible, by intentionally getting to know different networks, both formal (such as different religious groups) and informal (such as groups with "respectable" or "badly behaved" reputations). However, the research priority was to build trusting relationships with teenagers, particularly *MEMA kwa Vijana* trial participants. Sometimes adolescents did not associate with each other or disliked each other, such as children in a religious host family who disapproved of young people who attended video shows. In such instances, researchers tried to be diplomatic in meeting different individuals at different times, and being polite and respectful of all of them. If questioned about perceived alliances, fieldworkers explained that they needed to get to know as many different kinds of young people as possible in order to do their work well, while also stressing that anything anyone told them was confidential. In addition to cultivating relationships with young people in general, field researchers tried to observe and engage with *MEMA kwa Vijana* intervention implementers, such as peer educators, condom distributors, teachers, and health workers, as well as their control community counterparts.

Pairs of participant observation researchers often lived several kilometers apart from one another, and developed distinct and only occasionally overlapping informant lists. For a given visit, each researcher typically had twelve to fifteen key informants with whom they spent a great deal of time and discussed adolescent sexual health issues in depth. This usually included several household members, several other adolescent *MEMA kwa Vijana* trial participants, several single or married young adults in their late teens or twenties, and several thirty- to sixty-year-old villagers who engaged in activities of interest such as health services, traditional medicine, and teaching. Most of these people continued to be key informants in subsequent visits when new key informant relationships were also developed.

In the early years of participant observation, it was sometimes difficult for researchers to spend much time with *MEMA kwa Vijana* trial participants other than those in their host household, because many trial participants were still in primary school during the day. Even when they were out of school, it was not always easy to establish close relationships with trial participants, because it was unusual for people in their twenties to seek out youths of the same sex who were five to ten years younger to socialize with them. In addition, social division of the sexes was strongly established in rural areas. When researchers attempted to engage with the opposite sex, this was often interpreted as a kind of sexual negotiation. Researchers thus mainly spent time with older, out-of-school youth of the same sex, although they established relationships with trial participants whenever possible.

Data Collection and Recording

Participant observation data collection was guided by a detailed list of research topics. This guideline addressed broad aspects of village life, such as main economic activities, social divisions, kinship relations, and illness treatment beliefs and practices. Participant observation researchers were also instructed to record any observations and informant comments about the different components of the *MEMA kwa Vijana* intervention or trial surveys. This included formal and informal activities, and adult and adolescent perceptions of intervention teachers, peer educators, health workers, and condom distributors. Fieldworkers similarly collected data about health services, schools, and any other youth and/ or sexual health programs in trial control communities.

Participant observation data collection also focused on young people's social lives, such as their interactions while working within *rika* (youth peer groups), carrying out chores, or attending sport, video, or *ngoma* events. Data were also collected on young people's sexual and reproductive knowledge, attitudes, and behavior, and youth sexual culture, such as how young people negotiated sexual encounters or managed ongoing sexual relationships. Researchers collected sexual behavior data in multiple ways. For example, each researcher frequently witnessed couples discussing plans to meet for sex later, or an intermediary negotiating sex for a third person. Researchers were also sometimes present when young people prepared for, or returned from, sexual encounters. For example, in some villages, female researchers shared a room and a mattress with young women who snuck out of the house late at night to meet boys or men for sex at prearranged times. Similarly, researchers observed young men within their households preparing for clandestine sexual encounters at night, such as when a young man explained that he carried a mat with him each evening to use when having sex in fields.

At all times, field researchers carried a small notebook so that they could discreetly jot down notes soon after an event or a discussion of interest. These jottings facilitated recall and accuracy when they wrote lengthier notes in a larger notebook each day for one to two hours. These fieldnotes were entered as a series of short segments identified by number, codename of person, place, date, and time. Several measures were taken to prevent villagers reading confidential information in these notebooks: codes were used in place of informant names; the researcher always kept the master code list on him/her; the notebooks were locked inside a suitcase when not in use; and the graduate researchers wrote in English, a language that was rarely spoken or understood in rural Mwanza. Sukuma researchers instead wrote their participant observation field notes in Swahili.

Researchers conducted five Swahili and three Sukuma group discussions during participant observation visits, as well as sixteen Swahili and seven Sukuma formal individual interviews. For some of these, informants agreed to be audio-recorded. Informants usually spoke much less freely in the formal, recorded interviews than they did in informal discussions. The resultant cassette tapes were locked with the recorder in the suitcase during fieldwork.

Researchers did not take photographs during the first eighteen months of participant observation because of the possibility that this might draw undue attention to them. At the time, cameras of any kind were rare in rural Mwanza. During the last eighteen months of research, however, each pair of participant observation researchers carried one 35 mm camera with them, which they occasionally used to document typical aspects of village life. When not in a public setting, researchers requested verbal permission of their subjects before taking photographs. They offered to send a copy of photographs back to those subjects after the field work ended, and most people requested this. Fieldworkers were discreet in their photography, and during their two-month participant observation visits each pair of researchers only took forty photographs on average.

Each participant observation visit included a day-long debriefing meeting in Mwanza City with the research coordinator and other field researchers mid-way through and immediately after the participant observation ended. After each visit was completed, field researchers also wrote a summary report in English or Swahili, and compiled a list of all informants mentioned in their field notebooks, with a twenty-five-word profile of each. These meetings and reports were used to assess the research process, to identify and resolve problems that had arisen, to evaluate the nature and quality of the data already collected, and to revise the approach to subsequent data collection.

A saturation approach was employed for collection of data on general topics. For example, if sufficient sociodemographic information had been collected about a village on a previous visit, researchers did not seek out or record additional sociodemographic data in subsequent visits, unless important changes occurred. In contrast, researchers attempted to document all observations or discussions related to reproductive and sexual health and behavior throughout their participant observation research, including any mention of *MEMA kwa Vijana* or other sexual health interventions.

IN-DEPTH INTERVIEWS

As discussed in chapter 1, an in-depth interview usually involves an interviewer asking a respondent a series of open-ended questions based on a broad topic guideline. The interviewer tries to create an intimate and trusting setting during the interview, encouraging the respondent to carefully reflect and honestly answer questions even if they address sensitive or difficult topics. The respondent is asked to describe their particular world view in their own terms. The semi-structured nature of this approach allows respondents to raise unanticipated issues within a topic, which can then be explored in depth (Smith and Morrow, 1996; Price and Hawkins, 2002). In-depth interview findings are generally considered to be less representative but more accurate and meaningful than survey interviews (Parker, Herdt, and Carballo, 1991; Konings et al., 1995; Smith and Morrow, 1996; Messersmith et al., 2000; Larsen and Hollos, 2003).

Respondent Selection and Recruitment

HALIRA's pilot in-depth interviews were conducted from April to September 1999, both to train researchers and to improve the interview schedule and protocol. These interviews were conducted with twenty-six *MEMA kwa Vijana* trial participants randomly selected from both intervention and control schools. An additional fourteen pilot interviews were conducted with other rural youth, teachers, and village authorities.

After completion of the pilot interviews, field researchers conducted 184 formal interviews with ninety-two other trial members (table 2.2). In total there were four series of interviews which are numbered chronologically (table 1.1). These included three series which were conducted with the same respondents, specifically: first interviews with seventy-three respondents in 1999–2000 (the "first" series); second interviews with seventy-one of those individuals or a family member at the end of the trial in 2002 (the "second" series); and third interviews with twenty-three of those individuals who had been intervention participants, in conjunction with a trial follow-up survey in 2009 (the "fourth" series). In addition, nineteen other trial members were interviewed one time only, at the end of the trial in 2002 (the "third" series).

In-depth interview respondents were drawn from all *MEMA kwa Vijana* trial communities (figure 2.1). Just over half of the respondents in the first three series of interviews were intervention participants and all of them were in the fourth series (table 2.2). Most respondents were randomly selected from the general population, but some were selected because they were pregnant or they had a preliminary HIV-positive test result. Interviewers knew of these three selection categories, but did not know the reason why any particular in-depth interview respondent was selected. The selection process is described in detail below.

The First In-Depth Interview Series

The first series of HALIRA in-depth interviews took place in 1999–2000 (table 1.1). These involved pregnant, HIV-positive, and randomly selected pupils. One percent (32/4149) of the female participants in the 1998 survey tested positive for pregnancy, and three of them were randomly selected for this interview series. Twenty-three of 9,283 trial participants had preliminary HIV-positive results in the 1998 survey, of whom twenty were randomly selected for interviews. Later testing of those specimens and/or other specimens those individuals provided at later surveys determined that only seven (two male and five female) of the twenty were truly HIV-positive (table 2.2) (Plummer, Ross et al., 2004).

During analysis and in this book, those respondents who were initially selected because of an HIV-positive test result, but who later were confirmed to be HIV-negative, are included with those who were randomly selected from the general population. Specifically, in the first series of in-depth interviews, respondents were considered to be "randomly selected" from the

Table 2.2. In-Depth Interviews with *Mema kwa Vijana* Trial Members, by Series, Selection Status, Sex, and Intervention Status

| Year | Interview Series | Number of Trial Members (Number of Intervention Participants) | | | | | |
| | | Randomly Selected[a] | | Confirmed HIV-positive[b] | | Pregnant in 1998 | Total |
		Male	Female	Male	Female	Female	
1999	Pilot	13 (11)	13 (7)	0	0	0	26 (18)
1999–2000	Series 1	29 (13)	34 (20)	2 (1)	5 (3)	3 (1)	73 (38)
2002	Series 2[c]	29 (13)	33 (20)	1 (0)	3 (2)	3 (1)	69 (36)
2009	Series 4[d]	11 (11)	12 (12)	0	0	0	23 (23)
2002	Series 3	4 (2)	9 (4)	1 (1)	5 (4)	0	19 (11)
1999–2009	Total	46 (26)	56 (31)	3 (2)	10 (7)	3 (1)	118 (67)

[a]Randomly selected respondents are defined as: (1) pairs randomly selected from the same class in a school that had no HIV-positive trial participants; (2) individuals randomly selected from the same school and class as a trial participant who had a preliminary positive HIV or pregnancy test result; and (3) respondents who were selected for interview because of a preliminary HIV-positive result, but who subsequently were confirmed to be HIV-negative through a series of later tests.

[b]Two HIV-positive respondents from the first interview series died before the second series took place. During the second interview series, two semi-structured interviews were conducted with a guardian or parent for each of them; those interviews are not included in the figures above.

[c]The second interview series involved reinterviewing all respondents from the first series who could be located and who agreed to participate.

[d]In the fourth interview series, fifteen males and fifteen females were randomly selected from the thirty-three randomly selected intervention participants who had participated in the first two series. All of those who could be located and agreed to participate were interviewed.

general population if they were selected in one of three ways: (a) pairs randomly selected from the same class in a school that had no HIV-positive trial
participants in 1998 (n = 27); (b) one individual randomly selected from the
same school and class as each trial participant who had a preliminary positive
HIV or pregnancy test result in 1998 (n = 23); and (c) respondents who were
selected for interview because of a preliminary HIV-positive result in 1998,
but who subsequently were confirmed to be HIV-negative through a series of
later tests (n = 13) (table 2.2).

   In that first interview series, most respondents were found at school and the
remainder in their homes. Of the seventy-four individuals who were initially
selected, eight of those who were randomly selected were either not found
(n = 7) or refused to participate (n = 1), resulting in 89 percent compliance.
Randomly selected alternates replaced the eight missing people, but one of
their interviews was excluded from analysis after the respondent was found
to be using another child's name in school.

The Second In-Depth Interview Series

The second series of in-depth interviews involved reinterviewing respondents from the first series in 2002 (tables 1.1 and 2.2). In the two to two and
a half year interim, most respondents had left primary school and had begun
their lives as independent adults. This included some who had married and
moved to another village (mostly women), and some who were working in
occupations that involved travel, such as fishing, mining, or trade (mostly
men). Field researchers made intensive efforts to interview every original
respondent, to minimize the chance that particular types of individuals
might be excluded from repeat interviews. One randomly selected woman
refused to be reinterviewed, one HIV-positive woman could not be located,
and two HIV-positive youths (one male, one female) had died. In the event
that a respondent had died, researchers then interviewed a close family
member using a special interview guide.

The Third In-Depth Interview Series

For the third series of in-depth interviews, twenty new respondents were selected based on their preliminary HIV test results from the 2001–2002 survey
at the end of the trial (tables 1.1 and 2.2). At the time of selection, twenty-six
(three male and twenty-three female) survey participants had results which
suggested they had become HIV-positive since the 1998 survey. All three
males were selected and seven of the females were randomly selected for
in-depth interviews. An additional three males and seven females were randomly selected for interview from the same school and class lists as those

respondents. However, one of the HIV-positive men could not be located for interview. In addition, one man and two women in this series with preliminary HIV-positive results were ultimately found to be HIV-negative after later testing. In total, researchers interviewed nineteen respondents in the third series, six of whom were HIV-positive.

The Fourth In-Depth Interview Series

The fourth series of in-depth interviews was designed to complement the long-term cross-sectional survey evaluation of *MEMA kwa Vijana* intervention impact (table 1.1) (Doyle et al., 2010). Individuals were selected for the fourth series from the pool of intervention participants who had been randomly selected for the first interview series (n = 33). Specifically, fifteen males and fifteen females were randomly selected for this series, of whom eleven males and twelve females were located and agreed to participate (table 2.2). Most respondents were still living in rural Mwanza and were interviewed there. A few were interviewed where they were living in neighboring regions, and one who lived in Tanzania's commercial capital, Dar es Salaam, was interviewed by telephone.

Interview Protocol and Content

For the first two series of in-depth interviews, researchers traveled in same-sex pairs of one graduate researcher and one Sukuma researcher. For the third series, one male and one female Sukuma researcher traveled independently. For the fourth series, the male and female graduate researcher each traveled independently. Verbal consent was obtained from all respondents prior to interviews, and again immediately prior to the use of a tape recorder. For respondents who were still in school and/or living with their parents, verbal consent was also obtained from a head teacher and/or a parent.

The interviewers tried to spend one to two hours building rapport with respondents prior to interviews, taking walks with them, playing games, telling jokes, and sharing a snack with them. In the first and second series of interviews the pair of researchers did this with their two respondents together, which allowed them to identify which youth might most benefit from being interviewed in Sukuma. There was no occasion when both youths said that they would be unable or uncomfortable participating in an interview in Swahili, which would have required recruiting another randomly selected, Swahili-speaking youth. In the first series, forty-five (62 percent) interviews were conducted in Swahili, and twenty-eight (38 percent) in Sukuma, compared to forty-six (67 percent) in Swahili and twenty-three (33 percent) in Sukuma with a subset of the same respondents in the second series. In the third series the Sukuma researchers conducted nine (47 percent) interviews in Swahili and ten (53 percent) in Sukuma with the new set of respondents, while in the fourth series the graduate researchers conducted all nineteen interviews in Swahili.

Interviews were conducted away from home, school, and work settings, usually in an isolated, outdoor, shaded area where there was little chance of interruption or eavesdropping by passers-by. They usually took two hours. The HALIRA interview guides were initially drafted in English, translated into Swahili and Sukuma, back-translated into English, and then edited to promote conceptual equivalence in all three languages. They were further modified based on pilot study findings and tailored to the specific interview series. Respondents were first asked general background questions about their home life, family, school experiences, friendships, and paid and unpaid work. They were then asked their opinions about young people being sexually active, and about their own sexual experiences. Young people who reported they had never had sex were asked about their attitudes and decisions related to this. In the first interview series, respondents who reported experience of sex were then asked in-depth questions about their first sexual experience, including the circumstances that led up to it, how it was negotiated, characteristics of their partner, and the nature of any ongoing sexual relationship that resulted from it. They were also asked about other partners, and to estimate their lifetime number of partners and sexual encounters. However, discussion of these topics was sometimes constrained by limited time. The latter part of interviews in the first series focused on respondent opinions and experience of pregnancy, contraception (including condom use), abortion, circumcision, health care, and HIV/AIDS and other sexually transmitted infections.

The second, third, and fourth series of interviews addressed many of the same topics that were discussed in the first. New questions included those related to the respondents' older age and experience, such as end of primary school, experience of secondary school, work, travel, marriage, and/or children. These interviews did not focus on first sexual experience unless respondents had reported never having had sex in their first interviews. Respondents were instead asked to describe the circumstances surrounding their last sexual experience as well as broader behavior patterns, such as their experience of one-off encounters, partner change, and concurrent partnerships. In the final portion of these interviews, intervention participants were also asked about their experiences and opinions of the *MEMA kwa Vijana* intervention program. Specifically, they were asked for their opinions about each of the intervention components, the different program implementers, and the value and feasibility of the ABC behavioral goals.

Interview Process

During the pilot in-depth interviews it became clear that some respondents spoke little Swahili, even though they were in the upper years of Swahili language primary schools. This challenge was partially resolved by hiring Sukuma-speaking interviewers. In addition, some respondents had difficulty estimating their current age or clearly recalling an earlier age (e.g., age at first sex). The problem of frequent, large errors in age-related data has also been documented in other studies which have scrutinized age estimates in sub-Saharan Africa (Cohen, 1998; Żaba et al., 2009). Some respondents also had substantial difficulty estimating the timing of events (e.g., first sex with different partners), or calculating accurate summaries or frequencies (e.g., number of partners).

Such challenges led to a new technique to help clarify reports. If a respondent mentioned a sexual partner, the researcher might do a simple sketch of that individual with one or two identifying characteristics, such as shirt color, a fish (for fishermen), or a book (for school boys). A sequence of partners could then be drawn and referred to throughout the interview. This process allowed for revisions. For example, if the respondent corrected herself to report a partner prior to the first one mentioned, the new one would be added at the beginning of the series of drawings, or the order of partners could be rearranged. While this technique seemed to improve the accuracy of some reports, inconsistencies in estimated age and the other variables mentioned above continued to be a great problem for all of the research methods used in the HALIRA project and the *MEMA kwa Vijana* trial. Inconsistent reporting related to poor math skills and recall may have been exacerbated by the sensitive nature of many of the interview questions. For example, it was not unusual for respondents to have inconsistent reports about their age at first sex, or lifetime number of partners, in their first and second in-depth interviews. This inconsistency tended to go in one direction, with respondents reporting older ages at first sex or fewer numbers of partners in the later interview, suggesting it sometimes involved a social desirability bias. This pattern was particularly common for female respondents, and especially those who had married between their first and second interview.

Many in-depth interviews were awkward and respondents reticent, only answering questions with a few words and rarely making expansive contributions, particularly in the first interview series, when all respondents were still in primary school. These interviews thus rarely functioned as qualitative research is intended to, allowing respondents to describe their world from their own perspectives and not according to a structure and themes imposed by the researcher. Much of the first series of interviews was devoted to establishing basic information, such as whether a respondent had ever had sex, and then to understanding the circumstances surrounding his or her first sexual experience or relationship. Attempts to ascertain broader sexual behavior patterns were often superficial. Reports about frequency of sex or total number of partners sometimes changed within the course of the interview. In-depth interview respondents' reluctance to talk probably related to multiple factors, including: rarely, if ever, having been interviewed or asked to describe their lives in narrative form; the status difference between themselves and their interviewers; lack of trust in research confidentiality, particularly amongst school pupils; and for young women, the importance of discretion given stigma associated with premarital or extramarital sexual activity.

For a total of eleven pilot in-depth interviews or formal in-depth interviews in the first series, respondents were asked if they would like to identify a close, same-sex friend to participate in the interview with them. Paired interviews were attempted to see if young people were more comfortable or honest talking about sensitive issues in the company of a close friend. This seemed to be effective in a few cases in which truly close friends were selected, as respondents seemed to relax and openly discuss sensitive issues that they had already shared with one another. In a number of interviews, however, researchers found the respondent selected someone who was only a casual friend, and this did not become clear until the interview was well underway. Such paired interviews became uncomfortable when the respondents were asked about sexual behavior. Given the difficulty of identifying close friends in advance of the interview, this paired interview approach was rejected.

All interviews were audio-recorded. After each one, field researchers wrote a brief process report, describing their interactions with the respondent before, during, and after the interview, and any unusual events that occurred related to it.

GROUP DISCUSSIONS

Group discussions are intended to give study participants more influence over the research process than might occur during individual interviews. Researchers facilitate group discussion in a semi-structured way, using open-ended questions to prompt participants to engage with one another (Bernard, 1995; Mack et al., 2005). Ideally, group discussions are more inductive than in-depth interviews, allowing free-flowing informal exchanges that lead to the emergence of new issues which were not previously identified by the researchers (Madriz, 2000).

There are essentially two kinds of discussion groups: those composed of strangers and those of preexisting social groups. A possible advantage of group discussions between strangers is that they may not take their fellow participants' views for granted and so may clearly explain their opinions and experiences (Bloor et al., 2001). They also may be more comfortable expressing sensitive views because they do not have existing roles and relationships to maintain with other group members. Groups of existing friends or acquaintances, in contrast, are less artificial and more likely to mirror real life, because participants tend to present themselves to each other in the same way that they do in everyday life. They also may remind one another of shared experiences, or challenge one another if statements seem inconsistent with their prior knowledge of each other (Bloor et al., 2001).

The HALIRA project conducted two formal series of group discussions during the three years of fieldwork (table 1.1). First, discussions were held with intervention school pupils and class peer educators in 1999, to address their impressions of the *MEMA kwa Vijana* school curriculum and particularly peer education. Second, in 2000 a series of discussions were held with same-sex groups of out-of-school youth to better understand particularly sensitive sexual topics that had been difficult to investigate through other research methods. All group discussions were audio-recorded, and researchers wrote detailed summary reports on each series at the end of fieldwork.

Group Discussions with Primary School Pupils

The *MEMA kwa Vijana* primary school curriculum included a training course for pupil peer educators, who were taught to perform scripted dramas and otherwise support the teacher-led curriculum in class. Pupils from two intervention schools in each of the four study districts were randomly selected for one peer educator and one general pupil group discussion (figure 2.1). In total, four male and four female group discussions were held with six to eight pupils or peer educators, involving pupils in each year of the curriculum (Years 5–7). Head teachers and pupils gave verbal consent for the group discussions. Same-sex pairs of one graduate researcher and one Sukuma researcher led each discussion following a semi-structured question guide. Pupils were provided with a snack and chatted with researchers for five to ten minutes before discussions, which were held away from the school, usually outdoors or in an empty building. The discussions were planned and implemented in collaboration with the *MEMA kwa Vijana* intervention staff, as part of their ongoing, internal process evaluation.

All pupils were asked about material covered in their *MEMA kwa Vijana* classes (e.g., the content of what they had learned; what they liked or disliked; what was clear or confusing); how they felt about teachers teaching them sexual health information; and their perceptions of peer education and the curriculum drama series. The peer educators were additionally asked about any benefits or challenges of being a peer educator for their skills development, personal behavior, and reputations.

These discussions generated some useful information about the pupils' experiences and perceptions of the intervention, but they did not flow easily, and the researchers found it difficult to facilitate an open dialogue between participants. Thus rather than participants discussing topics between themselves, these sessions were effectively group interviews in which the researcher asked questions which specific individuals answered in turn.

Group Discussions and In-Depth Interviews with Young Adults

Following the first year of fieldwork, a series of three or four group discussions were conducted with each of six groups of out-of-school young people, to explore sensitive sexual topics which had been particularly difficult to investigate through participant observation or in-depth interviews. Generally, group discussions are used to examine broad social norms, not intimate, personal experiences or sensitive behaviors (Madriz, 2000; Mack et al., 2005). This sub-study was thus designed so that general opinions would be explored in the group discussions. However, when salient issues came up that warranted further, private exploration, they were addressed in follow-up individual interviews with two or three participants immediately after each discussion.

Three villages were selected to represent different types of rural settings: multiethnic lakeside fishing/farming, multiethnic interior farmland near a mine, and almost entirely Sukuma interior farmland (figure 2.1). The team of four researchers spent one week in each village. During the first few days they developed rapport with young villagers in public areas, such as markets and sports fields. The researchers tried to select and recruit preexisting same-sex groups of friends for discussions, in order to maximize group participants' confidence in discussing sensitive issues amongst themselves, and to minimize the artificiality of the interaction. Over the final two or three days, same-sex researchers then facilitated three to four two-hour discussions with a male and a female group on the following topics.

The first discussion explored girls' motives for sex, including affection, pleasure, coercion, and a desire or need for gifts or money. The second discussion investigated beliefs and practices related to pregnancy prevention, suspended pregnancy (a widely reported belief during participant observation), and induced abortion. The third discussion addressed the range, frequency, and contexts of specific sexual practices, including intentional lubrication or drying of the vagina; foreplay; vaginal intercourse; anal intercourse; oral sex on a man or a woman; male and female homosexuality; and masturbation. The fourth discussion examined condom use and beliefs about the causes and treatment of sexually transmitted infections.

The groups consisted of nine to twelve young people aged fifteen to twenty-seven years, with mean group ages of eighteen to twenty-one years. In two villages, the female groups were mainly single young women engaged in petty trading or farming, while in the third village they were mainly primary school girls or recent primary school leavers. Most of the male participants were farmers, fishermen, or cattle herders, although some petty traders and primary and secondary school students also participated. After each discussion, facilitators held fifteen- to thirty-minute individual in-depth interviews with two or three participants. These interviews were fairly brief and unstructured and focused on one or two specific topics which had arisen during the group discussion. In total, twenty-one discussions and fifty follow-up interviews were conducted.

The group discussions with young adults generally proceeded very well. Participants usually entered into lively discussions, and respectfully questioned and challenged each other based on their mutual familiarity. The facilitators were generally able to curtail individuals who dominated discussions by re-directing questions to less talkative members, and they sometimes interviewed those individuals afterward. Overall, this set of discussions was very effective in collecting information on highly stigmatized practices (e.g., anal intercourse), even when they were infrequent or illegal (e.g., induced abortion).

SIMULATED PATIENT EXERCISES

In simulated patient (also called "mystery client" or "dummy patient") exercises, trained local community members visit health facilities in the assumed role of clients, and then report on their experiences to researchers afterward. Simulated patients generally are not expected to undergo clinical examinations, so this method is best used to assess the quality of clinical interactions (Boyce and Neale, 2006). Simulated patient research is more objective and less biased than some other methods, such as clinician interviews or formal observation, because clinicians may not report or follow their normal practice in such conditions (O'Hara et al., 2001). However, one limitation of this method is that it usually depends on simulated patient recall of what they experienced, and memory can be inaccurate (Baddeley, 1979; Leiva et al., 2001; Joel et al., 2004; Boyce and Neale, 2006; Colvin et al., 2006; Oraby et al., 2008).

In 2000, HALIRA researchers collaborated with the *MEMA kwa Vijana* intervention team to conduct a process evaluation of the youth-friendly health services component of the intervention (table 1.1). Simulated patient exercises were attempted by trained rural young people in twenty trial health facilities (figure 2.1). Approximately six months before these exercises took place, all intervention and control health facilities were informed of, and agreed to, the possibility of such visits. All health workers were subsequently reminded of this possibility by a letter from the Regional Medical Officer. In each of the ten intervention and ten control communities, a health facility was randomly selected for a simulated patient visit.

The simulated patients were selected from eighty-four young applicants from a Sukuma village outside of the study area, based on their confidence, recall, creativity, acting skills, and youthful, rural appearance. Two male and two female fifteen- to seventeen-year-olds were trained to present themselves at health facilities as patients seeking condoms, contraception, or advice about a possible sexually transmitted infection. In case they were challenged, each simulated patient carried letters from the Regional Medical Officer and the *MEMA kwa Vijana* trial director explaining their role in the exercise. In addition, a clinically qualified supervisor was present in a nearby guesthouse when the simulated patient visited a health facility, and could be called on if necessary.

Three scenarios were developed for the simulated patient exercises. In the sexually transmitted infection scenario, the adolescent told the clinician that he or she had had sex with someone two days earlier, and then heard that the person had a sexually transmitted infection, so was concerned about exposure. If the clinician requested an examination, the adolescent was instructed to decline because there were no symptoms. In the condom scenario, the adolescent requested condoms, and at some point during the consultation asked whether new condoms have holes in them, as rumored. In the contraception scenario, a female adolescent requested birth control, and if given options, said that she preferred oral contraceptives. If the clinician requested to examine her, the adolescent was instructed to decline, saying that she was menstruating.

One intervention health facility was closed, so no simulated patient exercise was conducted there. Simulated patients carried a tape recorder to discreetly record clinical consultations. Three visits did not result in usable recordings, because one health facility did not have condoms available for a condom request and two recordings were inaudible. Immediately after each exercise, a clinical supervisor within the intervention debriefed the simulated patient using a semi-structured questionnaire. At the end of the fieldwork, the senior clinical supervisor wrote a summary report.

The simulated patient exercises generally proceeded well. The scripted scenarios provided adequate, plausible reasons for adolescents to obtain sexual health services from clinicians without an examination, although in a couple of instances the adolescents had to repeatedly refuse to be examined. The trained young people acted out their scenarios well, and came up with appropriate responses when they were asked unexpected questions, such as those about their sexual partners. None of the clinicians seemed to suspect that an adolescent was a simulated patient, although several clinicians seemed suspicious of the adolescent's motivations for other reasons. For example, some clinicians were concerned that a girl might have requested contraception to abort an existing pregnancy. The simulated patient transcripts were very useful when combined with debriefing questionnaires and the summary report.

OTHER RESEARCH METHODS

In addition to the main HALIRA methods outlined above, this book will also occasionally draw on data from other sources, including the author's fieldwork, the *MEMA kwa Vijana* intervention team's monitoring and evaluation data, and results from the *MEMA kwa Vijana* trial process evaluation surveys. First, from 1998 to 2002 the author observed teaching in intervention and control classrooms on many occasions, as well as specific intervention activities, e.g., four weeks of teacher, peer educator, and condom distributor selection and training courses. The author also participated in biannual reviews of the intervention during the trial, contributed to its ongoing formative evaluation and modification, and co-led the *MEMA kwa Vijana* impact and process evaluation surveys.

In addition, the *MEMA kwa Vijana* intervention team based at the African Medical and Research Foundation (AMREF) collected extensive monitoring and evaluation data on each of the intervention components throughout the trial (Wight and Obasi, 2003; Obasi et al., 2006; Larke et al., 2010). This included systematic and detailed data on program coverage and quality, such as the number of implementers trained, the number of young people who attended health facilities for treatment of sexually transmitted infections, and the proportion of curriculum sessions taught in schools. For example, the school component of the curriculum was evaluated during pre-scheduled and unannounced annual visits to every intervention school, at which time teachers were observed teaching intervention sessions and curriculum coverage was estimated, primarily based on a review of pupils' exercise books. At annual training courses, all intervention teachers also completed confidential pre- and post-training questionnaires, and subgroups of teachers participated in a series of group discussions with intervention staff.

Finally, two *MEMA kwa Vijana* trial process evaluation surveys were conducted in 1999 and 2000 with 250 government representatives and trial implementers at the district, ward, school, and health facility levels (table

1.1). This included interviews with clinicians from every intervention and control health facility as well as teachers from one randomly selected school in each trial ward. These surveys assessed a large range of variables, including attitudes toward adolescent sexual health education and services; school and health facility training, staffing, and supervision; clinical supplies and school teaching materials; the provision of adolescent sexual health education and services; collaboration between teachers and health workers; other intervention activities; and knowledge and opinions about the *MEMA kwa Vijana* intervention.

In this book, intervention staff monitoring and evaluation findings and trial process evaluation survey results will be cited as documented in published papers, conference abstracts, and unpublished reports.

DATA PROCESSING, ANALYSIS, AND WRITE-UP

Participant observation field notes and recordings of the first three in-depth interview series, the two group discussion series, and the simulated patient exercises were transcribed verbatim in their original Sukuma, Swahili, or English. Sukuma and Swahili transcripts were then translated into English. The quality of transcription or translation was randomly assessed for almost half of all documents by having a second transcriber or translator review them for accuracy. The full English language qualitative dataset consisted of 4.9 million words, 54 percent of which were trial participant in-depth interviews, 24 percent participant observation field notes, 13 percent young adult group discussions and follow-up interviews, 6 percent participant observation group discussions and in-depth interviews, 2 percent pupil group discussions, and 0.3 percent simulated patient exercises.

A coding frame of thirty-two broad categories was developed to organize the data by theme within NUD*IST 4, the Non-numerical Unstructured Data Indexing Searching and Theorizing Computer Program Version 4 (QSR International Pty Ltd, Melbourne, Australia). Sample transcripts from different research methods were used to pilot test and finalize the coding scheme. Five graduate researchers coded different sections of the dataset after each received training that included an evaluation of inter-coder reliability and resolution of differences.

Over twenty broad and sometimes overlapping topics were selected for analysis, such as cultural norms, first sexual experiences, concurrent partnerships, and process evaluations of each of the intervention components. Analysis took place using a thematic and grounded theory approach to generate hypotheses. Hypotheses were then tested against the data through repeated readings of the transcripts and discussion with other HALIRA researchers. For analysis of most topics, data organized under relevant NUD*IST codes were summarized within a few dozen pre-identified themes, as well as themes which emerged during analysis. Additional analysis then often included: comparison of findings with field summary reports; direct searching of the original transcripts using key roots or words; and/or reading all data for people mentioned within particular incidents or topics. This latter step was often critical to obtain a nuanced and full understanding of individuals and the particular contexts of their behaviors.

Analysis of the topic "condom use" provides one example of the process described above. Data which had been organized under the NUD*IST codes "condom distribution and access," "condom beliefs and attitudes," and "condom use" were summarized under thirty-one pre-identified themes, such as "shop access," "health beliefs," and "use in casual relationships." These categories were then analyzed and compared by trial intervention and control status. In addition, all data related to certain individuals were reviewed, such as all data for *MEMA kwa Vijana* condom distributors. Given the possibility of young people falsely reporting condom use, case studies of individuals who tried to use condoms (like case studies of those who tried to abstain, have few partners, and/or practice fidelity) were limited to individuals who provided detailed, plausible, and consistent reports of those behaviors. Where possible, such self-reported data were also compared to third-person reports, researcher observation, and/or biological markers.

The massive scale of the combined HALIRA dataset meant it was not feasible to analyze it in its entirety for some topics. The entire participant observation database was analyzed for most topics, but when analysis of a topic was particularly subtle, complex, and time-consuming, it was occasionally restricted to a pre-selected portion of the participant observation dataset. For example, a detailed analysis of the "cultural norms" topic was only conducted with the Sukuma researcher's participant observation field notes, since they had documented villagers' conversations whether they were in Sukuma or Swahili. In that case, the detailed findings were then compared to all field researchers' summary reports and other data sources to assess their generalizability.

For this book, the author analyzed all in-depth interview transcripts from the first three series for most topics, as well as select interview transcripts from the fourth series for two case studies. Primary analysis of data collected using other research methods only took place when the dataset was particularly relevant to the topic and time allowed. Sometimes this analysis involved a different protocol than that outlined above. For example, based on the simulated patient transcripts and debriefing questionnaires, measures of the quality of clinical consultations (e.g., confidentiality, respectfulness, privacy, and service) were ranked independently by two individuals: first by the assistant intervention coordinator (Bernadette Cleophas-Mazige), who was also the senior clinical supervisor for the simulated patients' study, and then by the author, who conducted the assessment blinded to the intervention or control status of the health facilities. There were few discrepant rankings, and for those the author again reviewed the relevant transcripts and debriefing questionnaires before deciding a final rank. In addition to the clinician above, one graduate researcher (Tom Ingall) conducted preliminary analyses on two topics in this book, that is, condom use, and the *MEMA kwa Vijana* school program process evaluation. The author closely guided his work and carried out additional analyses on those topics.

USE OF DATA AND TERMINOLOGY IN THIS BOOK

In this book words in *non-bold italics* are Swahili, while words in ***bold italics*** are Sukuma. In Tanzania there are seven Standards, or years, of primary school and six Forms, or years, of secondary school. In this book, to make the total years of schooling clear to readers who are unfamiliar with this system, primary school level is referred to by "Year" (such as "Year 7"), and secondary school level is referred to by both "Form" and "Year" (such as "Form 2, the equivalent of Year 9"). "Informants" refers to those who provided information during participant observation, "respondents" to those who provided information in in-depth interviews, and "participants" to those who provided information through group discussions, unless otherwise specified.

Many different terms have been used to describe individuals as they transition from childhood into adulthood, including "prepubescent," "adolescent," "youth," "young person," and "young adult." Each of these terms is open to varying definitions depending on physical, emotional, and cognitive development, as well as age, social status, and other factors. In this book, "prepubescent" children are those who have not yet undergone puberty (often children aged eight to eleven years), while "adolescents" are loosely defined as young people aged twelve to eighteen years, and "young adults" are loosely defined as those aged eighteen to twenty-four years. The terms "youth" and "young people" instead are used broadly to encompass both adolescents and young adults. Importantly, these are rough and overlapping definitions. For example, girls typically enter puberty twelve to eighteen months earlier than boys, and even within each sex the age at which individuals begin puberty can differ by several years. Similarly, young adulthood in rural Mwanza was often defined in terms of social status (e.g., out of school, married, working)

Table 2.3. Examples of Transcript Codes

Code	Explanation
PO-02-I-4-1m	2002 participant observation notes from intervention village no. 4, written by male researcher no. 1.
II-99-I-52-f	In-depth interview no. 52 conducted in 1999 with a female intervention participant.
GD-00-C-10-2f	Group discussion no. 2 conducted with female participants in control village no. 10 in 2000.
GDII-00-C-12-4m	In-depth interview no. 4 conducted with a male group discussion participant in control village no. 12 in 2000.
SP-00-I-21-7f	Simulated patient exercise in intervention village no. 21 conducted in 2000 by female simulated patient no. 7.

rather than chronological age. Thus villagers might treat a twenty-one-year-old primary school pupil as a child, but a married sixteen-year-old farmer as an adult. This will be discussed more in the next chapter.

Excerpts from participant observation field notes or summary reports used in this book are a researcher's reconstruction of what was said or observed previously. Informant and respondent names have been replaced with pseudonyms. When the original names were Christian, Muslim, Swahili, and/or Sukuma, common names of similar religious and/or ethnic origin were selected as pseudonyms. In in-depth interview excerpts, "I" refers to the interviewer and "R" to the respondent; in group discussion excerpts, "F" refers to the facilitator and "P" to the participant; and in simulated patient excerpts, "HW" refers to the health worker and "SP" to the simulated patient. After each excerpt, references in brackets first indicate method, year, trial intervention/control status, and village number. In addition, researcher number and sex are indicated for participant observation and simulated patient excerpts, while group discussion or interview number and sex are indicated for other methods. Examples are provided in table 2.3. All photographs used in this book were taken by the field researchers during participant observation, except for one photograph taken by the author and one taken by David Ross, the *MEMA kwa Vijana* trial director.

CONCLUSION

This chapter described the HALIRA qualitative study that is the basis for this book, including participant observation, in-depth interviews, group discussions, and simulated patient exercises. Before evaluating the *MEMA kwa Vijana* intervention in chapters 4–7, the next chapter will describe typical young people's lives and sexual relationships in rural Mwanza in the absence of a sexual health intervention.

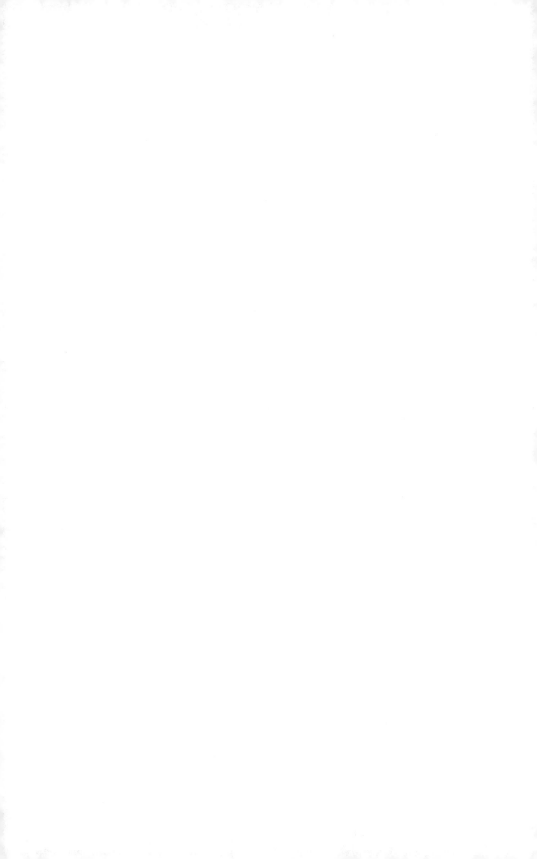

Chapter Three

Typical Young People's Lives and Sexual Relationships

Before examining this book's main question—how to better promote low-risk sexual behaviors with rural African adolescents—it is important to first consider the lives of typical young people in the absence of an intervention. That is the focus of this book's companion volume (Plummer and Wight, 2011), and its findings will be summarized in this chapter. Specifically, this chapter will review HALIRA findings on: general village life; children's relationships with parents, peers, and teachers; sexual norms and expectations; unmarried young people's sexual relationships; married young people's sexual relationships; reproductive beliefs and practices; HIV and other sexually transmitted infections; and contextual barriers and facilitators of sexual risk reduction.

GENERAL VILLAGE LIFE

Most *MEMA kwa Vijana* trial villages had a population of two thousand to three thousand residents. Each village were composed of five to eight sub-villages, each of which consisted of about fifty family compounds or homesteads. Outside of a village's center, homesteads were typically 100 to 300 meters apart, and the distance from one sub-village to another was 1.5 to 3 km. Households varied widely in their number of occupants, but most had six to eight adults and children.

With the exception of some fishing villages, agriculture was the core of economies in rural areas, and most families grew a mix of subsistence and cash crops. The main crops grown for household use were maize, sweet potatoes, cassava, sorghum, millet, bananas, bambara nuts, peanuts, beans, and lentils. The main cash crops were cotton, rice, maize, and cassava. Many families owned several acres or more, and it was not unusual for young

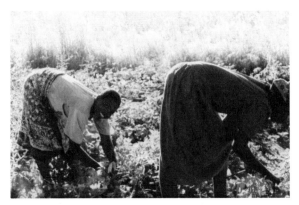

Figure 3.1.   A Sukuma researcher (right) harvesting sweet potatoes with a twenty-year-old.

people to have land which they cultivated separately from their parents, or for them to sell the produce for themselves, but they often required parental permission when they worked on their own plot rather than their family's plot. Almost all farming in study villages was still done by hand (figure 3.1). The main period of cultivation took place during the long rainy season from February to May. At that time, almost everyone in farming households worked from dawn until dusk on their farms, including many pupils who stayed home from school to help.

Cattle ownership was common and highly valued in rural areas because it provided economic security and social status. In one inland village, for example, a researcher estimated that 30 percent of families owned at least one cow, and the majority of those families owned from one to nine cows. Cattle were usually only sold or bartered in exceptional circumstances, for instance, to acquire land, to pay bridewealth, or to cope with a health crisis. Few parents sold their cattle to pay for their children's school fees. Cattle were owned by the heads of household, usually older men, but typically five- to eight-year-old boys herded them. Most of these boys had not yet attended school or had dropped out. Other animals that were widely kept were goats, chickens, and muscovy ducks. As children grew older, they sometimes were given a few such small animals of their own.

Some of the large study villages had permanent shops, but most relied on small seasonal and/or part-time kiosks. Kiosks generally were owned and run by young men and typically stocked limited quantities of cooking oil, sugar, wheat flour, rice, *dagaa* (a small fish similar to whitebait), candy, cookies, soda, soap, body oil, kerosene, matches, and bicycle spare parts. They also usually provided basic medicines such as antimalarials (e.g., choloroquine or sulfa drugs), headache tablets (e.g., acetaminophen or as- pirin), and antibiotics (e.g., co-trimoxazole).

Livelihoods

Non-agricultural livelihoods for men varied considerably according to the village's proximity to roads, urban settlements, fishing villages, or mines. Generally, the further villages were inland and away from main roads, the fewer non-farming occupations there were, and the poorer the populations were.

Most villages had a weekly market or had access to one in a nearby village. Petty trade was a common occupation, pursued primarily by young men who sold products by running a market stall, hawking in the village center, or staffing a more permanent kiosk or shop there. Other livelihoods for men included selling wood, burning charcoal, making bricks, building houses, carpentry, casual labor, bicycle taxi driving, bicycle repair, and traditional medicine (figure 3.2). Typically the only salaried positions were held by a few government officials, teachers, and health workers.

A small proportion of young men migrated to district towns or the regional capital, Mwanza City, to work as casual laborers. Some young men instead moved to other rural areas where there were mines, fishing villages, or remote fishing camps, because they could earn relatively high incomes in such settings over periods of months or years. Fishing and mining villages typically were larger than remote, inland villages; had more mobile and ethnically heterogeneous populations; had more money in circulation; and experienced more crime.

Many women worked almost exclusively carrying out domestic chores and subsistence farming for their husband's households, such as fetching water or firewood, washing clothes, cooking, cleaning, and weeding and harvesting crops (figure 3.3). If such women earned money, it was usually only on a small scale from petty businesses or selling crops. Village women had far fewer types of paid work available to them than to men, and these

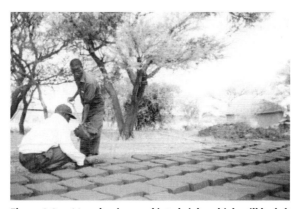

Figure 3.2.   Men shaping mud into bricks which will be left
to dry for two weeks before being used for house-building.

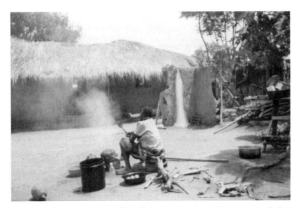

Figure 3.3. A young daughter-in-law cooking a meal for her household.

often were less lucrative than men's work. A minority of women staffed food stalls in the village center, and a minority brewed and sold home-made beer, particularly unmarried or separated women. In addition, a small minority of women migrated to mines, fishing villages, larger towns, or Mwanza City, usually to work in domestic service or food facilities. After marrying, young women typically reduced or stopped such external economic activities in order to focus entirely on domestic work and subsistence farming for their husbands' households.

Adolescent boys and girls were expected to help farm during the cultivation season. When they were not in school or farming, girls spent almost all of their waking hours engaged in domestic tasks. Boys sometimes had domestic responsibilities, but generally they had far more free time than girls. In many families, boys and girls were also expected to pay for some of their basic needs by their teen years, and increasingly to meet those needs themselves during their teens, including clothing, underwear, soap, body oil, and school fees and supplies. Boys had more opportunities to work for pay than girls, as they could engage in many of the types of work men did for pay. Girls who had time to work for pay instead were generally limited to hiring themselves out as farm labor, or preparing small food items to sell at the weekly market or in the village center in the evening (figure 3.4).

Material Living Conditions

Most residents in study villages lived in homesteads consisting of two or more houses built of wattle and mud walls, or occasionally fired brick walls. These homes usually had thatched roofs and no internal doors, and sometimes

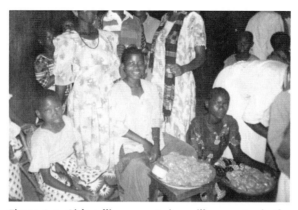

Figure 3.4. Girls selling peanuts in a village center in the evening.

also no external doors. Most households had pit latrines, but many were not used because they were in poor condition, in which case people relieved themselves in fields nearby instead.

Small children typically slept in the same room as their parents. Older children and adolescents of the same sex usually shared a sleeping room, either within their parents' house (mainly girls) or in a free-standing house in the same compound (either boys or girls). An important rite of passage for many young men in their late teens or early twenties was to build their own one-roomed hut within their parents' homestead. All household members slept on the earth floor, on a reed mat, sacking, cattle hide, or a homemade mattress stuffed with cotton.

Village men generally wore western style shirts or T-shirts and long trousers. Women typically wore simple dresses or a blouse and a *kanga* (a colored, patterned cotton cloth with a border and message) wrapped around the waist like a long skirt. The majority of villagers wore some kind of foot-wear, often flip flops or open sandals made from car tires, but in the poorest villages most people went barefoot. Young people had two or three sets of clothes, one for working, a neater set for public places and, if at school, the required uniform. Many could only wash their clothes once a fortnight or less frequently due to lack of soap or water. Soap was highly valued, as was body oil, which villagers considered essential to prevent unhealthy and unattractive dry and cracked skin. Girls and women used old cloths for sanitary towels. In the wet season most women walked one to two kilometers to fetch water for their household's drinking, cooking, and washing, often from a shallow pond dug where there was a high water table. Sometimes they walked twice that distance in the dry season. Firewood used for cooking was generally collected two or more kilometers away from homesteads.

Meals in rural households usually were gender segregated. When breakfast was available, it typically consisted of *ugali* (a stiff porridge staple made of millet, maize, or maize and cassava mixed) or another form of carbohydrate, such as roasted maize, sweet potatoes, or cassava. However, many families did not eat breakfast, and it was not unusual for a family to only eat two meals per day, one around 3 p.m. and the other around 8 p.m. Typically these consisted of *ugali* and a vegetable side dish that sometimes included beans, fish, or rarely meat, depending on affluence and proximity to Lake Victoria. Food was scarce in the cultivation season and then many families lived with hunger as a part of daily life and only had one meal in the evening each day. Girls and women were especially likely to be hungry when food was scarce as they generally received smaller portions of food than boys and men.

Most households in study villages did not own a bicycle, although many could borrow or hire one, which was very important for transportation, particularly of water. Few households had a radio, although perhaps one in ten young men did. Mobile telephone services did not yet reach rural Mwanza at the time of the HALIRA study. The only telephone service available was provided at public offices in large rural towns, so very few villagers had ever used a telephone.

Social Relationships

The main formal social differences within Mwanza villages were religious. In the 1998 *MEMA kwa Vijana* assisted self-completion questionnaire survey, 77 percent of school pupils reported that they were Christian, 13 percent said they had no religion, 9 percent reported they were Muslim, and 1 percent said they followed a traditional religion. Amongst Christians approximately one-half were Roman Catholic and one-half Protestant, the latter mainly of African Inland Church, Pentecostal (several different sects), and Seventh Day Adventist faiths. Rural Muslims instead were Sunni of varying sects. Religious belief and practice varied greatly, from those who rarely attended church or mosque to a small minority who prayed every day and attended services more than weekly. Villagers generally cooperated with each other without regard to religious affiliations.

Most productive and social activities in rural Mwanza were segregated by gender with the exception of very young children's activities. Men were generally more socially and economically powerful than women. As already described, men had more access to paid employment and they generally owned the land and the cattle. Any man in a household generally had greater authority than resident women and was responsible for major decisions.

Social Events

During evening hours some villagers, primarily male youths and adult men, strolled and mingled in the village center, and some regularly met to drink home-brewed beer there. Attending weekly markets, church, funerals, weddings, video shows, discos, holiday celebrations, or *ngoma* events were the main events at which people met informally outside of work. With the exception of Christian or Muslim events, men were more likely to drink alcohol and become intoxicated than normal at the social gatherings above, as were a small minority of women.

In most villages, a video show was hosted by traveling men from approximately 8 p.m. to 1 a.m. on market days or holidays. A diverse range of videos were shown, such as East African music videos, Chinese action films, and American pornography, the latter typically being shown late at night. Video shows mainly were attended by married and unmarried men.

Discos were less common than video shows, and seemed to draw fewer participants. Discos usually took place outside, mainly were attended by male youth and adult men, and were hosted by traveling disc jockeys who brought small groups of female dancers. Male villagers bid against one another to have a song and dance with the dancer of their choice. Both discos and video shows were held most frequently in fishing villages.

Ngoma events were important social occasions in most villages, particularly those in remote, almost entirely Sukuma settings. Unlike video shows and discos, *ngoma* events were attended by large numbers of male and female villagers of all ages, particularly before dark. In keeping with tradition, during these events two *ngoma* groups typically competed on opposite sides of a large, cleared area, and villagers paid to observe the performances (figure 3.5).

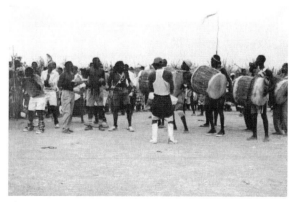

Figure 3.5.   A traveling *ngoma* (drumming-dancing) group performing at a *Saba saba* (July 7th national holiday) event.

Illness Beliefs and Practices

As noted above, most villagers identified as Christians or Muslims, but almost all also had traditional[1] supernatural beliefs and practices which contradicted those religions. Very few villagers felt conflicted about such pluralistic beliefs.

Beliefs about illness causation generally fell into five categories which were not mutually exclusive: natural/biological, chance, God's will, ancestral displeasure, and witchcraft. It was widely believed, for example, that one's ancestors influenced one's life, either through protection from illness, injury, or malicious forces, or by withdrawing protection and actively causing harm if they became angered. Most villagers also believed that some maladies were caused by witchcraft, particularly villagers in the overwhelmingly Sukuma districts. Witchcraft was linked to envy, as some villagers who accumulated wealth or other advantages feared that envious people might bewitch them, and people who experienced misfortune sometimes believed that they had been bewitched by others who envied them. In most study villages there were a few individuals—usually older women—who were reported to be witches by many of their fellow villagers.

Symptoms were very important in illness recognition, diagnosis, and treatment in rural Mwanza, and once symptoms resolved people generally believed that they were cured of an illness. The three major sources of treatment were home remedies (both traditional and biomedical), traditional healers, and biomedical health care providers (officially at health facilities, or less frequently at the providers' homes). Treatment-seeking was pluralistic and opportunistic, depending on factors such as the perceived cause, nature, and severity of symptoms, and the proximity, cost, and perceived confidentiality of care providers.

Traditional healers identified illnesses by diagnosing symptoms, dream interpretation, and/or performing rituals with special plants or animals. Treatment usually involved ingestion or external application of processed wild herbs, bark, and/or roots. Treatment sometimes also included rituals against what was believed to be the original cause of the condition, for instance, conducting a ceremony to appease a patient's ancestors, or casting a counter-spell to harm a suspected witch. Some traditional healers also performed minor surgery, such as incisions in the skin for application of a medicine.

Each government health facility in rural Mwanza served three to five villages, and private facilities were even less common. Most travel took place on foot, and villagers often had to walk three to ten kilometers to visit a health facility. Government health facilities had very limited staff, equipment, and medication stocks. Medical care mainly consisted of syndromic management of common illnesses and/or treatment of symptoms, such as fever, cough, bloody urine, and genital discharge. Government health services will be described in more detail in chapter 6.

CHILDREN'S RELATIONSHIPS WITH THEIR PARENTS, PEERS, AND TEACHERS

Parent-Child Relationships

The composition of families and households in rural Mwanza was quite variable. At the beginning of the *MEMA kwa Vijana* trial, approximately one-third of the sixty-three randomly selected in-depth interview respondents reported that they lived with parents who were in a monogamous marriage. One-quarter instead said their parents were in a polygynous marriage, and most of those respondents lived with their mother full-time and their father when he visited on a daily, weekly, or yearly basis. A few, however, lived in a household with their father, mother, and one or more co-wives. Another quarter of respondents said they lived with only one of their biological parents and possibly a stepparent, while the remainder said they lived with a grandparent, aunt, uncle, sibling, or, in one case, a husband.

In rural Mwanza, relationships between parents and their children were typically formal. From a young age children (and especially girls) were taught to be deferential toward adults and markedly so toward their parents. For example, when talking with their parents, and especially their fathers, children usually did not look them in the eyes, behaved demurely, talked quietly, and rarely joked. Parents might feel affection toward their children but were rarely demonstrative or direct in expressing it. Parental concern for their children's current and future welfare was often evident in the material support and practical training they provided, their general monitoring and regulation of their children's activities, and the primary care and advocacy they provided when their children were ill. Parents seldom worked alongside their children, apart from domestic work involving mothers and daughters or intensive periods of farm work. It was also rare to see parents spending their leisure time—something largely restricted to males—with their children, although parents sometimes ate meals with their children.

Parents generally did not discuss sexual issues with their children, except sometimes indirectly, as when admiring or criticizing others' behavior. Fathers were generally less approachable and stricter than mothers, so children feared their punishment more. It was considered acceptable for parents to use corporal punishment to train or discipline a child, including hitting or caning. However, in most families this seemed to be unusual and was rarely severe. Nonetheless, many adolescents told researchers that they hid forbidden activities specifically to avoid being beaten by their parents. Children's covert resistance of parental power was very common. The fieldworkers often recorded examples of adolescents disobeying their parents when unsupervised, such as planning sexual liaisons or attending a video show that had been prohibited.

Children's Relationships with Their Peers

Young boys and girls sometimes played together and shared tasks such as herding, but by the time they started school there was little opportunity for them to interact with the opposite sex publicly. Important exceptions were when young people were walking to or from school, on pathways when carrying out errands, and sometimes in the village center in the evenings when working or strolling there. Gender segregation was also relaxed when participating in church or political party choirs, mixed-sex *rika*, holiday festivals, and *ngoma* events. These conditions sometimes overlapped, as when a church group worked together on each other's farms, or a *rika* farming team performed together as an *ngoma* group when not engaged in cultivation (figure 3.6).

By school age, children in rural Mwanza thus mainly socialized with same-sex relatives, neighbors, and friends of roughly the same age. Outside of school, girls mostly engaged with other girls in the course of shared domestic or agricultural work. Boys typically shared agricultural tasks and leisure activities with each other, such as strolling in the village and playing soccer or other games.

Teacher-Pupil Relationships

Before describing teacher-pupil relationships in rural Mwanza, general primary school conditions will be outlined briefly below. General school conditions will then be examined in more depth in chapters 4 and 5.

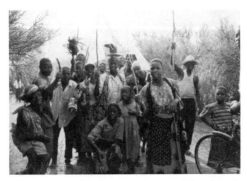

Figure 3.6.   A local *ngoma* group celebrating after winning a drumming and dance competition.

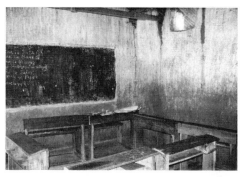

Figure 3.7. A primary school classroom with chalkboard and walls in typical condition. Desks usually are arranged in rows facing the front, but had been rearranged for a training course.

In the study area, rural primary school classrooms were constructed of earth or cement brick walls, iron-sheeted roofs, earth floors, and open doors and windows. They usually were equipped with a worn blackboard, chalk, and a limited number of two-person desks (figure 3.7). Teachers often managed with only one textbook for an entire class, and sometimes with none at all. Schools did not have electricity or running water, and to relieve themselves teachers and pupils used pit latrines or, occasionally, nearby fields. During the study period, annual school fees of Tshs[2] 2,000 ($2.40) were abolished, but villagers still reported spending Tshs 6,000–8,000 ($7.20–$9.60) per pupil per year for sports fees, running costs, paper, pencils, and school uniforms and shoes.

Primary school teachers' motivation seemed to vary considerably, ranging from those who were enthusiastic and strove to teach their pupils well despite working with few resources and in difficult circumstances, to those who seemed poorly motivated and who frequently complained about pay, conditions, and pupils. Teaching primarily focused on learning by rote, and there was little attempt to develop pupils' critical thinking skills or to have a mutual exchange of views and experiences. Teachers generally addressed pupils in an authoritarian way, and pupils would stand up to answer formally. When describing teachers they liked, in-depth interview respondents almost always mentioned a teacher's respect and fairness, often specifically saying that their favorite teachers used little or no corporal punishment.

The HALIRA study identified three areas where teacher-pupil relationships were problematic, including routine use of corporal punishment, occasional mandatory pregnancy examinations of older girls, and sexual abuse of female pupils by certain male teachers. In all study schools, corporal punishment was used routinely for minor and major infractions, such as being late for school, perceived disrespect to teachers, or passing notes in class. Corporal punishment in schools usually involved beating with a slender, flexible stick, but it could include other forms of physical discomfort, pain, or humiliation, such as being made to kneel silently in front of a classroom for an entire class period. Corporal punishment was so established that no teachers and few parents questioned it. Pupils also took it for granted and many considered it acceptable if used fairly and in moderation.

One reason pupils might be beaten severely was if they were found to have had sex. Sometimes this was revealed when a girl became pregnant. In some schools, teachers occasionally took groups of school girls to a local health facility for mandatory pregnancy examinations. Girls universally reported disliking these examinations. Pregnant school girls dropped out, sometimes without experiencing much stigma or punishment. However, in each of the four study districts there were also reports of a boy or man who impregnated a girl who then was forced to pay substantial amounts both to the girl's family and to her school teachers. In exchange, teachers falsified the girl's school records, for example, attributing her departure to another reason.

Within the HALIRA study there were also plausible first- and third-person reports of individual male teachers having sex with female pupils in eight of the nine participant observation villages and in one-third of in-depth interviews with randomly selected respondents. These reports involved recent cases of male teachers impregnating school girls, being caught having sex with pupils, and/or pressuring girls to have sex. Generally such sexual abuse involved the teacher isolating the girl and then threatening her with punishment and/or offering her special privileges to pressure her for sex. If a girl refused sex, some teachers made excuses to verbally abuse or beat her over subsequent months, interspersed with further attempts to seduce her. Sometimes adults seemed aware of a teacher's sexual abuse of a school girl but did not act to prevent it, because they lacked evidence, they felt little recourse, or they believed it did not affect them or their family personally. If parents had strong evidence that a teacher had a sexual relationship with a school girl, he typically transferred to another school on his own initiative, or that of an authority.

SEXUAL NORMS AND EXPECTATIONS

The HALIRA study found that some sexual norms and expectations in rural Mwanza conflicted with one another in seemingly contradictory ways. The term "norm" is used here to describe ideal standards of behavior shared by a social group which do not necessarily reflect actual behavior. Norms are not prescriptive in determining behavior, but people may draw on them to legitimize or criticize specific behaviors. Some norms and expectations were restrictive for young people in rural Mwanza, while others were relatively permissive. Those which were restrictive included heterosexuality; school pupil abstinence; women's sexual respectability; men's sexual respectability; taboos against the discussion of sex; and religious beliefs about sexual abstinence and fidelity. Permissive expectations were that male sexual activity is an essential drive central to masculine identity; that female sexual activity is a resource to be exploited; that sex is inevitable unless prevented; and that sexual restrictions are relaxed at festivals and social gatherings. Each of these will be discussed more below.

Restrictive Sexual Norms and Expectations

Heterosexuality was a widespread norm in rural Mwanza. Many villagers were not aware of the possibility of homosexuality, and within the research there were only rare, third-person reports of it. Villagers who were aware of homosexuality had usually been exposed to it through western media such as video shows. They generally found it repugnant and commented about it as a strange and alien practice. The tone of such comments was typically detached, amused, and/or disbelieving, rather than personally threatened or hostile.

One of the most fundamental sexual norms for young people in rural Mwanza, at least among adults, was that school pupils should not be sexually active. Parents tried to enforce this norm by prohibiting pupils (especially girls) from participating in unsupervised mixed-sex activities. Most pupils did not contest the ideal of school pupil abstinence in the presence of adults, but as they grew older the majority started to circumvent it. Notably, primary schooling often continued into the late teens and even the early twenties, especially for male pupils. In contrast, some children never went to school and approximately one-third to one-half of pupils dropped out before completing Year 7. For out-of-school youth in their teens, particularly boys, discreet premarital sexual activity was tolerated and even expected, although like adults they were expected to avoid sexual relationships with pupils. In addition, many teenage girls married soon after leaving primary school, whether they were in their mid or late teens. Thus the acceptability of young people's sexual activity often was judged by their school status, marital status, and adult responsibilities rather than their chronological age.

Sexual issues were rarely discussed publicly in rural Mwanza, and explicit discussion was regarded by some as obscene. Parents rarely provided sexual information to their children, and sometimes said a school-based sexual health intervention was unacceptable because it involved discussing sexual issues across generations and between sexes. Many were also concerned that such education might encourage sexual activity. There were, however, some notable exceptions to the cross-generational taboo of discussing sex, including older women who sometimes discreetly advised young women about contraception, or parents who advised their children about the treatment of sexually transmitted infections. Furthermore, in many homes small children shared sleeping rooms with their parents, where some witnessed their parents' sexual activity. Older children generally shared rooms with older, same-sex siblings and cousins, and many said they had observed sexual activity in that context as well.

In rural Mwanza both men and women frequently used sexual respectability to categorize each other, but it was particularly important for women. Monogamous married women generally had the greatest respectability, followed by unmarried young women living with their parents who were not known to have ever been sexually active, although it was difficult to maintain this reputation for more than a couple of years after leaving school. Almost all other never married, divorced, or widowed women of reproductive age, most of whom were mothers, were considered to be less reputable; these women were referred to by the term *wasimbe* and constituted about one-quarter to one-third of women in most villages. Women who were perceived to be very promiscuous had the worst reputations. Importantly, the categories above could be permeable and transient, particularly as it was not unusual for women to divorce and remarry at least once in their lifetimes.

Women primarily maintained their respectability by hiding out-of-wedlock sexual relationships. If a woman was known to have been sexually active, she could still promote her respectability by not openly initiating sexual encounters, not agreeing to sex too quickly, and not being known to have had several sexual partners. Other threats to a girl or woman's sexual respectability were accepting a low amount of money in exchange for sex, wearing immodest clothing, attending video shows, having a sexually transmitted infection, aborting a pregnancy, and living alone.

In contrast to women, high numbers of sexual partners and greater sexual activity often enhanced men's reputations amongst other men. Women generally did not admire this, however, and they might condemn particular men's sexual irresponsibility or faithlessness, particularly when men did not support their offspring.

Religion did not seem to have a prominent role in shaping sexual norms and practices in rural Mwanza. Formal religions were probably more influential in shaping ideals of sexual conduct and women's sexual respectability than in reducing young people's actual sexual activity. In the few very devout Christian or Muslim families, parents were unusually restrictive of their children and especially their daughters. However, some youths in strictly religious households said that close parental monitoring simply made them more secretive than other young people.

Permissive Sexual Expectations and Norms

The HALIRA study found that sexual desire and satisfaction were the overwhelming motivations for boys and men to have sex, and male sexual activity was perceived as an essential biological drive. Most young people reported that, once a young man had had sex, it was extremely difficult for him to abstain and maintain his mental and physical wellbeing. Young men enjoyed and were proud to be sexually "strong," for example, to have sex frequently. Many also were pleased to make their partners pregnant, even when this resulted in fines or punishments, because it demonstrated their potency and fertility. For almost all men, but particularly those not yet married or with children, sexual experience was prestigious and intertwined with their masculine identity.

However, participant observation data suggest that peer pressure might have been as important as sexual desire in motivating adolescent boys to start sexual activity. Boys older than fourteen who had not yet engaged in sexual activity were likely to be ridiculed by their more sexually experienced peers. The prestige of male sexual experience related to the ability to seduce many partners. However, young men had to balance the esteem of perceived sexual experience against the risk of jealousy and suspicion of unfaithfulness from sexual partners, and punishment from adult authorities. Rather than publicize the details of their sexual relationships, they thus often preferred a reputation of sexual experience based on rumor.

For young women, sex was regarded primarily as a resource that they could exploit, as girls and women received something in exchange for virtually all sexual encounters outside of marriage, unless they were physically forced, which was rare. Material exchange for sex was so established that almost any gift a young man gave to a young woman, such as a snack, soap, payment of video show entrance, or a "loan" of money, was seen by both parties as a contract to have sex. The size of the gift given for each sexual encounter varied according to the man's affluence, the woman's prestige, and their relative experience and negotiation skills. School boys with the least money typically gave sugar cane, soap, or Tshs 100-500 ($0.12–$0.60) per sexual encounter, while older men typically gave Tshs 500-2,000 ($0.60–$2.40). Many young women used their earnings for essential purchases, such as soap, clothes, or a small mid-day meal. However, young women often showed each other what they received from their sexual partners, and there was also evidence of female peer pressure to acquire commodities.

Gifts received in exchange for sex were generally concealed in order to hide relationships, but no one considered material exchange for sex problematic in itself. To the contrary, a girl or young woman who received a small gift, or nothing, was generally scorned and considered to lack self-respect, while unmarried women who had sex for free were condemned as sexually loose. The underlying logic of many comments about transactional sex was the principle of reciprocity, or mutual give-and-take. The continued provision of money or gifts for sexual encounters within a relationship was assumed to ensure a woman's fidelity, except with women who had reputations for promiscuity. If gift giving was not maintained or substantially diminished, relationships often ended quickly, or the young woman secretly found another boyfriend. The amount exchanged for sex generally fell during a relationship, giving young women an incentive to change partners.

Another permissive expectation in rural Mwanza was the assumption that social contact between members of the opposite sex would lead to sex unless it was prevented, so long as those involved were not related, young children, or old. Sexual activity was thus believed to be constrained primarily by externally imposed restrictions, particularly sexual segregation, rather than self-imposed discipline. A final, widely held permissive expectation was that normal restrictions on sexual activity should be relaxed at festivals and special social gatherings. This expectation primarily was maintained by young people, but often also seemed to be condoned by many older people. Four main factors seemed to underlie this: the sexual license sometimes had a symbolic or ritual function; adults felt a celebratory, permissive mood which led them to indulge their children; the usual social controls were not as effective given the crowds, movement, and/or darkness after nightfall; and/or young men had more money than normal, which facilitated greater alcohol use for some and sexual activity for many. Almost all social gatherings were associated with greater youth sexual activity, as were special events, such as sports competitions and annual parties for *rika* members.

UNMARRIED YOUNG PEOPLE'S SEXUAL RELATIONSHIPS

In both *MEMA kwa Vijana* surveys and HALIRA research it was challenging to collect accurate data on whether young people had begun to have sex, and if they had, what their age was at sexual debut and how many total partners they had had. In surveys, it was not unusual for pupils to report they had never had sex. However, those reports often conflicted with what the same individuals reported in interviews held during the same time period, or with their pregnancy or sexually transmitted infection test results (Plummer, Ross et al., 2004; Plummer, Wight et al., 2004). Similarly, unmarried adolescent girls who reported sexual experience in in-depth interviews, and who then went on to marry a new partner, often subsequently denied they had ever had a sexual partner other than their husbands. It seems likely that only a minority of young people truly remained abstinent until mid-adolescence, and only a very small minority did so until late adolescence and/or marriage. The motivations and experiences of such young people will be examined in chapter 8.

When data from all research methods are considered together, they broadly suggest that over half of fifteen-year-old boys and girls in the study population had had vaginal intercourse. Those methods also suggest that, at that age, a larger majority of girls than boys were sexually active, and many—if not most—sexually active girls had sex frequently (e.g., weekly), while sexually active boys typically went for many weeks or months between sexual encounters. By their late teens, a large majority of both unmarried young men and women were sexually active, had had several sexual partners, and typically had sex on a weekly basis. By their early twenties most unmarried young men and women had had more sexual partners.

The HALIRA study identified three types of sexual relationship which school pupils and out-of-school youth commonly experienced. These were relationships which involved onetime encounters; those which involved occasional opportunistic encounters within an open-ended timeframe; and those which were steady, sometimes semipublic partnerships which involved more frequent encounters. For each of these types of relationship, sexual encounters increased around special events. Onetime encounters and opportunistic relationships often involved a partner who was a visitor to the village, or alternatively, someone a villager met while traveling elsewhere. Open-ended and opportunistic sexual relationships were usually, but not always, casual. If the couple did not actively end the relationship—as might occur if bad feelings developed between them—and if the right circumstances occurred again after a period of weeks, months, or years, then they might readily have sex again. In such circumstances, mutual attraction and familiarity could make sexual negotiation with a previous partner much easier than with a new partner.

The extent and nature of each of these types of relationship varied depending on gender and school status. This will be described more below for prepubescent children, school boys, school girls, out-of-school young men, and out-of-school young women.

Sexual Relationships in Preadolescence, Adolescence, and Young Adulthood

Many villagers reported that their earliest experience of vaginal intercourse took place while they were "playing" at sex in their preadolescent years, particularly while herding livestock. This was often described as exploratory, game-like imitation, in which children pretended to be their fathers and mothers, or other relatives who they might have seen having sex in a shared bedroom. Such prepubescent sexual relationships differed from later partnerships in several ways: it was not unusual for the girl to be one or two years older than the boy; boys typically did not give girls money or gifts in exchange for sexual encounters; and boys often did not ejaculate or experience pleasure, and sometimes experienced pain if it was their first experience of intercourse. Most boys who described such experiences reported that, once they began school, three to six years passed before they again had intercourse in their early to middle teen years.

Adolescent and Young Adult Males

Many early adolescent school boys reported frequently approaching girls to try to negotiate sex, but rarely succeeding. School boys had little money or gifts to offer a girl in exchange for sex, so they typically invested a lot of effort in wooing and declaring their liking or love for a girl during prolonged periods of negotiation, using peer intermediaries, letters, and a direct approach. In their early teen years, school boys had the greatest chance of having a sexual relationship with girls who were the same age or younger than them, because such girls typically were inexperienced and expected relatively little in exchange for a sexual encounter. These sexual relationships usually involved one or a few brief, rushed, and opportunistic sexual encounters.

In their early to mid-teens, it was not unusual for sexually active school boys to only have sex once or twice per year, but by their mid-teens they might have sex about once per month, and by their late teens about once per week. As school boys grew older, their experience, confidence, and access to cash usually also grew, as did their pool of potential partners, because the number of sexually active girls of the same age or younger increased as they aged. As a result older school boys were more successful in directly negotiating longer term sexual relationships which involved regular sexual encounters, and also in finding new partners soon after a break-up.

After leaving school, young men typically began to have sex more often and with more partners than they had before. Some said they did not want to commit to one sexual partner because they found it exciting to seduce new ones. Seduction went hand in hand with young men's new earning abilities after they had finished schooling, as well as their main forms of entertainment and relaxation, such as hanging out in the village center in the evening, or attending videos, discos, *ngoma*, or holiday events. It was not unusual for unmarried young men to have a series of partners in close succession or to maintain open-ended, concurrent relationships. The durations of their sexual relationships were highly variable, as were the frequency of encounters within them. Sometimes a young man had an out-of-school partner with whom he had a discreet but semipublic relationship, so that the two were recognized as a couple within a broader group of peers.

Adolescent and Young Adult Females

In their early teen years, school girls often had their first sexual relationships with same aged or slightly older school boys, as described in the section above. As they grew older, however, adolescent girls learned from other girls and out-of-school youths and men that more could be obtained from a relationship with someone out of school, and they often began to pursue such relationships instead or as well as those with school boys. Older and/or out-of-school partners could usually provide more money and gifts in exchange for a particular sexual encounter, and could do so on a regular basis, contributing to longer-term relationships with more frequent sexual encounters than school girls had with their male classmates. These out-of-school men were typically a couple of years to a decade older than their school girl partners.

The vast majority of young women were sexually active by the time they left school, and it was common for those who were not married to have a steady sexual partner who they met for sex once or twice per week. If such a relationship ended, there was usually only a short gap (such as one week) before a new one began. As for out-of-school young men, it was not unusual for an unmarried young woman who had been out of school for a couple of years to have a discreet sexual relationship that was commonly known but not publicly acknowledged. Couples in such relationships could be somewhat open and develop a kind of routine, for example, spending time together when mingling in a group of mixed sex peers at *ngoma* events or the village center in the evening. However, such activity could negatively affect a woman's reputation and her potential to marry.

The Emotional Nature of Relationships

Adolescence and young adulthood were times of great exploration, discovery, and transition for young people in rural Mwanza, as elsewhere in the world. Often sexual relationships began in an opportunistic and exploratory way with neither partner having a clear expectation that it would end or continue beyond their first sexual encounter. The mutual attraction that led a couple to have an initial sexual encounter could evolve into a longer term sexual relationship. Whether such a relationship involved occasional or frequent sexual encounters depended on how strongly the couple liked one another and their specific circumstances, such as how convenient it was for them to meet, whether either partner already had a steady partner, and whether the young man could offer money or gifts on a frequent basis.

When young people were asked to describe their emotions or attraction for a partner, they often simply said, "I liked/loved him/her" using the terms *kupenda* and **kutogwa**, both of which can be translated as "to like" or "to love." Sometimes it seemed clear in the context of a statement whether someone meant "like" or "love," but often this was ambiguous. The emotional nature and intensity of unmarried young people's sexual relationships varied. Sometimes unmarried girls or women seemed to be neutral or indifferent toward particular partners, maintaining a sexual relationship for the sole purpose of material support. The extent to which a woman liked a man was often the deciding factor in her choice between suitors who offered the same amount of money, or in her choice to have sex with a particular suitor even if he had little to offer her in exchange.

The very limited nature of one-to-one contact beyond sexual encounters meant that unmarried couples usually had limited knowledge of one another and little opportunity to become emotionally close through non-sexual contact. In addition, the secretive nature of premarital sexual relationships meant that there was little scope for peers to strengthen a couple's relationship through social recognition and, conversely, less risk of sanctions if one had other sexual partners. The greatest potential for an unmarried couple to develop emotional intimacy seemed to occur if they met at night on multiple occasions over weeks or months, particularly young adults who spent many hours together after dark. However, unmarried young people rarely expressed a wish to get to know someone of the opposite sex other than to arrange and to have sex. Sexual intercourse also rarely seemed to have symbolic significance as an expression of a couple's emotional intimacy.

Nonetheless, there was considerable evidence of possessiveness and jealousy in some premarital relationships. Young men and women in steady relationships usually felt strongly about being their partner's sole sexual partner, and discovery of a partner's infidelity often led to break-ups. However, it was much less common for a young person to perceive a certain partner as his or her "one and only," even in steady relationships. Many young people were emotionally attached to a particular partner and hoped to eventually marry him or her, but they did not seem to romantically idealize that partner as the *only* person with whom they could perceive having a sexual relationship and a shared future. Even in such relatively committed sexual relationships, young people might still have other, less serious relationships which fulfilled a particular desire for sex or money, or which served as a kind of marital "back-up" in case the main relationship did not work out.

Multiple Partnerships and Sexual Mixing Patterns

Villagers often criticized people—particularly women—who were believed to have multiple sexual partners out-of-wedlock. However, certain types of concurrency were socially acceptable and even admired in rural Mwanza, particularly formally within polygynous marriage or informally amongst men in general. Indeed, the HALIRA findings suggest that secretive, overlapping sexual relationships were not unusual amongst young people, especially by their late teen years.

Sometimes young people had concurrent sexual relationships but did not recognize them as such. For example, some adolescents initially said they had never had overlapping relationships but then acknowledged having had one or more onetime sexual partners while still in the midst of a longer-term, open-ended relationship. There were many other instances, however, when youth knowingly had concurrent relationships, as when young adults with one main relationship occasionally or regularly had more secretive sexual relationships. The open-ended and hidden nature of many young people's sexual relation-ships helped foster spontaneous and opportunistic concurrency.

Male and female informants involved in concurrent relationships rarely seemed to view the overlapping nature of their relationships as inherently wrong or immoral. However, they usually strove to hide them to avoid pos-sible jealousies, break-ups, and (especially for girls and women) stigma they might experience if they became public knowledge. The discretion that young people practiced to hide sexual relationships from parents and older villagers often also effectively hid them from other young people, which was important in maintaining concurrency.

In each village, mill workers, shopkeepers, bicycle taxi drivers, and other young men who provided needed goods or services, earned an above average income, and had high contact with girls and women typically had more sexual activity—and more partners—than other young men. It was more difficult to identify groups of unmarried young women who were particularly likely to have many partners or to engage in concurrent sexual partnerships. Generally, however, material exchange was an important motivation for young women who reported this, whether as a means to access entertainment and gifts or to meet subsistence needs.

Unmarried young villagers who traveled for school or work were more likely than other villagers to maintain concurrent partnerships in different loca-tions. Young men who traveled for work usually earned sufficient money and had ample opportunity to have sex frequently, because many young women who worked in guesthouses, food kiosks, and bars supplemented their income through sex with customers. Figure 3.8 illustrates sexual negotiation in such a

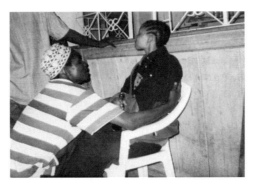

Figure 3.8. A man trying to seduce a bar maid in a bar in a large village.

setting, as it shows a man trying to seduce a bar maid in a bar of a large village. In addition, some men had sex with prostitutes while traveling, particularly in male-dominated locations such as mines or fishing camps. There were also reports of men having sex with other boys or men in isolated fishing camps. Importantly, when young men and women returned to their home villages after an extended period away, they often were seen as desirable sexual partners because their experiences beyond the village were considered exciting and interesting. Such individuals were often admired for their *kisasa* (modern) clothing and hair styles, especially returning women, and the returning men frequently had more cash than local men.

When a young person's sexual partner traveled away from the village, it also was not unusual for the person remaining behind to have a different partner during their absence. Young women usually did this to supplement their income, but attraction and other factors could also play a role. Men who traveled might commonly have onetime encounters with strangers, as noted above, but women who remained behind in the village seemed more likely to have open-ended relationships with someone known to them, possibly resulting in long-term concurrent relationships when the traveling partner returned and/or traveled again.

These findings highlight distinct networks or populations which were "bridged" by individuals who had sexual partners in different groups. One example is older men and younger women who bridged predominantly same-aged sexual networks about five to ten years apart. Another is individuals—usually young men—who traveled for work or school and had sexual partners both inside and away from a village. Regular travel could take a range of forms, including daily (e.g., bicycle taxi drivers), weekly or monthly (e.g., traders or fishermen), or yearly (e.g., people working in towns or cities). There were also a small number of men with homes in urban areas who traveled to villages on a onetime, occasional, or frequent basis, such as bus drivers, video show hosts, *ngoma* performers, and people who were visiting relatives in the village.

Having described broad, macro-social aspects of unmarried young people's sexual relationships above, the next two sections will now consider interpersonal, micro-social aspects of them, including sexual motivation, negotiation, coercion, and practices.

Sexual Negotiation and Exchange

The vast majority of young men reported that they had involved peers or others as intermediaries in their sexual negotiation, particularly when they were first becoming sexually active. Intermediaries passed information between the partners and often negotiated on behalf of one of the partners while discussing the gifts or money to be exchanged. When two potential partners directly negotiated sex with one another, this was usually initiated by the boy or man, although girls and women sometimes discreetly encouraged it. Most often the boy began by saying, "I like/love you," and he would immediately accompany this with some reference to what he had to offer, in order to persuade a girl or woman to have sex. Subsequent negotiation often involved explicit bargaining about specific gifts or amounts of money to be exchanged.

Sometimes young women reported multiple motivations to start a sexual relationship, including sexual desire, peer pressure, wishing to conceive, or wanting to convince a man to marry. However, such motivations were widely considered to be relatively minor compared with the common and overriding motivation of material gain. In many cases, transactional sex was motivated by a young woman's extreme poverty, so that she could procure essential clothing, hygiene requirements, food to stave off hunger, or school necessities. Most unmarried young women did not reveal to their parents the gifts they received for sex, but a few mothers or grandmothers tolerated or encouraged young women to engage in transactional sex if it helped support their household.

Although many young women had sexual relationships to meet such subsistence needs, some also or instead engaged in transactional sex to gain beauty products or clothes which were not essential for survival, such as attractive clothes or scented body lotion. It is difficult, however, to distinguish between the motivation to seek money or gifts for subsistence rather than for non-essential consumption. In practice the two motivations were sometimes inseparable, since for a young woman to attract a sexual partner to meet her subsistence needs, she might need clothing and beauty products to look attractive. Young women's desire for commodities and their readiness to have sex to acquire them was also influenced strongly by shared expectations amongst female peers, whether they were family, friends, or acquaintances. Some girls who had not had sex borrowed nicer clothes and lotion from their sexually active friends, but their peers rarely were prepared to share their possessions for long if they felt a girl could obtain them herself through her own sexual activity.

Sexual Coercion

Young women in rural Mwanza often exercised some degree of choice and agency in negotiating whether or not to have sex and how they would be materially rewarded, even if their bargaining position was compromised by their particular attributes or circumstances. However, there were various ways in which men sometimes manipulated girls' or women's circumstances to strengthen their negotiating position, used threats, or, occasionally, resorted to physical coercion to have sex. The HALIRA data suggest there were several forms of sexual coercion which most women in rural Mwanza would have recognized, including: bullying and tricks; pressure by higher status third parties; teacher sexual abuse of pupils; coercion when drunk or drugged; forced sex other than that labeled "rape"; and publicly recognized rape. Importantly, none of these categories are mutually exclusive, and many reported incidents fell into two or more of them.

Most threats or force to make a young woman have sex occurred when she was thought to have reneged on an explicit or implicit agreement to have sex in return for a gift. Occasionally, men were also reported to bully women into agreeing to sex by fabricating stories about prior gifts and threatening to shame them publicly. Another common trick was for a man to use an intermediary to give a young woman a gift while misleading her about who gave it to her until she could no longer return it. Sometimes an intermediary in a sexual negotiation was someone older than the girl who was in a position of authority, such as an elder sister, aunt, employer, or parent, and the young woman might only agree to have sex out of trust, respect, or obligation toward that person.

It is difficult to estimate how widespread such practices were using the qualitative data alone. Based on their cumulative participant observation research, female field researchers tentatively estimated that 20 to 30 percent of sexually active young women had received gifts and then been blackmailed or pressured into having sex, and about half had been coerced into having sex through intermediaries. Male fieldworkers in turn estimated that about 60 to 70 percent of sexually active boys lied to trick a girl into having sex, for instance, saying he would marry her or give her money at a later date when he did not intend to do so.

As noted earlier, there were also plausible reports of male teacher sexual abuse of female pupils in many trial villages. Most school girls were not sexually abused by a male teacher, but there was strong evidence that a minority in almost all study schools were. With respect to overtly violent coercion, however, school girls were generally less vulnerable than out-of-school women, because men were afraid of school girls' parents and the possibility of quasi-judicial punishments.

In almost every participant observation village there were also reports of a local man or men sexually assaulting a drunken woman at some point in the past. If the woman had been drinking with the man before the assault—particularly if he had paid for her drinks—then villagers often considered her partly responsible for any subsequent sexual encounter. During participant observation, researchers learned of numerous other incidents of sexual violence which the girls or women did not make public. There were two important reasons why they might not disclose such assaults. First, there was the concern that the girl or woman might be blamed for the incident. In one example, a girl was assaulted violently while working and delivering food to a man's house, but she did not tell her parents because she thought they would blame her for going to his house. The second factor discouraging disclosure was that sometimes an authority figure, an older relative, or trusted friend had acted as the intermediary in incidents of forced sex.

The examples above generally were not described as "rape" by study participants. An event was more likely to be perceived as rape by villagers, and thus be the focus of judicial or quasi-judicial proceedings, if the victim had no prior sexual relationship with the man, if she was prepubescent or in early adolescence, if she had not received any gift from him, if the man was a close relative, if he was believed to have raped women before, and/or if he was mad, drunk, or high on illegal drugs at the time, and the woman was not. In contrast, if the man had a good reputation then people were more likely to assume the woman contributed to the incident. When an assault was likely to be perceived as rape, the man typically fled the village, and if caught soon afterward he typically was beaten. Usually village authorities and communal decision-making played a role in resolving such incidents, sometimes through a conciliatory process in which the rapist was made to formally apologize to the woman's family and to pay them a fine. In each of the participant observation villages there were reports that such a publicly recognized rape had occurred within the last two to three years, and researchers were resident in villages several times when rapes were reported to have happened. Nonetheless, during participant observation, there was only one reported case of a man going to prison after being accused of rape. In the entire study, there were few reports of incest, and similarly few reports of sexual abuse of small, prepubescent children.

Sexual Practices

Although the AIDS epidemic has been severe in sub-Saharan Africa, and HIV is believed to primarily be transmitted through sexual activity in general African populations, very few African studies have examined what people actually do during sexual encounters. This is probably due to several interrelated factors, including: the widespread norm that it is improper to talk about sex explicitly; researchers' reluctance to investigate beyond the standard measures of sexual behavior for fear of being seen as intrusive or prurient; and concern that research findings would be perceived as offensive. However, detailed knowledge of sexual practices is important for several reasons. First, it is critical to understanding people's exposure to sexually transmitted infections and their experience of conception, and also to interpreting why the AIDS epidemic has been so virulent in sub-Saharan Africa. Second, detailed information about sexual practices helps us understand how the power imbalance between the genders works itself out in sexual encounters, and why some people might be motivated to change their sexual partners. Third, such knowledge is important in assessing what kind of biomedical or behavioral change might be most realistic and effective within interventions.

In rural Mwanza, several common genital hygiene practices were said to make sex more enjoyable, including washing the genitals shortly before sex; occasionally shaving pubic hair with a razor or cutting it with scissors; and avoiding intercourse during menstruation. Less commonly, a minority of young men chose to be circumcised for this reason. Genital cleanliness could not be insured prior to sex, however, because water, soap, and toilet paper were often quite limited in rural areas. For example, most people were not able to use anything to clean themselves after urinating or defecating, or they used a leaf taken from a nearby bush. If possible, young people liked to bathe once per day using soap and water that had been carried to the household from a local water source. Typically they tried to clean their genitals more often if they were menstruating (for women) or sexually active (before and/or after intercourse).

In terms of sexual activities, data from all of the HALIRA research methods suggest that young people considered vaginal intercourse to be the only normal form of sex. It was unusual for a couple to have a sexual encounter that did not involve vaginal intercourse, and many encounters only involved vaginal intercourse, with very little other contact between the partners. Unmarried young men ideally liked to have multiple orgasms during one sexual rendezvous, for example, to have vaginal intercourse and to ejaculate two to four times in the course of several hours spent with a partner at night. However, it is not clear how often they actually achieved this.

Sometimes young people reported that, prior to intercourse, they engaged in sexual foreplay, that is, non-penetrative sexual activity such as caressing different parts of the body. However, kissing on the mouth or sucking of any part of the body was unusual. Foreplay was most often reported by older youth and young adults who were more sexually experienced than early to mid-adolescents. Many young people said that foreplay helped to arouse and naturally lubricate a woman in a desirable way. Villagers reported that it was optimal for a woman to be moderately lubricated during intercourse, and attempts to artificially increase or decrease natural lubrication were rare.

In the young adult group discussions, participants described occasional circumstances when a man and woman might engage in sexual activities without also engaging in vaginal intercourse, such as when a woman was menstruating. This usually involved rubbing against one another, or, rarely, oral sex on the man. However, both oral sex and anal sex usually were perceived very negatively by villagers. All of the data sources suggest that heterosexual anal intercourse was rare in remote, Sukuma villages, and was practiced only by a very small minority in larger, multiethnic villages, particularly fishing villages. The few women who reported personal experience of anal intercourse described their partners as either coercing or forcing them to engage in it, and they said the experience was painful.

During the HALIRA research, both male and female villagers occasionally made implicit or explicit references to women's sexual comfort and pleasure, but only a small minority believed that women primarily had sex for this reason rather than for material gain. Experience of orgasm during sexual encounters seemed to be highly variable between women and for individual women at different times or with different partners. Adolescent girls were reported to be least likely to experience it. Female participants in each of the young adult group discussions also mentioned various techniques that women occasionally might use to reduce or satisfy their sexual desires alone.

The different data sources suggest that male masturbation was not uncommon in rural Mwanza, especially among adolescent boys. In the group discussion series, some male youths seemed to see masturbation as natural and normal if a boy is unable to have sex with a girl, although unlike sexual intercourse it was not something they would normally discuss with their peers. If masturbation was mentioned in casual conversation, it was usually disparaged. Few young men seemed to perceive it as sinful or immoral, but many perceived it negatively, associating it with weakness, shame, and lack of discipline. Some reported that masturbation was physically harmful and could cause impotence or sterility. Some believed it is more safe and healthy to have unprotected intercourse than to masturbate.

As noted earlier, in most villages male and female homosexuality seemed to be very rare. Almost all accounts of men having sex with one another involved the following contexts: fishing villages/camps, prisons, or unusual circumstances in people's homes. Both prisons and remote fishing camps were largely or entirely male settings where rape and sexual coercion of boys and men were said to occur. Accounts of homosexual activity in those contexts usually described situations in which the penetrative partner was unable to have vaginal intercourse, which was his first choice for sexual satisfaction, and the receptive partner was coerced and was believed to lose sexual prowess in the course of the act. The prevalence of such practices at fishing camps may have contributed to the male homosexual activity and heterosexual anal intercourse that were rumored to occasionally happen in fishing villages, but almost never in other villages. There were only isolated, third-person accounts of a man or an older boy attempting to have sex with a younger boy in other participant observation villages, as well as isolated third-person reports of consensual homosexual activity between adolescent girls.

MARRIED YOUNG PEOPLE'S SEXUAL RELATIONSHIPS

Before marriage, when young men described a desirable sexual partner they often mentioned physical characteristics, but when describing a desirable wife they also mentioned a hard-working nature, politeness, and good behavior, such as sexual fidelity. Like men, young women often desired physical attractiveness in a husband, but also said that he should be faithful and hard-working. Many young women also valued a man with personal wealth, achievement, and status, such as owning a kiosk or being a community leader. The more gifts or money men provided in premarital sexual relationships the more desirable they usually were considered to be as potential husbands.

Of sixty-three Year 5–7 pupils who were randomly selected to participate in in-depth interviews at the beginning the *MEMA kwa Vijana* trial, two of twenty-nine men and seventeen of thirty-three women were married when reinterviewed two to three years later. At that time one of the men and five of the women already had one child, and some other women were pregnant. The participant observation research found that most young men wanted to be economically independent before marrying, so they typically did not marry until they had been out of school for several years.

The Process of Marrying

For both young men and women, marriage usually represented a welcome transition to adulthood and its anticipated independence, security, status, and comfort. Sex also played an important part in the decision to marry, as a way to have unlimited and exclusive sexual access to a desired partner (particularly for men) and as a way to legitimately have children (particularly for women). Many young people married after having had varied and complicated premarital sexual relationships, and a few expressed hope that mutual marital fidelity would reduce their sexual health risk. Indeed, it seems likely that, in the first months and years after marrying, many young people (particularly wives) had fewer sexual partners and/or became more faithful than they had been prior to marriage, although this behavior change may not have been maintained long-term. Chapter 9 will examine the motivations and experiences of young people who intentionally limited their partner number and/or practiced fidelity, before or after marriage.

At the end of the trial, most married in-depth interview respondents reported that they had met their spouse for the first time about one month before marrying, regardless of whether they married by engagement, elopement, or simply moving in together. Often it did not seem necessary to know a partner well before marrying, but what was critical was for both individuals to be at a point in their lives when they wanted to marry. Very few villagers in rural Mwanza had a legally registered marriage. For young women who had recently left school, the most common forms of marriage were either formal engagement, when a man proposed to a woman's parents and negotiated bridewealth in advance, or elopement, when a couple ran away together and a lesser elopement fine was paid by the husband to the woman's family after the fact. Half of the in-depth interview respondents said they had been engaged before marriage, but only a small minority had had formal Christian, Muslim, or traditional weddings. Notably, two women from different districts who had formal Protestant (African Inland Church) ceremonies were required by their church to be screened for infectious illnesses with their husbands before marrying.

Eloping was less costly and time-consuming than a formal marriage, and it did not require the active involvement and approval of both sets of parents, which was important for couples who feared parental opposition. Often elopement happened fairly spontaneously based on a couple's appeal for one another and general desire to marry. In some cases a girl's parents reacted angrily to her elopement, particularly if she was young, if the parents had expected to receive ample bridewealth, and/or if they disapproved of her partner. However, the act of eloping effectively forced their hand, and the elopement fine that was negotiated afterward was usually about half of what they would have expected in bridewealth.

It was unusual for young men to marry within the first one or two years after leaving school, and usually this reflected atypical circumstances, such as the young man being extraordinarily affluent or having a pregnant girlfriend. Occasionally, a young woman who recently had left school became pregnant and married the man simply by moving in with him. In such cases the man either did not compensate her parents or paid them a relatively small traditional fine for having caused a pregnancy out-of-wedlock. Some young men and women specifically sought a pregnancy in the hope that it would lead to marriage with a particular partner. In almost every participant observation village there were also plausible first-person accounts of women who publicly attributed a pregnancy to the sexual partner who they most wanted to marry, even though a different partner was equally or more likely to be the biological father.

Once young women had been out of school for several years, almost all marriages happened either by elopement or simply by moving in together, and the woman's parents usually did not receive bridewealth, an elopement fine, or a pregnancy fine. Indeed, at that stage of life the informal and transient nature of many marriages meant that a couple might be perceived as married by some villagers but not by other villagers, and sometimes even the members of the couple themselves perceived the nature of their union differently. A couple's marital status could be unclear, for example, when a man traveled away from the village for extended periods for work, or when he was known to have a formal wife elsewhere.

Married Life

Young couples gained status, privileges and responsibilities when they married, for example, moving from shared same-sex housing into a house of their own within the husband's family homestead. The transition to married life involved the greatest change for young wives, as it often meant living in a new home with a largely unfamiliar husband and sometimes his entirely unfamiliar family and village. A young wife typically held many domestic and farming responsibilities and was expected to obey her husband's wishes and those of his parents. Young wives often also had less freedom of movement than they had had before marriage. Many young wives seemed comfortable and satisfied with this role, but some were not. Some young married couples lived in the husband's parental homestead long-term, while others moved away, either within the village or to a more distant village or town to pursue new livelihoods. The status of those who stayed within a homestead typically grew over time as they cultivated their own agricultural plots in addition to the family's, built small businesses, and increasingly contributed to the economic welfare of the homestead and family.

Married couples usually spent little time together in the course of their daily lives, for both economic and social reasons. Participant observation researchers occasionally observed married couples laughing together as they worked, but joint work was the exception rather than the rule, and usually it was restricted to the most intensive periods of the agricultural cycle. In public places, husbands and wives rarely walked together or chatted with each other. At night, wives were expected to be sexually available to their husbands except in certain circumstances, such as when they were menstruating or they had recently delivered a child. After marriage a man usually did not provide money or gifts to his wife in exchange for a specific sexual encounter, but his material support was still a very important part of the marital relationship. In fact the most common reason why women were reported to have extramarital relationships, or to end a marriage, was inadequate financial support from a husband. Husbands typically provided the most for their wives early in a marriage. Long-term, wives often had to pay for many household expenses and buy their own clothes, shoes, and body lotion.

Most young women were expected to conceive a child within a year of marriage, so it was very rare for a couple to consider contraception before their first baby. After having one or more children some women did wish to practice contraception, particularly to space out their subsequent pregnancies. However, men typically did not wish to prevent conception within marriage, and women were expected to follow their decisions.

If a wife refused to have sex with her husband or was discovered to use contraception against his wishes, this could lead to public conflict and divorce. Participant observation suggested that it was unusual for men to use physical force to assert their will over their girlfriends and wives, but it did happen on occasion, most commonly with men who were heavy drinkers. Indeed, in the two group discussions with unmarried women in their early twenties, about half said they had experienced physical violence within a sexual relationship at some time. When this occurred, it usually was not condoned by others and it could be considered adequate justification for a woman to leave her husband. Nonetheless, there were occasional instances when a husband was perceived as justified in hitting his wife, such as when he had evidence that she was unfaithful.

Polygyny

According to Tanzanian law, a registered traditional marriage can have an unlimited number of wives, while a Muslim marriage can have no more than four, and a Christian or civil marriage can have only one. However, as noted earlier, very few marriages of any kind—either monogamous or polygynous—were legally registered in rural Mwanza, and many men who identified themselves as Christian also had multiple wives.

There were several ways in which polygynous marriages formed in rural Mwanza. Sometimes a man who wanted an additional wife due to sexual attraction or a desire for more children simply moved her into his household and identified her as a junior wife. Often the new wife was younger than the man and his preexisting wives, came from a relatively poor family, and/ or had already been married or had a child, so her family did not expect much or any bridewealth. Co-wives in the same household often cooperated with one another, especially if both wives had been aware and willing when entering into the polygynous marriage. They typically spent more time together than with their husband, as they shared many domestic and farming responsibilities. Some co-wives seemed to like one another and get along well, while others struggled with resentment and anger for one another.

Most polygynous marriages in rural Mwanza involved co-wives who lived in separate households, and such co-wives often had little or no contact with one another. This kind of polygynous marriage often came into being after a husband's clandestine extramarital relationship with a woman evolved into a more openly acknowledged, long-term relationship. In such circumstances, a man's first wife sometimes felt betrayed by his lack of fidelity, or resentful and angry about loss of income. However, if she did not want to divorce her husband she usually resigned herself to another wife.

Extramarital Relationships

In most participant observation villages there were first-person and third-person reports of many young husbands and a few young wives having secretive extramarital sexual relationships. Those data suggest that most men experienced at least one—and sometimes many—such relationships by the time they had been married for several years. Secrecy was equally or more important in extramarital relationships than in premarital ones, especially for women. Fidelity seemed to be most common during the first months and years of a marriage, when husbands enjoyed novel, nightly sexual access to their wives, and wives often had their material needs met and were monitored closely within their husband's household. Men sometimes began extramarital sexual relationships when they traveled, when their wives were in late pregnancy or were recovering from delivery, or simply when they desired a different sexual partner than their wife. As with premarital relationships, a man's extramarital affairs could take a number of different forms, including: one-off, spontaneous sexual encounters (for example, around a celebrative event); repeated clandestine, opportunistic encounters with a particular person; and semi-open, long-term relationships that might eventually result in offspring and a formal marriage. Again, many wives seemed to be aware of their husbands' infidelity and this often led to conflict within the marriage, but if the couple did not separate then wives typically resigned themselves to it.

Women's extramarital sexual relationships mainly seemed to consist of secretive, open-ended, and sometimes long-term involvement with one or two familiar men, rather than one-off encounters with strangers. Married women most often reported taking lovers to support themselves or their families, particularly if their husbands were drunkards, had traveled for extended periods, divided limited income between different households (as in polygynous marriages), or did not contribute sufficiently to a household for some other reason. There were also occasional reports of women who had extramarital relationships due to sexual desire, or because they believed their husbands to be sterile and they wanted to have a child.

Divorce

Marital separation and divorce were not unusual in rural Mwanza, including amongst young people. In all participant observation villages there were accounts of couples who ran away together, were considered married, and then ended the relationship within a few days, weeks, or months. Some couples who hardly knew one another before marrying quickly separated after they found they did not like or love each other enough to stay married, or that their marriage was unacceptable for some other reason. Marriages were most commonly reported to end because of insufficient economic support (from husbands), infidelity (particularly by wives), difficulty having children, and general disagreements, such as whether to use contraception. Other factors which were reported to cause a divorce included incomplete payment of bridewealth, a spouse's drunkenness, a husband's violence, tensions between a wife and her husband's family (including a co-wife), and geographic separation (as when a husband left for work and never returned).

Just as many marriages happened informally, separation and divorce could be similarly informal in rural Mwanza, usually simply signified by one member of the couple moving out of a shared residence. Most typically a young woman moved back into her parents' or a relative's household, but sometimes she might move into a household with one or more other single women. If bridewealth or an elopement fine had been paid, the couple had not been married for long, and there were no offspring, then the woman's family was expected to repay the man's family.

Many villagers shifted between being unmarried and in a monogamous or polygynous marriage repeatedly over the course of one or two decades, depending on their particular experience of separation, divorce, widowhood, and new marriage. Just as marrying sometimes resulted in a reduction in risk behaviors for some, separation and divorce sometimes involved a shift to higher risk behaviors, as men and women sought new partners for sexual satisfaction, material support, or potential marriage.

REPRODUCTIVE BELIEFS AND PRACTICES

Contraception

In rural Mwanza, having children—especially many children—was almost universally viewed as a source of pride, accomplishment, and security in one's old age. Many men and some women considered pregnancy to be desirable in any circumstances. Nonetheless there also were many accounts of unmarried adolescent girls and young women who did not want to become pregnant for fear of the stigma, punishment, and hardship sometimes associated with out-of-wedlock pregnancies. Some did not try to prevent pregnancy because they did not know how to do so, or they believed that they could not become pregnant (e.g., due to young age) or that contraception was alien or harmful. Some school girls and childless young women instead used traditional contraceptive methods that were unlikely to be effective, such as wearing charms or drinking solutions made of wood ashes. It was very rare for school girls to use modern contraceptives. Even if they were aware contraception was available at health facilities, they were very unlikely to try to obtain it because of distance to facilities and fear that health workers would judge them and discuss their visit with other villagers. Such concerns were often warranted. For example, in half of the *MEMA kwa Vijana* control communities, health worker comments to simulated patients were ranked as moderately to extremely judgmental, and they provided those young people with little or none of the appropriate information.

Young mothers, whether married or not, generally had more access to modern contraceptives than childless young women, because they attended health services for prenatal check-ups and their children's health care, and health facility staff specifically targeted them with contraceptive advice. However, only a minority of young mothers used modern contraception consistently, sometimes without their sexual partners' awareness. The most popular choices were quarterly Depo Provera hormonal injections, followed by daily oral contraceptives. Many informants voiced wariness of hormonal methods, particularly oral contraceptives, because they were widely rumored to have negative side effects, such as weight loss or gain, continuous or sporadic menstrual bleeding, reproductive cancer, and infertility. One of the most commonly cited concerns about both traditional and modern contraception was that they might harm a woman's long-term fertility.

Many villagers in *MEMA kwa Vijana* control communities had heard of condoms through radio programs, public meetings, or informal discussions. People generally associated condoms with the prevention of sexually transmitted infection, not contraception. Condoms were available for free in government health facilities, and they usually could be purchased in kiosks for Tshs 50 ($0.06) for a pack of three. However, condom availability and access was very limited in rural Mwanza, especially for youth. This will be described more in chapter 6.

Few villagers had ever seen a condom outside of its packet or had a clear understanding of how one was used. Generally, condoms were perceived very negatively. The vast majority of informants reported many reasons why they would not use condoms, including: a belief that condoms reduce sexual pleasure; not being "used to" condoms (particularly men); not having a say in the decision to use condoms (particularly women); not wanting to prevent conception; willingness to leave HIV exposure to chance or God's will; perceiving no personal risk of acquiring HIV/AIDS or other sexually transmitted infections; trust in a partner; fear of stigma, rejection, or punishment; and suspicion that new condoms might have holes, contain HIV, or be harmful in other ways. For example, a small minority of villagers reported that blocking a man's semen from entering a woman during intercourse was unnatural and dissatisfying, because semen was believed to enhance a woman's beauty and health, and/or it symbolized the man's sexual conquest of her, however temporary. However, a reduction in pleasure seemed to be the main reason many men perceived condom use as unacceptable, even if the other concerns listed above were resolved. Outside of marriage, men generally felt entitled to set the terms of sexual encounters once they had provided a woman with a gift or money, and most considered condom use to be poor value for their money. For most women, in turn, the overwhelming determinant of condom use was whether their partners wanted to use them.

The most common circumstance in which men reported that they might use a condom was if they suspected a partner of having many other partners, or of having a sexually transmitted infection. Indeed, a small number of men selectively used condoms with partners who they perceived to be high risk in these ways; their motivations and experiences will be examined in chapter 10. However, most men did not use condoms, even when they suspected a partner of being at high risk of infection. The association of promiscuity with condoms may have contributed to a fear of stigma among some potential condom users, particularly women. Broaching the issue of condoms also raised uncomfortable questions about a partner's infidelity, or one's own, potentially offending and alienating a partner.

Christian and Muslim leaders rarely opposed hormonal contraception in rural Mwanza, but their attitudes and advice about condom use were quite variable, ranging from leaders who voiced adamant opposition to it, to some who discreetly endorsed it, for example, by hosting an AIDS awareness workshop.

Abortion

In most countries of sub-Saharan Africa, induced abortion is illegal unless the woman's life is in danger, and in Tanzania abortion for almost any other reason is punishable by fourteen years of imprisonment for the person administering the abortion, seven years for the woman, and three years for anyone who knowingly supplied materials used to induce abortion.

In HALIRA participant observation villages, the vast majority of informants opposed induced abortion as illegal, dangerous for the woman, morally wrong, and particularly unacceptable if the man who caused the pregnancy did not consent. In each of the four study districts there also were villagers who reported that ancestral spirits in some Sukuma clans opposed abortion and would kill any female members, and particularly the sexual partners of any male members, who attempted it. Men were perceived as entitled to their potential offspring, and some men were outraged that this right might be undermined through induced abortion. Less frequently reported reasons why people opposed abortion were that it was disrespectful (e.g., insulting to infertile individuals), or unwise (e.g., reducing the number of children who could care for a woman in her old age).

Although most informants said they were opposed to abortion, some were also sympathetic, acknowledging that girls and women usually terminated pregnancies because of difficult life circumstances. A minority of informants did not condemn abortion when the topic came up. These tended to be women who had attempted to end a pregnancy themselves, or who had friends who had done so. This group ranged in age from young to middle-aged, and included women of different social status, for example, women who were single and considered somewhat disreputable, single and socially respected women, and married women. Informants commonly reported interrelated reasons why a girl or woman might terminate a pregnancy, including being in school and still living with her parents, being unmarried and unsupported by the baby's father, experiencing financial hardship, being afraid to jeopardize marriage prospects, and/or wanting longer intervals between children.

Overall, the HALIRA study found that induced abortion was highly stigmatized, hidden, and infrequent. Nonetheless, several participants in the female discussion group based in the largest village reported their own or a close acquaintance's abortion attempt. In addition, in most participant observation villages female researchers heard a few first-person accounts of abortion attempts; several relatively discreet and plausibly detailed stories about a friend's or relative's abortion attempt; and widespread rumors about one or more women who were believed to have recently terminated a pregnancy with dramatic consequences.

The most widely and frequently reported abortion method was ingestion of particular materials, mainly wood ashes in solution, certain other plant solutions, high doses of chloroquine, and/or a solution of "Blue," a brand of laundry detergent sold in tablet form. A few villagers reported that a woman could terminate her pregnancy manually, using a twig. A few believed that certain villagers (usually older women) were experienced at performing manual abortions, using unknown instruments in their own homes. However, most young people who talked about manual abortions described them as being performed by health facility staff, typically costing Tshs 10,000–15,000 ($12–$18) per procedure.

A number of women reported secret abortion attempts which failed, from which they had no apparent consequences and then carried their pregnancies to term. Of the women who reported having terminated a pregnancy, most said that at a minimum they had short-term negative health consequences (e.g., severe pain and bleeding for days or weeks), but none mentioned regretting the decision later. Other negative consequences women experienced after induced abortion included opposition from their sexual partners, sexual exploitation by practitioners, health problems (often requiring a follow-up visit to a health facility), social ostracism, and quasi-legal sanctions.

Fertility Protection and Promotion

Protection and promotion of future fertility was paramount for young, unmarried women in rural Mwanza, even if they did not want to become pregnant in the near future. Thus if unmarried girls believed that contraception or an induced abortion might affect their long-term fertility, they would generally rather risk immediate pregnancy and childbearing than later infertility. Once a woman married, her priority quickly shifted to becoming pregnant. Infertility and miscarriage were widely attributed to physical causes (e.g., sexually transmitted infections, contraception, or abortion history for females; "cold" sperm or one testicle for males) as well as supernatural causes (e.g., God's will, witchcraft, or ancestral punishment).

If a married couple did not conceive within one or two years, the woman was almost always assumed to have fertility problems. Typically, a man was only considered to be infertile if he had had multiple long-term sexual relationships with women who did not conceive, particularly if the women were known to have conceived children with other men. As noted earlier, some wives of infertile men were believed to have secret extramarital partners specifically to become pregnant, and this was a rare instance when discreet female infidelity was considered understandable and even warranted. There was very little opportunity for biomedical treatment of infertility in rural Mwanza, with the exception of treatment of sexually transmitted infections, which indirectly could protect or promote fertility. Active attempts to treat infertility were almost always traditional in nature, usually consisting of specific herbs or roots that were prepared for the woman to ingest.

HIV AND OTHER SEXUALLY TRANSMITTED INFECTIONS

Sexually Transmitted Infections

A large proportion of young villagers knew that sexually transmitted infections such as syphilis and gonorrhea are contracted through sexual intercourse. Notably, the term for "sexually transmitted infections" in Swahili—*magonjwa ya zinaa*—literally means "illnesses of fornication/adultery." It is based on the Arabic word "zina," which means unlawful sexual intercourse as defined by Islamic law, including premarital sex or extramarital sex. The Swahili term for sexually transmitted infection thus not only suggests the mode of infection but also has an inherently negative connotation.

In the HALIRA study, many people reported that individuals who have multiple sexual partners out-of-wedlock are in danger of getting sexually transmitted infections. On a few occasions informants specifically mentioned that sexually transmitted infections are caused by small organisms. However, some villagers had symptoms of sexually transmitted infection which they did not recognize as such, and which they instead attributed to non-sexual causes, such as stepping on contaminated material that had been left on a pathway by someone attempting to rid themselves of the same illness.

At the end of the *MEMA kwa Vijana* trial, 14 percent of male participants (average age nineteen) tested positive for one or more of the five infections tested for males, while 45 percent of female participants (average age eighteen) tested positive for one or more of the six infections tested for females (Helen Weiss, personal communication). The proportions were similar for young people who had been randomly selected for the first in-depth interview series, as at the end of the trial 7 percent of those male respondents and 42 percent of those female respondents tested positive for one or more infections. In addition, a few in-depth interview respondents who tested negative for all infections during the trial surveys reported in their second in-depth interview that they had had a sexually transmitted infection that had been treated at a health facility. Of the female respondents, fewer of those who were married (five of seventeen) than single (nine of sixteen) tested positive for an infection in the final trial survey, but two of the married women had two sexually transmitted infections, whereas none of the unmarried women had more than one.

Treatment of sexually transmitted infections in rural Mwanza was opportunistic and pluralistic, similar to treatment of other illnesses. However, there was greater stigma associated with sexually transmitted infections, so if people suspected they had one their fear of stigma could delay them from seeking treatment. Almost all reports of treatment initially involved traditional home remedies. When villagers had persistent symptoms they often consulted a traditional healer or someone else who was believed to have expertise in traditional medicine. Treatment of sexually transmitted infection by traditional healers was not limited to solutions which were drunk or applied topically, as there were also reports of traditional healers using razors to cut off genital growths which may have resulted from a sexually transmitted infection, such as genital warts.

Kiosk staff reported that some men but very few women purchased medication to treat sexually transmitted infections from them. Health workers instead reported that women were more likely than men to seek such treatment from health facilities. Health workers stipulated this was because health facility treatment was free, and pregnant women and mothers of young children already attended the facilities for prenatal or pediatric care. However, most health workers also reported that women were shyer than men when seeking sexually transmitted infection treatment.

Young people and older adults who had received treatment for sexually transmitted infections at health facilities generally spoke positively about the experience and were very grateful if their symptoms resolved. However, some symptomatic young people—especially girls—feared that they would be verbally abused if they sought treatment at a health facility and that their consultation would not be kept confidential, so they did not seek treatment even if their symptoms intensified. As was the case with girls who were afraid to seek contraception, concern about health worker judgment and lack of confidentiality also seemed warranted in this area.

HIV and AIDS

At the time of the *MEMA kwa Vijana* trial and the HALIRA study, only very limited HIV testing services were available at district or regional hospitals in Mwanza, and villagers rarely knew of or used such services. Antiretroviral therapy was not available anywhere in Tanzania, so medical treatment of AIDS amounted to treatment of opportunistic infections, at best.

The HALIRA study found that the majority of villagers in rural Mwanza had heard about AIDS from the radio, public meetings, fellow villagers, and/ or school. The common term for AIDS in Tanzania is the Swahili acronym, *UKIMWI.* Many people in rural Mwanza knew this term but did not know its full meaning, that is, reduction/lack of protection for the body (*Upungufu/ Ukosefu wa Kinga ya Mwili*). In all villages, many people also reported hearing about someone in the village having AIDS, although some said they had never heard this. A small proportion of villagers said that AIDS, like many other illnesses, is simply a result of chance or bad luck. However, the main causes attributed to AIDS were natural (biological) and witchcraft.

In terms of natural causes, most informants reported that AIDS could be contracted through sexual intercourse, a blood transfusion, or contact with a sharp, infected object, such as razors. People especially associated AIDS with sex, and many informants said that promiscuous women spread AIDS in the villages through their sexual activity. In Swahili, the term for HIV (*virusi vya UKIMWI*) literally means "AIDS virus," but few villagers knew that HIV causes AIDS, and those who did usually did not understand the term "virus" or its relationship to immune deficiency and opportunistic infections. Some villagers knew that a person could be infected and infectious but not yet show signs of AIDS, but even they typically were confused about the length of the asymptomatic period and the diverse illnesses that a person with AIDS might eventually have. A few informants also believed that AIDS could be spread through natural means which in fact do not transmit HIV, such as touching or sharing food with a person with AIDS.

In addition, many people in all participant observation villages reported that individuals rumored to have AIDS might in fact have had an AIDS-like illness that was caused by witchcraft. These informants typically believed in both a "real" (natural) AIDS, which leads to certain death, and a similar illness caused by witchcraft, which could be cured by traditional medicine. There were several reasons reported for why a person might be bewitched with an AIDS-like illness, including envy, punishment for an offense, and revenge on someone in authority. Only a minority of villagers in the study doubted whether witchcraft could cause an AIDS-like illness.

The in-depth interviews with the seven young people who were HIV-positive at the start of the *MEMA kwa Vijana* trial suggest that some of them contracted HIV from their mothers in utero, at birth, or through breast milk. In contrast, most or all of the six in-depth interview respondents who became HIV-positive in the course of the trial probably contracted HIV sexually. The one young man in this group reported an extraordinarily high number of sexual partners, i.e., eleven partners in the three years prior to the interview. He said none of those relationships were concurrent, but there had only been gaps of about one week between them. The female respondents in this group did not report unusually high numbers of partners or experience of concurrent partnerships. Instead, their interviews suggest they were exposed to HIV by a partner who was likely to have had many partners, like a truck driver or a cotton ginnery operator, or while they were living in settings with relatively high HIV prevalences, such as Mwanza City, a district capital, or large villages on major truck routes.

In rural Mwanza, many signs and symptoms of AIDS-related opportunistic infections were similar to those of other common illnesses, such as diarrhea, fevers, skin rashes, or chest infections. Villagers thus often treated them in the same way, initially trying home remedies and then increasingly paying for care from traditional healers and health care facilities as the conditions worsened. Some people with AIDS seemed to pursue traditional treatments for longer than biomedical treatment because traditional treatments offered them hope of a cure, especially as some traditional healers claimed that they could cure people who had "false" AIDS.

CONTEXTUAL BARRIERS AND FACILITATORS OF SEXUAL RISK REDUCTION

The findings presented in this chapter illustrate many contextual factors which made it difficult for young people in rural Mwanza to avoid risky sexual behaviors, as well as some which could potentially facilitate sexual behavior change and risk reduction. Some contextual barriers to risk reduction can be categorized as economic and some as sociocultural, but in practice those dimensions were deeply intertwined. Economic barriers included women's lower status and economic dependence on men; sex being an important economic resource for women; and the poor quality of formal education and health services. Sociocultural barriers included contradictory sexual norms and related secrecy; sexual activity being perceived as central to young men's identities; a belief in the inevitability of sex once initiated; misconceptions and ambivalence about contraception; low salience of, and perceived susceptibility to, HIV/AIDS; and quick and arbitrary decision-making and fatalism.

In contrast, some contextual factors seemed to have a potential to promote young people's sexual risk reduction in rural Mwanza, including restrictive norms (e.g., that school pupils should be abstinent, or that couples should be faithful), and parents' concern for their children's health and welfare. Dominant community values thus both discouraged adolescent sexual activity (e.g., women should not have many sexual partners) and encouraged it (e.g., sex is a resource for women to exploit). Young people managed such contradictory

influences by concealing their sexual activity, contributing to short-term relationships with fast partner change, and/or long-term overlapping relationships,
both of which contributed to young people's sexual health risk.

CONCLUSION

This chapter described the typical lives and sexual risk behaviors of young
people in rural Mwanza in the absence of an adolescent sexual health intervention, largely by drawing on HALIRA findings from *MEMA kwa Vijana* trial
control communities which are described in detail in this book's companion
volume (Plummer and Wight, 2011). Importantly, these findings suggest that a
minority of adolescents actively tried to abstain throughout their school years,
and a minority also or instead tried to have long-term, mutually faithful sexual
relationships before marriage, although they often did not succeed in this. Many
adolescents aspired to be abstinent or faithful because these were widely shared
social ideals, particularly for girls. In contrast, condom use was viewed negatively in rural areas, and the qualitative research suggests that only a very small
minority of young people ever tried to use condoms once or twice, and almost
none had used them consistently.

The focus on typical village life in this chapter provides the context for the
book's main topic: the promotion of low-risk sexual behaviors with young
rural Africans. Chapters 4–7 will now examine this topic by evaluating the
process and impact of the *MEMA kwa Vijana* adolescent sexual health program as implemented in Mwanza Region from 1999 to 2002. Chapters 8–10
will then return to the broader qualitative findings to examine the motivations
and experiences of atypical young people in the study population who practiced low-risk sexual behaviors.

NOTES

1. The term "traditional" is used here to describe local, non-Western beliefs and
practices that were reportedly handed down from prior generations. However, it is
likely that some of these were more recently introduced, or had been substantially
modified over time (Wijsen and Tanner, 2002).

2. During the HALIRA study from 1999 to 2002, the exchange rate was approximately Tanzanian Shillings (Tshs) 1,000 to US $1.20. The official minimum monthly
wage was Tshs 30,000, but many laborers made far less than that. During the fourth
series of in-depth interviews in 2009, the exchange rate was approximately Tshs
1,000 to US $0.80, so the later exchange rate is applied to amounts mentioned in
those interviews.

Part II

INTERVENTION EVALUATION

Chapter Four

MEMA kwa Vijana
Intervention Overview and
Community Mobilization

This chapter will provide an introduction and overview of the *MEMA kwa Vijana* intervention, which was the adolescent sexual health program that was evaluated from 1997 to 2002 in the *MEMA kwa Vijana* community randomized trial described in chapter 1. The main component of the *MEMA kwa Vijana* intervention was a primary school program, so the chapter begins with an overview of primary education in Mwanza Region and Tanzania at the time when the intervention was developed. It continues with a description of Tanzanian national guidelines on HIV prevention in primary schools, and then reviews HIV prevention activities in Mwanza Region in the 1990s, prior to the start of the *MEMA kwa Vijana* intervention. This will be followed by a background and overview of the intervention, describing its four components, its theoretical basis, and its behavioral goals. The development and design of the school curriculum will then be described, including pre-test, pilot test, modification during the trial, and final content. The chapter will conclude with a description and process evaluation of community-wide activities within the *MEMA kwa Vijana* intervention, which largely consisted of community mobilization at the start of the trial.

PRIMARY EDUCATION IN RURAL MWANZA
AT THE TIME OF THE STUDY

At the beginning of the twenty-first century, national school systems in sub-Saharan Africa faced many challenges, including limited enrollment and completion rates, and low levels of knowledge and skills even among those who did complete school (Johnson, 2008; Lloyd and Hewett, 2009). In several African countries, less than half of fifteen- to twenty-four-year-old women could read a simple sentence after three years of primary school; even many of those who reached lower secondary school could hardly read or write (World Bank, 2006). Within that context, the Tanzanian education system was considered to be particularly challenged. Indeed, Cooksey and Riedmiller (1997, 123) described it as "a very late developer," characterized by extreme underfunding, bureaucratic inefficiency, corruption, and one of the smallest secondary and tertiary education sectors in the world.

When the *MEMA kwa Vijana* intervention was first implemented in 1999, for example, only 29 percent of men and 26 percent of women in Tanzania had completed Year 7, the final year of primary school, and only 5 percent and 4 percent respectively had gone on to secondary school (National Bureau of Statistics and Macro International, 2000). At that time over half of boys (51 percent) and girls (56 percent) of official primary school age (seven to thirteen years) were registered as attending primary school. Notably, higher proportions of girls than boys attended school at the ages of seven to ten years, but by the age of thirteen this shifted to higher proportions of boys than girls, and a large proportion of the primary school population was older than that. In 2003, for example, over half of Year 7 pupils were fifteen to seventeen years old, because many had only started school when they were nine or ten years old and many had repeated school years (Partnership for Child Development, 1998; Bommier and Lambert, 2000; United Republic of Tanzania, 2003). At that time, only 19 percent of Year 7 pupils went on to secondary school (Palmer et al., 2007).

As noted in chapter 3, material conditions in Tanzanian primary schools were also very poor during the *MEMA kwa Vijana* trial, particularly in rural schools, which rarely had running water, electricity, or other basic facilities (Arthur, 2001; O-saki and Agu, 2002; Towse et al., 2002; Nilsson, 2003). Primary school teachers had quite variable levels of training. Most of those trained in the 1970s and 1980s had only completed Year 7 of primary school themselves, and then had one additional year of teacher training college (Bennell and Mukyanuzi, 2005). In the 1990s the national government set a goal for new teachers to have four years of secondary school and one or two years of teacher training college, but when the *MEMA kwa Vijana* intervention began only 54 percent of Mwanza Region primary school teachers had those qualifications (United Republic of Tanzania, 1999). Many teachers perceived teaching as a "last resort," low-status, low-paid job, and they particularly wanted to avoid the isolation and hardship associated with rural settings (Towse et al., 2002). Rural Mwanza thus had some of the most underqualified and understaffed schools in the country, and only a minority of teachers were female (Bennell and Mukyanuzi, 2005).

In terms of teaching practice, primary school teaching in Mwanza and elsewhere in Tanzania consisted almost entirely of lecturing, formal question-and-answer sessions, recitation, and having pupils copy sentences from the chalkboard (Cooksey and Riedmiller, 1997; Arthur, 2001; O-saki and Agu, 2002). Emphasis was placed on memorizing information to pass national examinations, rather than the development of critical thinking, knowledge application, or problem-solving skills. As noted in chapter 3, it was common for primary school teachers and the children who they appointed as prefects to practice corporal punishment, that is, to intentionally inflict pain to discipline a pupil, usually by hitting or caning them. Nonetheless, in the absence of more progressive teacher training, some Tanzanian teachers employed creative, interactive approaches which were rooted in local culture, such as games involving riddles and proverbs (Barrett, 2007).

When the *MEMA kwa Vijana* intervention was first developed and implemented there were 931 primary schools and 40 secondary schools in Mwanza Region. The primary schools had an average of 675 registered pupils and nine teachers per school (United Republic of Tanzania, 2003). Class sizes and teacher-to-pupil ratios have worsened since then. For example, class sizes of 100 to 200 pupils per teacher have become typical in the first two years of primary school (Benson, 2006; Barrett, 2007).

TANZANIAN NATIONAL GUIDELINES ON HIV PREVENTION IN PRIMARY SCHOOLS

Given a large proportion of adolescent Tanzanians were in primary school in the late 1990s, and very few went on to secondary school, primary schools were the only way to systematically reach large numbers of adolescents with HIV prevention interventions. The situation has improved since then, but the general pattern remains true. For example, in the 2010 Tanzanian Demographic and Health Survey, 69 percent of male and 71 percent of female fifteen- to nineteen-year-olds had completed primary school, but only 39 percent and 35 percent respectively had completed secondary school (National Bureau of Statistics and ICF Macro, 2011).

In 1993, the Tanzanian government outlined a brief national AIDS curriculum for teachers to implement in primary schools. It was intended to provide pupils with basic information about HIV and other sexually transmitted infections and to promote abstinence until marriage (Schapink, Hema, and Mujaya, 1997). This curriculum permitted acknowledgement of condom use as a way to reduce sexual risk, but visual depiction of condoms, condom demonstrations (i.e., when a condom is unrolled over an object while the steps of proper use are explained), and exercises to develop condom negotiation skills were not allowed in school. Teachers were supposed to participate in an in-service course to become competent in teaching this curriculum, but there were insufficient funds to systematically carry out the training course. In the end, few teachers actually participated in the intended training, few teaching guides and books were distributed, and few schools implemented the curriculum even when teachers were trained (Schapink, Hema, and Mujaya, 1997).

In 1996, the Tanzanian Ministry of Education and Culture published new guidelines for HIV education in primary and secondary schools (United Republic of Tanzania, 1996). These guidelines stipulated that basic education about HIV and other sexually transmitted infections should be integrated within the broader curriculum for Years 5–7. Given an acute shortage of textbooks, the guidelines encouraged individuals and non-governmental organizations to develop teaching materials which, if approved by the government, could be taught to teachers in pre-service and in-service education courses. The guidelines specified that one-half of HIV education teaching time should focus on promoting responsible behaviors, which were defined as delaying sex or having protected sex for those youth who were sexually active. The guidelines further noted that, "education for proper use of condoms will be given and promoted yet the distribution of condoms in schools will not be permitted" (United Republic of Tanzania, 1996, 14–15).

In addition, in 2000 the Tanzanian Ministry of Education and Culture issued brief policy guidelines identifying a need for a broad school health curriculum that integrated family life, life skills, nutrition, hygiene, and AIDS education (United Republic of Tanzania, 2000). However, due to lack of funding this was not implemented on the ground (Bornemisza, 2001).

In 2004, the national guidelines for HIV education in primary and secondary schools were revised (United Republic of Tanzania, 2004). The new guidelines were intended to integrate HIV education with broader life skills education, but there was little actual change to the content of the previous guidelines. The new version specified that education about the proper use of condoms should be provided in both teacher training colleges and schools, but condoms could not be demonstrated or distributed in either location.

In a recent review of the 2004 guidelines and the broader national curriculum for different school subjects, Mkumbo (2009) argues that the primary school social studies and science syllabi address some basic HIV prevention information, but not other aspects which are internationally recognized as important for education about sexuality and HIV prevention, such as sexual relationships, skills development, perceived risk, self-efficacy, attitudes, and values. Even at the secondary school level, where family planning is listed within the reproduction sub-topic of the biology curriculum, the meaning and importance of family planning is mentioned but there was no reference to contraception (Mkumbo, 2009). Mkumbo (2009) notes that his review only examines the national guidelines and curricula without assessing actual teaching, and highlights a need to evaluate how such recommendations are implemented in practice. He concludes that sexuality education in the national curriculum and guidelines is disorganized and scattered across different subjects, "to the extent that they can hardly be said to constitute a meaningful . . . programme" (Mkumbo, 2009, 624).

HIV PREVENTION IN RURAL MWANZA
AT THE TIME OF THE STUDY

In the 1990s, HIV prevention efforts in Mwanza Region were extremely limited. Efforts were underway to reduce HIV transmission during medical care, including testing blood before using it for transfusions and ensuring needles and syringes were sterilized. However, the possibility of transmission via those mechanisms was not eliminated. The blood supply was limited, so it was not unusual for family members or friends to provide untested blood when a patient needed a transfusion; indeed, this often was expected (Berege and Klokke, 1997). In addition, people often perceived injections as more powerful and fast-working than oral medications, so injections may have been over-used in health facilities, and traditional healers and lay people also sometimes used them in local, unregulated practices (Vos et al., 1992; Gumodoka, Favot, and Dolmans, 1997). As noted in chapter 3, during this time period only very limited HIV testing services were available at district and regional hospitals, and villagers rarely knew of or used such services. Approximately half of fifteen- to forty-four-year-olds who were admitted to medical wards of the regional referral hospital were HIV-positive (Kaluvya et al., 1998). However, antiretroviral therapy was not available anywhere in the country, so medical treatment of AIDS amounted to treatment of opportunistic infections, at best.

During this period, HIV education for the general public in Mwanza Region was mainly limited to national radio programs, billboard messages, brief mention in public meetings, and a few small-scale, short-term health promotion interventions (Boerma et al., 2002). Since 1993, a national radio soap opera—*Twende na Wakati* (literally "Let's Go with the Times")—had addressed HIV prevention, family planning, economic development, and other health issues in twice-weekly broadcasts (Vaughan et al., 2000; Macdowall and Mitchell, 2006). Population Services International was engaged in social marketing and distribution of subsidized condoms to private distributors, wholesalers, and retail outlets in urban areas (Agha and Meekers, 2004; Eloundou-Enyegue, Meekers, and Calvès, 2005). Condom distribution in rural areas was rudimentary and informal, so that only a small number of condoms were available in some shops and kiosks in large villages.

Within Tanzania, District AIDS Control Coordinators were expected to organize educational activities at the district level, but in rural areas they had very little funding and typically lacked transportation, so outreach was extremely limited and focused on clinical services (Bornemisza, 2001; Changalucha et al., 2002). For example, in one Mwanza district of more than three hundred thousand people, the Ministry of Health could only afford one staff member with a motorcycle to supply free condoms and provide HIV education to all government health facilities (Boerma et al., 2002). At that time there were some small-scale HIV education programs implemented by non-governmental organizations in a few villages in the region, but these typically were not well defined and were mainly intended to support existing government activities (Boerma et al., 2002). For example, a program led by the Tanzania Netherlands Project to Support HIV/AIDS Control (TANESA) in one semi-rural ward consisted of community mapping of high-risk places, the establishment of village AIDS committees, community campaigns against AIDS, the formulation of village by-laws to reduce high-risk sexual behavior (e.g., the creation of curfews for young people), and teacher implementation of the national AIDS curriculum with additional peer education (Plummer and Maswe, 1998; Mwaluko et al., 2003). However, a series of community surveys found that that program did not have an impact on HIV incidence or self-reported sexual behavior and risk perception, leading program implementers and evaluators to recommend that more intensive HIV prevention efforts be undertaken (Mwaluko et al., 2003).

During this period the Tanzanian National AIDS Control Program had plans to conduct adolescent sexual and reproductive health education at a district level in Mwanza Region, but due to lack of funds this did not occur (Bornemisza, 2001). However, in the late 1990s two non-governmental organizations, TANESA and the African Medical and Research Foundation (AMREF), each independently developed and implemented a primary school HIV prevention program which was intended to supplement the national AIDS curriculum in rural Mwanza (Schapink, Hema, and Mujaya, 1997; Obasi, 2001). These were small in scale and mainly relied upon adolescent peer educators to convey reproductive health messages from a peer educator workbook.

Formal evaluation of both programs found that relying on primary school pupils or recent school leavers to be the main intervention implementers was problematic, for several reasons (Plummer and Maswe, 1998; Obasi, 2001).

The evaluations found that pupils—especially girls—were socialized to be very subservient to those in authority, and peer educators had difficulty planning and carrying out activities without the close involvement of trainers or teachers. The evaluations further found that peer educators had difficulty understanding and conveying key concepts to other pupils in an accurate and clear way. For example, peer educator questionnaires completed before and after one training course indicated that some pupils' knowledge improved, but a large minority still could not answer basic HIV-related questions taken directly from their workbook (Plummer and Maswe, 1998). Going into the training courses, pupils typically had extremely low literacy and only very rudimentary understandings of biology and mathematics. This could make it challenging for them to fully understand basic concepts about disease transmission (e.g., an asymptomatic person can be infectious for years) or sexual networks (e.g., a sexual partner may have been indirectly infected by his or her prior partners' partners).

Ongoing pupil turnover was another challenge faced by these peer education programs, as the required annual training was difficult to sustain, even on a small scale. Finally, in one of the programs the main trainer and field supervisor was found to have coerced some female peer educators to have sex with him, while punishing or firing those who refused, indicating that a peer education program in that setting required more intensive external monitoring and supervision (Plummer and Maswe, 1998).

BACKGROUND OF THE *MEMA KWA VIJANA* INTERVENTION

In 1997 researchers at the Mwanza branches of AMREF and the Tanzanian National Institute for Medical Research, together with researchers from the London School of Hygiene and Tropical Medicine in the United Kingdom, obtained funding and permission to conduct the *MEMA kwa Vijana* trial. As noted in chapter 1, this randomized controlled trial was designed to evaluate an adolescent sexual health intervention in four rural Mwanza districts (Missungwi, Kwimba, Sengerema, and Geita), the core of which was to be a primary school sexual and reproductive health curriculum (Hayes et al., 2005). The *MEMA kwa Vijana* intervention and research began in 1997 and have continued in different manifestations since then, as shown in table 1.1. This book only describes the trial that took place from 1997 to 2002, which overlapped with HALIRA project qualitative research.

MEMA kwa Vijana intervention design, implementation, and scale-up was led by Angela Obasi, who began the work as a British medical doctor with Master's degrees in epidemiology and anthropology. She was employed by the London School of Hygiene and Tropical Medicine during the trial. In 1997 she conducted a situation analysis to identify existing adolescent health and education services in Mwanza and broader Tanzania (Obasi et al., 2006). During the same period she led a small team of Tanzanians from AMREF in the development of an intervention framework and the first draft of the *MEMA kwa Vijana* teacher's guide. The name "*MEMA kwa Vijana*" was created as an acronym for "*Mpango wa Elimu na Maadili ya Afya kwa Vijana,*" which is Swahili for "Health Education and Ethics/Morals Program for Youth." However, "*mema*" also means "good things" in Swahili, and the program has almost always been referred to by the acronym *MEMA kwa Vijana,* meaning "Good Things for Youth."

The initial school curriculum drew on adolescent intervention programs and epidemiological studies in Mwanza and other parts of Africa; consultations with local government, health, and education authorities; guidelines from the Tanzanian Ministries of Health and Education and Culture; and international "best practice" reviews and recommendations (e.g., Kirby et al., 1994; Plummer, 1994; WHO and UNESCO, 1994a; WHO and UNESCO, 1994b; WHO and UNESCO, 1994c; United Republic of Tanzania, 1996; Fuglesang, 1997; Grunseit, 1997; Klepp et al., 1997; Kinsman et al., 1999; Shuey et al., 1999). In 1998 the draft school curriculum was tested and modified, and the intervention's community mobilization and health facility components were designed and tested. During that year the AMREF intervention team also met with government representatives at regional, district, division, ward, and village levels throughout the study area; carried out week-long community mobilization events in each of the ten trial intervention communities; and trained health workers, teachers, and pupil peer educators in intervention implementation.

In late 1998 all Year 4–6 pupils in *MEMA kwa Vijana* trial schools were invited to join the trial, and those who consented participated in a baseline survey (table 1.1). At that time, the ages of pupils in Year 4–6 recorded in school registers ranged from nine to twenty-two years for boys and nine to twenty years for girls (Todd et al., 2004). During the trial, however, most Year 7 participants ranged from fourteen to eighteen years of age (Obasi et al., 2006).

OVERVIEW OF THE INTERVENTION

Intervention Components

During the period studied in this book, the *MEMA kwa Vijana* intervention had four components (Obasi et al., 2006). First, *community-wide activities* consisted of an initial mobilization visit, annual youth health weeks involving interschool competitions and performances by local youth groups, twice-yearly youth health days at health facilities, and quarterly educational video shows and discussions open to all community members. Second, the most intensive intervention component was the *teacher-led, peer-assisted primary school program* that in its final version consisted of ten to eleven forty-minute sessions per year for pupils in Years 5–7. Third, two to four health workers from each government health facility were trained for one week in the provision of *youth-friendly sexual and reproductive health services*, and then were supervised quarterly. Finally, *community-based condom distribution for young people* was conducted by four to five out-of-school youth per village, who had been elected by their peers and trained in the social marketing of condoms. The community-wide activities are described and evaluated later in this chapter. Chapter 5 provides an in-depth description and evaluation of the school component, as chapter 6 does for the health facility and condom distribution components. Many original *MEMA kwa Vijana* intervention and evaluation materials can also be accessed online at memakwavijana.org or globalhivarchive.org.

The *MEMA kwa Vijana* intervention was delivered within Tanzanian government schools and health facilities in order for it to be cost-effective, sustainable, replicable, and feasible to scale-up. All teachers, health workers, and other government officials received allowances during out-of-station training and supervision activities to cover the costs of their meals and accommodation. However, no additional salaries or allowances were paid for implementation activities, such as the teaching of classroom sessions, reciprocal visits between schools and health facilities, or participation in the annual youth health week activities.

In January 1999, the *MEMA kwa Vijana* intervention began in the sixty-two primary schools and eighteen health facilities of the ten intervention communities. The Tanzanian school year begins in January, so the *MEMA kwa Vijana* curriculum was introduced at the start of the school year for Years 5, 6, and 7. The intervention was implemented for three years during the trial. During that time it was modified based on ongoing evaluation by the AMREF intervention team, the HALIRA project staff, and external health and education professionals. By 2002, a total of 189 teachers, 62 head teachers, 1,496 peer educators, 54 health workers, and 228 condom distributers had completed *MEMA kwa Vijana* training courses, each of which took place over two to six days (Obasi et al., 2006).

During the trial, annual costs of the intervention dropped from $16 per child in the first year (1999) to $10 per child in the third year (2001) (Terris-Prestholt et al., 2006). This included costs related to intervention development, start-up, and initial implementation. In contrast, the estimated cost of maintaining the intervention after an approximately ten-fold scale-up was $1.54 per pupil per year (Terris-Prestholt et al., 2006).

Theoretical Basis

The *MEMA kwa Vijana* intervention was based on the two behavior change theories introduced in chapter 1, the Theory of Reasoned Action and the Social Cognitive Theory (Fishbein, 2000; Michie et al., 2005). The Theory of Reasoned Action emphasizes the importance of a person's intentions in determining their behavior (Aarø, Schaalma, and Åstrøm, 2008). It focuses on the influence of personal factors on behavior, but it also takes into consideration subjective, interpersonal influences, particularly a person's perceptions of their sexual partner's expectations. The Social Cognitive Theory instead emphasizes the importance of a person's self-efficacy and outcome expectations in determining their behavior (Bandura, 2004). This theory postulates that human functioning results from a dynamic interaction between personal, behavioral, and environmental factors. Personal factors include cognition, affect, and biological influences on behavior, while environmental factors include social, cultural, and economic facilitators and impediments of behavior (Bandura, 2004).

The *MEMA kwa Vijana* intervention addressed theoretically identified behavioral determinants in multiple ways. For example, knowledge about the risks and benefits of different behaviors was promoted through teacher explanations, disease transmission simulation exercises, flipchart illustrations, stories that were read aloud, and peer educator dramas in the classroom. Self-efficacy was promoted through condom demonstrations at health centers and pupil roleplays focused on negotiation and problem-solving skills. Pupils were encouraged to anticipate outcomes of their behavior and to set goals for themselves in reflective exercises. The peer education component was intended to facilitate behavior change through observational learning and modeling. Real and perceived environmental impediments to accessing condoms and other contraceptives, or treatment for sexually transmitted infections, were addressed through class visits to health centers and out-of-school condom promotion and distribution.

Behavioral Goals

The goals of the *MEMA kwa Vijana* intervention were: to provide young people with the knowledge and skills to delay sexual debut, or to abstain after they had already become sexually active; to reduce sexual risk-taking by sexually active youth (including reducing partner number and using condoms); and to increase the appropriate use of sexual health services for contraception and sexually transmitted infection treatment (Obasi et al., 2006). This book focuses on the promotion of low-risk sexual behaviors, so the goal of increasing appropriate use of sexual health services is not examined in depth.

The *MEMA kwa Vijana* intervention addressed these behavioral goals in different ways within each intervention component, and the extent to which they were addressed also varied over the course of the trial within some of the components. For example, representatives of the Tanzanian Ministry of Education and Culture instructed intervention developers that abstinence promotion must be the main focus of the school curriculum. Abstinence before marriage was thus strongly promoted in every school year, and the curriculum could be categorized as an "abstinence-plus" intervention, as described in chapter 1 (Dworkin and Santelli, 2007; Nixon et al., 2011). In contrast, Tanzanian government guidelines expressly forbade condoms to be visually depicted or shown in primary schools. In order to teach pupils how to use condoms correctly, intervention developers thus provided step-by-step verbal instructions about how to use a condom in a preliminary draft of the curriculum. However, when this draft was reviewed by the Mwanza Region Education Officer prior to pre-testing, he specified that—given the ambiguity of the national guidelines on teaching information about condoms in the classroom—that part of the curriculum and the flipchart page that related to it must be removed (Obasi, 2001).

The curriculum used for all class years during the first year of the intervention thus only superficially addressed condom use. Process evaluation findings and further advocacy with government authorities during the trial led to increased attention to it in later versions of the curriculum, although even this was limited. Given government restrictions about teaching condom use in schools, intervention teachers were instructed to schedule visits to government health facilities with their classes, where intervention health workers showed condoms to young people, provided condom demonstrations, and explained that condoms were available there for free. In addition, the out-of-school youth condom distribution component was designed at the end of the first year of the trial specifically to improve youth awareness of and access to condoms.

CURRICULUM DEVELOPMENT AND DESIGN

It is widely agreed that sexual health curricula should be designed and tailored to the particular cultural settings where they are implemented, to ensure that they appropriately address local people's understandings and experiences (e.g., Gallant and Maticka-Tyndale, 2004; UNAIDS, 2007; UNESCO, 2008; Harrison et al., 2010; Michielsen et al., 2010). While few would argue with this in principle, realizing it in practice can pose great challenges, for multiple reasons. First, in-depth research may be necessary well in advance of curriculum development to fully understand cultural attitudes and practices related to sensitive sexual behaviors, but often there is neither sufficient time nor resources to do this well. Second, there is a delicate balance in designing curricula which are both culturally appropriate and potentially replicable, so that they may eventually be implemented on a large scale as needed in many African contexts (Gallant and Maticka-Tyndale, 2004; UNAIDS, 2007; Bertozzi et al., 2008; Padian et al., 2011). Third, many rural African communities have diverse ethnic and linguistic populations, and local peoples may not speak national languages fluently, let alone the languages in which international "best practice" curricula are drafted (e.g., Klepp et al., 1997; Visser, Schoeman, and Perold, 2004; Harrison et al., 2010). This may result in programs being taught in languages which pupils do not fully understand (e.g., Kinsman et al., 1999), and/or long and complicated processes of translating and back-translating curricula and training guides during intervention development and testing. Despite the great challenges posed by these issues, they are rarely acknowledged in published evaluations of school-based sexual health programs in sub-Saharan Africa. Instead, most published evaluations have described intervention development and implementation superficially, at best (Michielsen et al., 2010).

The following sections will describe the process of designing the *MEMA kwa Vijana* intervention in a multilingual context; the development, pretesting, pilot testing, and modification of the in-school curriculum during the trial; and the content of the final teacher's guides and resource book.

The Multilingual Context

The *MEMA kwa Vijana* intervention team faced linguistic challenges in the development and ongoing modification of the in-school curriculum and other intervention materials. Both Swahili and English are officially recognized national languages in Tanzania. In primary school, classes are supposed to be taught in Swahili and in secondary schools they are supposed to be taught in English. In practice, however, few Tanzanians speak any English, and in remote rural areas local languages are often more commonly spoken than Swahili (Brock-Utne and Holmarsdottir, 2004; Brock-Utne, 2007).

At the onset of the *MEMA kwa Vijana* trial—and as of this writing—most international HIV prevention guidelines and model curricula are drafted in English. At the start of the trial, the *MEMA kwa Vijana* intervention coordinator and other senior staff were native English speakers whose understanding of Swahili ranged from beginner to intermediate levels. None spoke Sukuma, the main local language, which is a tonal language with virtually no history in written form (Gleason, 1961; Abrahams, 1967; Wijsen and Tanner, 2002).

Senior Tanzanian intervention staff were fluent in Swahili and spoke English from beginner to advanced levels. Few spoke any Sukuma. Swahili was the main language spoken by villagers in large, multiethnic villages and towns in Mwanza Region, but many Sukumas and members of other, smaller ethnic groups spoke other languages in their homes. Most remote villages had almost exclusively Sukuma populations and few villagers in such areas understood Swahili well. Often children in rural Mwanza thus did not begin to learn Swahili until they entered primary school. In the most remote villages, it was not unusual for children to reach the upper levels of primary school with only a very limited understanding of Swahili.

These multilingual circumstances meant that the *MEMA kwa Vijana* intervention team needed to frequently check the accuracy and understanding of materials when translating them between different languages. Many *MEMA kwa Vijana* intervention materials were initially drafted in English and/or were adapted from existing English language materials. By the start of the trial, however, most of the working training guides and curriculum drafts were written and taught in Swahili. During the trial, the subsequent review and modification of those materials primarily took place in Swahili.

The First Teacher's Guide

In the first year of formal intervention implementation (1999) one teacher's guide was used to teach all participants in Years 5, 6, and 7. It provided detailed instructions in how to use different participatory teaching methods and addressed basic information about sexual and reproductive biology, including male and female anatomies, puberty, the menstrual cycle, how pregnancy occurs, the transmission of diseases within networks, sexually transmitted infection symptoms, the importance of seeking medical treatment for them, and the relationship between HIV and AIDS. The guide also included exercises intended to promote personal risk perception, communication, and assertiveness skills. As noted earlier, the teacher's guide primarily promoted abstinence, but partner reduction, fidelity, and condom use repeatedly were acknowledged as low-risk practices for sexually active youth.

While developing the school curriculum, the intervention team considered holding entirely same-sex sessions to avoid offending young people and adults who felt sexual discussions should not take place in mixed company, and out of concern for gender discrimination which led boys to dominate classroom discussions. This idea was rejected, however, because limited time, teacher number, and classroom space meant it would have been logistically difficult to implement on a large scale. However, many specific curriculum activities were designed for same-sex groups.

The next two sections draw upon AMREF intervention team monitoring and evaluation data to describe the pre-testing and pilot test of the first draft teacher's guide (Obasi, 2001).

Pre-Test of the First Teacher's Guide

In March 1998, the draft teacher's guide was pre-tested to assess the acceptability and appropriateness of each session. This involved AMREF staff teaching the curriculum over a three-week period in four urban Mwanza primary schools. AMREF intervention team observation in the classroom found that teachers and pupils were enthusiastic to attend the pre-test sessions and appreciated the novel participatory teaching methods. However, pupils initially were reluctant to participate in roleplays and generally were more comfortable in roleplays involving two people of the same sex. It became clear in the course of the pre-test that pupil knowledge of reproductive biology was very poor, even in urban Mwanza schools which were likely to have higher teaching standards than rural schools.

A total of 69 teachers and 1,922 pupils completed one-page questionnaires after different pre-test sessions (Obasi, 2001). Almost all teachers reported that they enjoyed the sessions they observed. The majority felt the content was age-appropriate and said they would be happy to teach it after training. In a small number of questionnaires, teachers reported the material was too embarrassing for pupils, the pupils were too young for it, the pupils should be separated by gender, the language was inappropriate, or the discussion of condoms made them uncomfortable. In the vast majority of pupil questionnaires, pupils reported that the content was age-appropriate and they enjoyed the sessions and the participatory methods, particularly the stories and dramas acted out by AMREF staff. Approximately two-thirds said they would be comfortable with their normal teacher teaching the subjects. Of those pupils who requested an additional topic, the most frequent request was for additional material on menstruation, puberty, and other aspects of reproductive biology.

Pilot Test of the First Teacher's Guide

The curriculum was revised based on pre-test findings, including restructuring sessions to ensure they did not run over time, re-designing flipcharts so they were clearer and easier to read from a distance, and modifying dramas to make them more realistic and to improve the clarity of their delivery. In May 1998, the revised curriculum was pilot tested to assess the acceptability, feasibility, and effectiveness of training teachers and peer educators to implement it (Obasi, 2001). Two teachers from each of six schools (including three which had been involved in the pre-test) participated in a one-week training in the use of the teacher's guide, and two pupils from each school were trained to assist teachers in class, which mainly involved performing scripted dramas. Teachers then taught a unit of four to six curriculum sessions to their classes over a four-week period. Classroom observation found the quality of teaching to be highly variable, as three teachers were ranked as excellent, three as good, four as average, and two as very poor. Problems encountered among poorer performers included insufficient use of participatory methods, inappropriate terminology, and one teacher using corporal punishment while teaching her sessions. In an effort to promote abstinence, many teachers also over-emphasized the possible negative consequences of sex and discouraged pupils from using condoms, saying that condom use was good for adults, but pupils were not allowed to use condoms because they should not yet be sexually active.

In total, 495 pupils completed questionnaires which assessed their sexual and reproductive health knowledge before and after the pilot test. After the pilot test, a higher proportion of pupils answered each of the fifteen questions correctly than had done so at baseline, and for ten of the questions this was a statistically significant improvement. Peer educators all reported that they enjoyed acting in the dramas. However, when asked which characters they would most like to perform, they only selected those who were positive role models.

In focus group discussions, teachers reported positive experiences implementing the curriculum, including coming to see initially embarrassing material as similar to other topics they taught, pupils enjoying the sessions, and pupils becoming more open and trusting of the teachers. Several teachers also recommended that all teachers within each school be trained in the curriculum, because many teachers did not know the information themselves and wished to know more, while some others were hostile because they believed it promoted adolescent sexual activity. Some teachers reported they did not understand some factual material within the curriculum well enough to teach it, such as information about the menstrual cycle or sexually transmitted infections. In addition, the teachers who had taught the condom-related sessions reported they found it challenging to promote abstinence and condom use in the same curriculum, because they found the two contradicted rather than complemented each other. A number of modifications were made to the teacher training and the curriculum based on these findings, including greater focus on teacher ambivalence to teaching condom-related information; more practice of participatory methods; and the provision of a detailed glossary of reproductive health information.

Modification of the Curriculum during the Trial

At the onset of the *MEMA kwa Vijana* trial, the Swahili language curriculum acknowledged several of the social, cultural, and economic factors influencing young people's sexual behavior, including material exchange for sex, peer pressure to have sex, and negative attitudes toward condoms. The school curriculum also met the "best practice" criteria recommended by the World Health Organization and other reviews of school-based HIV-prevention programs at the time (Kirby et al., 1994; WHO and UNESCO, 1994a; WHO and UNESCO, 1994b; WHO and UNESCO, 1994c). For example, it involved: relatively young adolescent participants; integration in the school curriculum; a cascade approach to teacher training; use of peer educators as well as teachers; multiple participatory approaches; and implementation over a prolonged period of one year or more.

As noted earlier, during the three years of the trial the curriculum was modified based on process evaluation by the AMREF intervention team, HALIRA researchers, and external evaluators (Guyon et al., 2000; Kirby, 2001; Lugoe, 2001). Each year new versions of the teacher's guides were drafted, pre-tested, and pilot tested. Pre-tests involved AMREF intervention staff teaching all sessions to pupils from two rural schools. Pilot tests involved each session being taught at least once in each of three districts by different teachers.

The topic of transactional sex provides an example of how the school curriculum was modified over the course of the trial based on ongoing research. The first version of the curriculum recognized that boys and men frequently offered girls materials in exchange for sex and pressured girls to have sex. To address this, stories, dramas, roleplays, and skills-building exercises focused on developing girls' resistance and refusal skills. This curriculum repeatedly discouraged girls from accepting gifts or money from boys and men, but stressed that if a girl did indeed accept something from a boy or man, she was not obliged to have sex.

During the trial, HALIRA research suggested that transactional sex was an even more entrenched and complex phenomenon than suggested in that first version of the curriculum. This research found that transactional sex was central to most adolescent girls' lives as a way to obtain very basic necessities, such as underwear, soap, or required shoes for school, and as a way to obtain small luxuries, such as an occasional soda, a holiday dress, or entrance to an *ngoma* event. It further found that there were deeply embedded beliefs about material exchange, reciprocity, and self-respect in rural Mwanza, as described in chapter 3. Importantly, the vast majority of villagers believed that a girl who received a gift from a boy or man was indeed obliged to have sex with him, and moreover, sexually active girls who did *not* receive something in exchange for sex were perceived to have little self-respect. Later versions of the curriculum were modified somewhat based on such findings. In the final curriculum, for example, a drama and story series addressed how girls sometimes pressured one another to have sex to obtain money or gifts, and how abstaining from sex meant a girl might experience short-term sacrifices relative to her peers (such as being poorly dressed), but how ultimately such sacrifice may be necessary to protect one's sexual health.

The first draft of the teacher's guide, which was used to teach all participants in Years 5, 6, and 7 during the first year of the intervention, consisted of eleven forty-minute sessions and two eighty-minute sessions. As noted earlier, this version of the curriculum taught basic information about reproductive health; focused on developing participants' skills in risk perception, self-efficacy, sexual refusal, and future planning; and promoted abstinence. Monogamy and condom use were only briefly mentioned, mainly during a game that illustrated how diseases spread through sexual networks. That exercise illustrated that being monogamous may not be protective against infection, because a partner may have unknown partners. It also explained that consistent condom use offered greater protection. The use of one in-depth curriculum for Years 5, 6, and 7 during the first year of the trial partly resulted from logistical constraints, particularly insufficient time to tailor grade-specific curricula in advance of the trial. However, this curriculum was also intended to maximize the material received by Year 7 pupils during the first year of the trial, because they would only receive one year of the curriculum before leaving primary school.

In the second year of the intervention (2000), the same teacher's guide described above was used for the incoming Year 5 class. However, a new teacher's guide consisting of eleven forty-minute sessions was used for pupils in Years 6 and 7. The new teacher's guide reviewed much of the earlier material on reproductive biology and HIV and other sexually transmitted infections. It also had new sessions addressing family planning and abortion, and included new exercises focused on gender equality, respecting others' decisions, and resisting peer pressure. Abstinence was again the main behavior promoted within this teacher's guide, although partner reduction, monogamy, and/or condom use were also repeatedly acknowledged as low-risk sexual behaviors.

In the third year of the intervention (2001), the two guides described above were used for Years 5 and 6, respectively, and a third, new guide was used for Year 7. This new guide consisted of ten forty-minute sessions which reviewed earlier material and further addressed reproductive biology, risk perception, decision-making, self-efficacy, sexual refusal skills, and future planning. In addition, one new session focused specifically on partner reduction, fidelity, and the risks related to serial monogamy, and the final session focused specifically on condom use.

The Final Teacher's Guides, Resource Book, and Flipchart

Based on AMREF intervention team and HALIRA process evaluation during the third year of the intervention, revisions were made to each of the three teacher's guides before finalization. The completed, post-trial curriculum consists of ten to eleven forty-minute sessions for each of Years 5, 6, and 7.

In these teacher's guides, learning objectives are outlined at the beginning of each session, and appropriate review questions are presented at the end. Some objectives of the program are distilled into simply worded, key messages which are repeated as slogans throughout the curriculum. These include: "abstinence is the only completely safe practice"; "you can't tell just by looking [who has a disease]"; "even one time [even one sexual encounter can result in pregnancy or infection]"; "even me, even today"; "giving a gift does not mean entitlement to sex"; "there are many ways to refuse"; "don't be persuaded"; "sex can have life-long consequences"; "it is not enough to be monogamous"; and "condoms protect." Appendices 1–3 show the titles, teaching methods, objectives, and key points for each session in the final Year 5–7 teacher's guides.

The final Year 5 teacher's guide primarily provides information about reproductive and sexual biology, HIV/AIDS, and other sexually transmitted infections (Obasi, Chima, Cleophas-Frisch et al., 2002a; Obasi, Chima, Cleophas-Frisch et al., 2002b). Most mention of sexual behavior focuses on abstinence and related decision-making and assertiveness skills. The final Year 6 teacher's guide reviews and increases information about reproductive biology, HIV/AIDS, and other sexually transmitted infections, and also emphasizes abstinence and related life skills (Obasi, Chima, Cleophas-Frisch et al., 2002c; Obasi, Chima, Cleophas-Frisch et al., 2002d). However, the final session focuses on condom use, including an explanation of the benefits of condom use, a verbal description of condoms and their use, and information about where condoms can be obtained in rural areas. The final Year 7 teacher's guide reviews and increases information taught about reproductive biology, but also has specific sessions on abstinence, fidelity, and condom use, as well as sessions on decision-making and planning for the future (Obasi, Chima, Cleophas-Frisch et al., 2002e; Obasi, Chima, Cleophas-Frisch et al., 2002f). The final teacher's resource book provides teachers with additional, detailed information on symptoms of sexually transmitted diseases, family planning methods (including condom use), and frequently asked questions (Obasi, Chima, Cleophas-Frisch et al., 2002g; Obasi, Chima, Cleophas-Frisch et al., 2002h).

Within each of the final teacher's guides, teaching methods vary from session to session, including structured questions and answers, story reading, letter reading, guided discussions, small group work, games simulating disease transmission within networks, personalization exercises, knowledge competitions, quizzes, explanation of flipchart illustrations, scripted dramas, and informal roleplays. Several of these methods are described briefly below.

Within the *MEMA kwa Vijana* curriculum, trained pupils perform the *scripted dramas* as a prompt for teacher-led discussion of low and high-risk behaviors and their potential consequences. Those dramas will be described in detail in the next chapter. For *roleplays*, small groups of pupils instead develop and perform their own skits to practice different life skills, such as assertiveness and communication. The 60 × 42 cm *flipcharts* provide detailed illustrations of physical changes during puberty; internal and external reproductive anatomy; a person transitioning from initial HIV infection to AIDS; and activities which do or do not transmit HIV. During the trial, teachers in rural Mwanza only had chalkboards to use as visual aids, and often they did not even have chalk, so these flipcharts provided important, factual illustrations to support them in their teaching. *Network simulation games* convey to pupils how an infection can pass from one individual to many others through a few direct and indirect links, highlighting the risks involved in multiple partnerships and the protectiveness of condom use. An example is provided in box 4.1. Intervention developers found that girls were often inhibited in participating in class-wide discussions, so group work typically involves separating pupils into groups of five to eight girls or boys to discuss specific topics before reporting back to the larger class. In *knowledge competitions*, for example, *small same-sex groups* work together to answer a set of questions in a specified time frame. Finally, in *personalization exercises* pupils close their eyes and are asked a series of questions intended to prompt reflection about the gravity of a particular problem, the possibility of being affected by it themselves, and practical strategies to avoid it.

BOX 4.1. *MEMA KWA VIJANA*
NETWORK SIMULATION GAME[a]

The "Handshake Game" is an interactive exercise used to illustrate how a disease can spread from one individual to many within a sexual network, and how condom use can reduce that spread. The following instructions direct the teacher in how to lead the game. Within the Year 6 curriculum (Appendix 2), this game is followed by a teacher-led discussion and exercises which illustrate the local prevalences of sexually transmitted infections amongst youth and adults.

(continued)

THE HANDSHAKE GAME, PART ONE:
DISEASE TRANSMISSION WITHIN NETWORKS

1. Invite five girls and five boys to come forward to play a game.
2. Ask them to walk around for a few seconds and then tell them to stop.
3. Tell each boy and girl to shake hands with one other person in the group. Tell them to remember that this was the first person with whom they shook hands.
4. Ask them to walk around the room again, and then to stop and shake hands with someone different than the person they shook hands with the first time. Again they should remember this was the second person with whom they shook hands.
5. Ask them to walk around the room one more time and to stop and shake hands with someone different than the two they shook hands with previously.
6. Now ask the ten participants to stand in a line and face the class.
7. Choose one participant. This should be someone who is self-confident and popular with the other pupils. Ask this person to stand in a separate place in front of the class. Tell the class that this person will be called "X" in this game.
8. Explain that we will pretend that two things are true:
   a. That shaking hands with somebody in this game represents having sex in real life.
   b. That person X has a sexually transmitted infection that, in this game, can be transmitted through shaking hands.
9. Ask person X to name the three people with whom they shook hands. Ask those three to stand next to person X. In the same way, ask those three pupils to call forward everyone they shook hands with, to stand next to person X.
10. Ask the whole class the following questions:
    a. *What may have happened to the people who were called forward?*
       —Since they shook hands with person X or somebody who had done so, they could be infected with the infection that person X has, because, in this game, we are pretending that it can be passed from one person to another by shaking hands.
    b. *What was the goal of this game? (Encourage as many pupils to try answering this question before sharing the following explanation.)*

(continued)

—Since shaking hands in the game represented having sex in real life, the game showed how quickly sexually transmitted infections can spread from one person to many people.

—Person X was infected at the beginning of the game; therefore Person X may have infected the three people he/she had contact with. If those three people later shook hands with others, they may have infected those others.

c. *How are sexually transmitted infections spread?*

—By having sex without using a condom.

—People do not have to have penetrative sexual intercourse to become infected. The germs that cause sexually transmitted infections can be found in all sexual fluids (such as semen and vaginal fluid). So if any sexual fluids from an infected person come into contact with the genitals of another person, then he/she may become infected as well.

—A mother who is infected with a sexually transmitted infection may pass her infection to her child in the womb, or infect the infant's eyes while giving birth, causing blindness.

Key Points:

a. EMPHASIZE that shaking hands CANNOT pass a sexually transmitted infection from one person to another. Sexually transmitted infections are spread by having sex without using a condom.

b. Also emphasize that the pupils who participated in the game were pretending and DO NOT have a sexually transmitted infection as a result of being in the game. However, young people like them can get sexually transmitted infections if they have sex without using a condom.

THE HANDSHAKE GAME, PART TWO:
CONDOM USE WITHIN NETWORKS

1. Invite five boys and five girls to come forward as in the previous part of the game, only this time give five of them something to wear on their right hand, like a glove, sock, plastic bag, or envelope.

(continued)

2. Ask each participant to move around the room and shake hands with three different people. Each time they should shake hands with a new person as before. Ask them to remember each person with whom they shake hands.
3. Then ask all the participants to stand in a line facing the class.
4. Choose one of the participants who did not wear anything on their hand and name that person "Y." This should not be the same person as person X but should also be someone who is self-confident and popular with the other pupils. Ask this person to stand in a separate place in front of the class. Tell the class that this person will be called person Y in this game.
5. Explain that we will pretend that three things are true:
   a. That in this game person Y has an infection that can be transmitted through shaking hands.
   b. That shaking hands with somebody in this game represents having sex in real life.
   c. That in this game a glove/bag/envelope/sock (refer to what you used to cover the hand) represents a condom.
6. Ask person Y to name the three people with whom they shook hands. Ask them to stand next to person Y. If any of these three people are wearing something on their hand, tell them that they should rejoin the main group.
7. In the same way, ask the pupils who are still standing next to person Y to call forward everyone they shook hands with, to stand next to person Y. Again, if any of these new people are wearing something on their hand, ask them to rejoin the main group.
8. Explain that the people who wore something on their hand could neither get nor pass on the infection.
9. Compare the number of people who were infected in the first part of the game with the number who were infected in the second part of the game (the second number should be smaller).
10. Ask the whole class the following questions:
    a. *What may have happened to the people who shook hands with person Y?*
       —Since they shook hands with person Y or somebody who had done so, they could be infected with the person Y's infection, because it can be passed from one person to another by shaking hands.

(continued)

b. *What was the reason for separating those who had "gloves"?*
—Even though they came into contact with somebody who was infected, they did not get infected because they used gloves (or whatever they were using to cover their hands), which represent condoms and protect people from the infection.

c. *What was the goal of this game? (Encourage as many pupils to try answering this question before explaining the following.)*
—Shaking hands in the game represented having sex and wearing a "glove" represented using a condom in real life, so the game showed how people can protect themselves from getting sexually transmitted infections by using a condom. In doing so they reduce the spread of the sexually transmitted infection.

—Person Y was infected at the beginning of the game therefore he/she could have infected any of the people with whom he/she shook hands. However, those wearing gloves were not infected because they were protected. They also did not infect anyone else they had contact with. Because of this the infection spread to fewer people overall.

—Some of those who did not wear a "glove" (did not use a condom) may not yet have been infected, if they were lucky enough not to have shaken hands with someone who was already infected. However, they are in danger of being infected in the future if they continue having sex without protecting themselves.

d. *If we repeated this section of the play, what would you do as a participant?*
Either:
—I would not shake hands with anyone.
Or:
—I would not shake hands with anyone who is not wearing a "glove."
And:
—I would not shake hands with anyone unless I was wearing a "glove."

(*continued*)

Key Points:

a. EMPHASIZE that shaking hands CANNOT pass a sexually transmitted infection from one person to another. Sexually transmitted
   infections are spread by having sex without using a condom.
b. Also emphasize that the pupils who participated in the game DO
   NOT have a sexually transmitted infection as a result of being in
   the game.
c. All pupils should be aware that they can get sexually transmitted
   infections if they have sex without using a condom. Condoms protect against sexually transmitted infections and HIV infection, and
   pregnancies.
d. Nevertheless, not having sex at all is the only way to protect yourself completely.

[a]Excerpted from the teacher's guide for Year 6, Session 3: "How sexually transmitted infections are spread" (Obasi, Chima, Cleophas-Frisch et al.,
2002c, 15–19). Used with the authors' permission.

The next section summarizes how abstinence, partner reduction, fidelity,
and condom use are addressed in each of the final teacher's guides.

Abstinence

As noted earlier, the Tanzanian Ministry of Education and Culture instructed
MEMA kwa Vijana intervention developers that abstinence promotion must
be the main focus of the intervention within primary schools. Thus abstinence
(*kutokufanya mapenzi kabisa*, literally "to not make love at all") is strongly
promoted in all three years of the final curriculum, as can be seen in the
teacher's guide outlines in Appendices 1–3. This includes primary abstinence
(*kusubiri kufanya mapenzi hadi hapo utakapokua zaidi*, literally "to wait to
make love when one is older/physically mature") and secondary abstinence
(*kuacha kufanya mapenzi kabisa*, literally "to completely stop making love,"
for those who have already had sex).

To promote abstinence, the curriculum emphasizes the possible negative
consequences of unprotected sexual activity, encourages pupils to identify
and focus on their future goals, and fosters boys' and girls' skills to resist
peer pressure, and girls' skills to refuse unwanted sexual advances. However,
the curriculum only superficially addresses boys' overriding motivation to
have sex, i.e., sexual pleasure, and it does not acknowledge masturbation as a
safe way to satisfy sexual desire. Similarly, the curriculum only superficially
engages with girls about their main motivation to have sex, that is, material

exchange. The curriculum acknowledges that transactional sex is common and that girls who abstain might have less than their peers, but it does not address the centrality of transactional sex in girls' lives or offer them alternative ways to obtain basic necessities, such as underwear and soap.

Being Faithful

Reducing partner number (*kupunguza idadi ya wapenzi*, literally "reducing number of lovers"), monogamy (*kuwa na mpenzi mmoja,* literally "to have one lover"), and/or fidelity *(kuwa mwaminifu,* literally "being faithful/ trustworthy") were promoted as relatively low-risk sexual behaviors from the onset of the intervention. However, they received less focus than either abstinence or condom use, particularly in early versions of the curriculum. In the first years of the trial, messages about fidelity were particularly simple. However, preliminary HALIRA research suggested that many youths considered themselves to be monogamous and low risk even if they had a series of brief, monogamous sexual relationships involving rapid partner change, while others maintained secret, concurrent sexual relationships. Later versions of the curriculum thus included dramas and/or stories which illustrated the risks specific to concurrency, serial monogamy, and fast partner change.

In the final Year 5 teacher's guide (Appendix 1), risk related to sexual partner number is addressed through an exercise that illustrates how one person could transmit an infection to several people (directly or indirectly), even if each person only had two partners. Teachers also are instructed to explain that monogamy does not guarantee protection, as a partner can bring an infection into a relationship from a prior relationship.

In the final Year 6 teacher's guide (Appendix 2), the importance of monogamy and/or having few partners is addressed through another disease transmission simulation exercise, a drama, and a story. The exercise (box 4.1) is a slightly more complex game than the one in Year 5 that illustrates the nature of disease transmission within networks. The story is about two married couples, one of which is mutually monogamous and healthy, and the other which is not because the man has other partners, becomes infected with HIV, and ultimately infects his wife. Finally, the drama focuses on a young woman who becomes HIV-positive after having one or two new partners in succession each year for several years. Teacher-led discussions draw upon each of these activities to illustrate the potentially protective importance of monogamy and partner reduction.

In the final Year 7 teacher's guide (Appendix 3), one session specifically focuses on fidelity. It tells a story of a young woman who was faithful to her fiancé even when she is tempted by another man, as well as a story of a young man who has a series of monogamous sexual relationships and contracts a sexually transmitted infection. The teacher draws on these stories to illustrate the importance of monogamy being mutual and long term to reduce sexual health risk. However, that session also emphasizes that it is difficult to be certain of a partner's HIV status and fidelity, so even when practicing monogamy it is safest to use condoms.

Years 6 and 7 of the final curriculum also address partner selectivity to an extent, and particularly the relatively high risk involved if girls have older (rather than same-aged) sexual partners, as adult men are more likely to have contracted an infection from earlier relationships. However, in the final curriculum there is little discussion specifically about the risks involved in concurrent sexual relationships, and particularly those which overlap long-term. There also is little focus on strategies to negotiate and practice long-term, mutual monogamy either before or after marriage. For example, there are no skills-building exercises on how to discuss risk and negotiate mutual fidelity with a sexual partner.

Condom Use

As discussed earlier, at the time of the *MEMA kwa Vijana* trial, national curricula and guidelines stipulated that condoms should be promoted as an HIV prevention method in Tanzanian primary schools, but they were not to be visually depicted, demonstrated, or distributed there. Initially the Mwanza Region Education Officer—the highest regional authority within the government school system—interpreted these guidelines to mean that proper condom use should not be explained verbally in the classroom setting. During the trial, however, the AMREF intervention team continued to advocate for more detailed condom information being included in the school curriculum. The Mwanza Region Education Officer closely reviewed each of the curriculum drafts developed during the trial and for the final version agreed that the last session of Year 7 could include an optional, in-depth verbal discussion of condom use (*kutumia kondom*). This was considered acceptable because soon after that session most pupils would be leaving primary school and beginning their adult lives.

The final teacher's guides thus provide more information on condom use than had been allowed in earlier trial versions, but the content is still very limited and does not include any illustrations of condoms. Throughout the Year 5, 6, and 7 teacher's guides, teachers are repeatedly instructed to tell pupils that condoms prevent pregnancy and the transmission of infections, and that condoms must be used correctly every time to be effective. However, in the Year 5 sessions the description of condoms is limited to: "A condom is made of rubber. It is worn on the genitals and prevents two people's sexual fluids from mixing during sex. In this way it prevents HIV transmission" (e.g., Obasi, Chima, Cleophas-Frisch et al., 2002a, 13).

Each of the final Year 6 and 7 teacher's guides has a session specifically focused on condom use. In the session in Year 6 (Appendix 2), teachers are instructed to tell pupils the *Salama* condom brand name (which literally means "safety"), and to explain that detailed instructions and illustrations of how to use a condom can be found inside of *Salama* condom packets. For that session, teachers are also instructed to review detailed information on correct condom use in their resource books and to "make sure [pupils] know how to use condoms correctly" (Obasi, Chima, Cleophas-Frisch, et al., 2002c, 56). The extent of detail provided in such sessions is left up to the teacher's discretion.

For the final session in Year 7 (Appendix 3), teachers are instructed to choose between two sessions: the recommended session (box 4.2), in which the steps of correct condom use are discussed in detail, and the more superficial session, which essentially repeats the same general points made in the Year 6 session on condom use. In the recommended session, small groups of same-sex pupils are given a scrambled list of steps involved in condom use and are instructed to order them correctly, after which the teacher reviews the correct steps with the entire class. There are no other skills-building activities specific to condom use in the curriculum, for example, exercises which develop pupils' skills to communicate about and negotiate condom use with a partner.

BOX 4.2. *MEMA KWA VIJANA* CORRECT CONDOM USE GAME[a]

The "Correct Condom Use Game" is an optional exercise that follows a brief skit and teacher-led discussion about the value of condoms in the final session of the Year 7 curriculum (Appendix 3). Earlier in the curriculum, condom use is repeatedly acknowledged as an effective way for sexually active youth to prevent disease and pregnancy. Pupils who participated in class visits to health facilities also may have seen condoms and condom demonstrations on those occasions. However, this session represents the first time that condoms are described and discussed in detail in the classroom setting. Educational authorities did not allow condoms to be shown or visually depicted in schools, so this game was limited to verbal and written information. The following instructions direct the teacher in how to lead the game.

(continued)

1. Divide the groups in to same-sex groups of up to eight pupils. Tell them that you will now talk about the proper use of condoms.
2. Remind the pupils that male condoms are made of rubber, and that a condom rolls on to a penis. Tell them condoms fit a penis like a sock fits a foot.
3. Put up the flipchart sheet titled "Using Condoms—INCORRECT ORDER OF STEPS."
4. Tell them that these sentences explain the proper steps for using male condoms, but they are not in the correct order.
5. Give each group a blank sheet of paper.
6. Tell the groups that they have fifteen minutes to finish this assignment.
7. Tell them to put the following sentences in the correct order for condom use, starting from the first step until the last step. Each group should write the correct list on a piece of paper.

"USING CONDOMS—INCORRECT ORDER OF STEPS":

A. *Soon after the man ejaculates, he should withdraw his penis from the vagina while holding on to the condom at the base of his penis, to prevent sperm from falling out.*
B. *Open the packet holding the condom carefully. Do not use your teeth or nails when opening it.*
C. *Remove the condom, wrap it in paper if possible, and throw it down a pit latrine.*
D. *Use a new condom and make sure it has not expired.*
E. *The man should remove his penis from the vagina before his penis becomes soft.*
F. *While continuing to pinch the nipple of the condom, place it on the tip of the penis, and unroll it all the way to the base of the penis.*
G. *Distinguish between the inside and outside parts of the condom.*
H. *Discuss the use of condoms with your lover.*
I. *Pinch the nipple of the condom (the top part) to take out any air and to prevent any new air from entering it.*
J. *Start having sexual intercourse.*

8. Make sure that every pupil in every group participates.

(continued)

9. After fifteen minutes, ask each group to share their answers and write them down on the blackboard. In order to save time, write the responses by using the letters of the sentences. The correct order for this flipchart should have been:

H-D-B-G-I-F-J-A-E-C

10. Put up the next flipchart, "Using Condoms—CORRECT ORDER OF STEPS", and go through them one-by-one with the pupils.

"USING CONDOMS—CORRECT ORDER OF STEPS":

1. *Discuss the use of condoms with your lover.*
2. *Use a new condom and make sure it has not expired.*
3. *Open the packet holding the condom carefully. Do not use your teeth or nails when opening it.*
4. *Distinguish between the inside and outside parts of the condom.*
5. *Pinch the nipple of the condom (the top part) to take out any air and to prevent any new air from entering it.*
6. *While continuing to pinch the nipple of the condom, place it on the tip of the penis, and unroll it all the way to the base of the penis.*
7. *Start having sexual intercourse.*
8. *Soon after the man ejaculates, he should withdraw his penis from the vagina while holding on to the condom at the base of his penis, to prevent sperm from falling out.*
9. *The man should remove his penis from the vagina before it becomes soft.*
10. *Remove the condom, wrap it in paper if possible, and throw it down a pit latrine.*

11. Now ask each pupil to write all the sentences in the right order in their exercise books.

[a]Excerpted from the teacher's guide for Year 7, Session 9a: "Protecting yourself: Correct use of condoms" (Obasi, Chima, Cleophas-Frisch et al., 2002e, 52–54). Used with the authors' permission.

This concludes the detailed description of *MEMA kwa Vijana* school curriculum content, which was the core component of the broader intervention. The next section will describe and evaluate activities undertaken to raise awareness and support for the school program and the broader intervention in rural communities. Chapter 5 will then return to the school program to evaluate implementation of the curriculum during the trial.

RAISING COMMUNITY AWARENESS AND SUPPORT

Community Mobilization

As noted earlier, *MEMA kwa Vijana* intervention staff met with educational and other government authorities at regional, district, division, ward, and village levels to involve them in intervention development, to ensure they were fully informed about its final design, and to enlist their support and participation during community mobilization. Community mobilization was a relatively small component of the intervention program, because most resources were invested in developing and implementing the school program. However, community mobilization was the first step of intervention implementation in rural areas, so it will be described here first.

Community mobilization initially consisted of a one-week visit to each of the ten intervention communities for introductory meetings with local leaders, teachers, and parents. The objectives of these visits were to raise awareness of adolescent sexual and reproductive health problems, discuss community concerns and intervention ideas, introduce the *MEMA kwa Vijana* intervention, and form a local advisory committee to oversee the intervention at the ward level. During each one-week visit, AMREF intervention staff met with authorities and representatives at the division level on the first day, at the ward level on the second and third day, at the village level on the fourth day, and at the ward level again on the fifth day to train fifteen to twenty-two advisory committee members. In each one-week visit, an estimated four thousand participants from six to eight villages participated in mobilization meetings.

Key points which intervention staff made during community mobilization meetings were that many adolescents were sexually active and many had sexually transmitted infections, which suggested sexual health education was necessary in early to mid-adolescence. Concerns villagers commonly voiced included beliefs that sex education (and particularly condom promotion) encourages adolescent sexual activity, that condom use is harmful or dangerous, and that some teachers are questionable intervention implementers because they themselves may have sex with female pupils. Intervention staff addressed these concerns as they were voiced.

By the end of each week of community mobilization, many adult villagers who participated in the meetings expressed support for the intervention. One Village Executive Officer explained that parents had accepted the *MEMA kwa Vijana* school program for their children because they were concerned about AIDS:

> *R*: When the intervention was introduced there was no problem. No one tried to argue against it. . . . They don't think of *MEMA kwa Vijana* as a bad thing, because AIDS has spread everywhere and they see AIDS as something that . . . somehow brings evil to the children. Therefore they accept [*MEMA kwa Vijana*] as a way to protect their children. (II-99-I-7-m)

During community mobilization, villagers across the study area requested a similar education program for adults. In multiple meetings, for example, participants played on the name "*MEMA kwa Vijana*" (Good Things for Youth) and said there was an equal need for a "*MEMA kwa Wazee*" (Good Things for Elders) program, meaning a program for adults.

The community mobilization component of the intervention seemed to be broadly effective in informing local leaders and some pupils' parents about the intervention and the trial. After these visits, very few parents or leaders ever refused to allow their children to participate in either the intervention or the trial.

Ongoing Activities for the Broader Community

In the first year of the intervention, preliminary findings of HALIRA and the AMREF intervention team suggested that adult villagers' understanding of HIV, AIDS, and general sexual health was so poor that they might undermine the intervention's effectiveness with school pupils. For example, parents who did not understand their children's risk of HIV and other sexually transmitted infections might discourage them from using condoms if they were sexually active; this was also a concern for school girls' older, out-of-school sexual partners. There were very little resources available for additional intervention work with adult community members. A basic, low-cost option was thus developed involving quarterly public HIV-related video shows and discussions at the village level, which AMREF staff conducted when visiting communities for supervision of the condom distribution initiative. These were conducted throughout the second and third year of the intervention.

Given few villages had an electric supply, the equipment (e.g., generator, television, large screen, VHS cassettes) that was necessary for these video shows was brought to villages by vehicle. Preexisting Swahili language HIV prevention programs were shown in the evening in an open, central area, such as a market place, a bus stand, or a sports field, and were followed by a facilitated discussion afterward. These programs were fairly superficial but they reached a large number of people, as each show was usually attended by several hundred villagers. These video shows were received very favorably and those who attended them often said they provided important information which villagers would not otherwise receive. The following two examples were provided by former intervention participants from different districts; the first by a farmer in an inland village, the second by bicycle repairmen in a fishing village:

> *R*: Even in the village there are some people who use condoms, even those who are uneducated, because of the training they received. . . .
>
> *I*: Where have they received that training, if they haven't been to school?
>
> *R*: The year before last there was a *Mema kwa Vijana* meeting there at the market. They taught how to use condoms, so even an uneducated person was able to learn how to use them. (II-02-I-298-m)

> [Some young bicycle repairers] said *MEMA kwa Vijana* came to promote condoms on two different market days. They said they taught people how to use condoms and also gave away a small quantity of condoms. The youths said this was helpful, because people otherwise feel shy to ask for instructions about how to use condoms. (PO-01-I-7-5f)

In all aspects of the intervention and research, the occasional receipt of free materials or services (such as video shows, T-shirts, sports balls, and medication) was extremely well received by implementers, young people, and adult community members. Often these relatively small items seemed to play a major role in people's motivation and participation. Intervention teachers and peer educators were given *MEMA kwa Vijana* T-shirts, and these were also provided to intervention participants who won special events. The visibility of the *MEMA kwa Vijana* name and logo on T-shirts and vehicles seemed to make some people in the broader community at least superficially familiar with the *MEMA kwa Vijana* name.

However, some intervention topics remained controversial within communities throughout the trial, such as adolescent premarital sexual activity or condom use, and occasionally opposition to the program became public. For example:

> [A twenty-year-old teacher's wife] said one day a priest came to this village for a worship service and noted one of the young men wore a *Mema kwa Vijana* T-shirt. . . . She said that during the service the priest told people that *Mema kwa*

Vijana was a bad project because it taught children about sex before they had discovered it themselves. (PO-01-I-1-2f)

When the AMREF intervention team became aware of such public opposition to the program, they spoke with those involved and arranged public meetings to address concerns. The most extreme example involved a religious group that severely disrupted implementation of the program in one community by condemning the discussion of sexual matters in class and ceremonially burning a *MEMA kwa Vijana* T-shirt. However, after discussion with AMREF intervention staff, a senior member of the group agreed to participate in some of the *MEMA kwa Vijana* activities and became an active supporter of the intervention (Wight and Obasi, 2003).

The AMREF intervention team seemed effective in responding to such public controversies with respect and clarity, conveying the urgent need for an intervention, and ultimately winning the support of those most vocally opposed to it. However, many adult villagers were ambivalent or had negative attitudes toward the program but did not voice this publicly, and their concerns remained largely unaddressed. This will be discussed more below.

Adult Awareness and Attitudes toward the Intervention

Despite *MEMA kwa Vijana*'s initial and ongoing intervention activities in the broader community, overall in-depth interviews and participant observation found that many pupils' parents and other adult villagers did not know about the *MEMA kwa Vijana* program. For example, when a nineteen-year-old secondary school girl and former intervention participant was asked about villagers' opinions of the intervention, she replied, "In fact, I don't know if the villagers even knew that there was such a class as *Mema kwa Vijana*. Only very few used to know about it, but . . . I never heard what they said about it." (II-02-I-287-f)

Of the adults who knew about the intervention and its subject matter, a minority were consistently positive about it—particularly government representatives, health workers, teachers, and parents who were in the local *MEMA kwa Vijana* advisory committees. Similarly, a few in-depth interview respondents reported villagers universally approved of the intervention. For example, a twenty-one-year-old married, former intervention participant:

> R: I have never heard anything bad about *MEMA kwa Vijana*. . . . These are things they speak well about. They say *MEMA kwa Vijana* is—is a very good subject and they should continue teaching it, so that we people are educated. Because some of us don't know what causes many diseases. (II-02-I-288-f)

Occasionally parents seemed to be fairly well informed and positive about the intervention, and said they had discussed intervention content with their children. For example, a fifty-year-old Sukuma woman with eleven children:

R: The *MEMA kwa Vijana* people came here to the school and explained what the pupils are supposed to do, and the children came to tell us. . . . They brought home some papers/pamphlets. . . . Actually, we parents didn't go to the school. I haven't met any adult who went there to ask what they teach about. . . . [Later] I asked my daughter, "What is it that you are being taught in *MEMA kwa Vijana* lessons?" She said, "We are taught about unintended pregnancies while still in school, and to protect ourselves against AIDS."

I: Do you think the *MEMA kwa Vijana* lessons are good and important, or should they be discontinued?

R: I . . . actually, since I don't know about it in detail, I can't say for certain. But I also talked to the teacher about it once, and he/she explained . . . pupils are told the consequences [of sexual activity] and they see them in the dramas. For example, I think a school child became pregnant [in one drama storyline] and her father gave her this and that consequence. . . .

I: What if a pupil has already started having sex. Would it be acceptable to teach him/her to use a condom?

R: Actually, in my opinion I would just forbid him/her to have sex, because he/she is still a pupil, so he/she can't be involved in sexual activity while still schooling. (II-99-I-13-f)

In each of the study villages, numerous adults expressed concern that the *MEMA kwa Vijana* program might teach or encourage seduction and promiscuity. The following examples are from three different districts:

The wife of the political party secretary was complaining that her daughter, who completed primary school last year, is running around with men without even caring about AIDS or sexually transmitted diseases. . . . She said, "Even those who bring condoms don't do anything other than accelerate the frequency of sexual intercourse. In fact, nowadays there is a lesson at the school that teaches children to have sex." . . . She suggested that if I have time I should ask for a pupil's *MEMA kwa Vijana* exercise book to see for myself. (PO-01-I-7-5f)

[A man in his forties] said "*MEMA kwa Vijana* is just ruining the children." He said one day he looked at his son's exercise book and discovered that they were being taught matters concerning old people which even the other adults in the village were not aware of. He said that teaching those things to children makes young people know about those things and do them to test what they have learned. He went on to say that the youths perform dramas which teach them how to seduce. He believes that young people have more sex now than they did before they participated in the program. (PO-02-I-1-3m)

[A twelve-year-old in Year 5] explained to some family members that they are taught about AIDS, other sexually transmitted infections, and unintended pregnancies in *MEMA kwa Vijana* classes. She said that when they first were taught about it they really laughed a lot, but nowadays they have become used to it. . . . [Her father's thirty-year-old junior wife] was surprised and said, "Eh! Do you mean these *MEMA kwa Vijana* people teach such serious matters to Year 5 pupils, and even give them condoms and contraceptive pills? They are ruining the children! That is not the way to teach." [The twelve-year-old] said, "No, they are not ruining the children, they are helping whoever follows the instructions to abstain from sex, or to use condoms or contraceptive pills if they have sex." (PO-01-I-4-5f)

In in-depth interviews and participant observation, many intervention participants mentioned that their parents first learned about the content of the *MEMA kwa Vijana* curriculum after seeing their exercise books, and that their parents usually reacted negatively. As one young man explained, "If you take it home with you then your parent tells you, 'Let me have look at your exercise books.' You can't give him/her that exercise book and neither can you just sit there and not do so. I mean, words like 'penis' are mentioned in the exercise book, and they may make many parents believe that the organization is not teaching well." (GD-02-I-1-36m)

In isolated cases, villagers expressed their distrust of the program by modifying the name *MEMA kwa Vijana* (Good Things for Youth) and referring to it instead as "*Mabaya kwa Vijana*" (Evil Things for Youth) or "*MEMA kwa Wahuni*" (Good Things for the Misbehaved). However, as noted earlier, the adults who were reported to have the most negative beliefs about the intervention rarely seemed sufficiently concerned or assertive to voice public opposition to it, so intervention staff rarely responded to them directly.

During participant observation, many villagers suggested that the *MEMA kwa Vijana* program would have been more widely accepted and effective if more intervention work had been done with adults in the broader community. The following two examples were provided by a health inspector and a health worker in different villages:

He said that most villagers have received this program positively, although a few still reject it. He said that the few who reject it do so because they don't understand the *MEMA kwa Vijana* teachings and believe they encourage *uhuni* (socially disapproved of behavior, such as promiscuity). He said that there should be further mobilization and education of the parents, for example, that parents should be gathered for public meetings in each sub-village and the intervention dramas should be explained to them. He said that when the program started the content of the teacher's guides was not clearly explained, and furthermore intervention representatives only met with ward officials for one day instead of many days, which would have helped people understand their activities better. (PO-01-I-1-2f)

He said he was surprised that they only call doctors, nurses, education officers, and teachers for training courses. . . . He said, "Instead of giving that money to people at seminars, they should slaughter some cows and cook some rice, so people would gather there to eat and be given education at the same time. Such education should be given to people of all ages, not just children or young people." He said the projects are making a mistake as the message doesn't reach those concerned. (PO-02-I-4-5f)

DISCUSSION

At the beginning of the *MEMA kwa Vijana* trial, intervention developers knew that an adolescent sexual health program was more likely to be effective if it were integrated within a broader, intensive community-wide intervention. Given financial and logistical constraints, however, intervention developers prioritized the school component of the intervention and engaged in relatively superficial community mobilization. The community intervention component achieved its basic objectives of raising awareness of adolescent sexual health problems, introducing the *MEMA kwa Vijana* intervention at public meetings, forming local advisory committees, and addressing public opposition to the program when it arose. However, during the trial many pupils' parents, siblings, and out-of-school friends and sexual partners only had marginal exposure to the intervention and were poorly informed about it. Many did not understand the value of the promoted behaviors and thus did not support pupils adopting them. Given adolescents had a very low social status in rural Mwanza, it may have been too difficult for them to challenge powerful social norms and expectations by adopting low-risk sexual behaviors, particularly girls with older, out-of-school partners who typically determined the conditions of sexual encounters.

These findings suggest that adolescent sexual health programs may have little or no impact if they are implemented "in a vacuum," that is, if similarly intensive HIV prevention is not also conducted with adults in the broader community. Such community-wide intervention work may be especially important in African cultures where decisions and behaviors are often collective and individualism is discouraged (Airhihenbuwa and Obregon, 2000). In the face of severe resource constraints, community-level intervention may at first seem like a luxury, but if an adolescent sexual health program is to succeed, it may be a necessity. Chapter 11 will return to this issue by reviewing promising community-based interventions for youth and adults which have been developed and tested elsewhere in sub-Saharan Africa.

The next chapter will provide an in-depth process evaluation of the school component of the *MEMA kwa Vijana* intervention, while chapter 6 will detail process evaluations of the health service and condom distribution components. The findings from these three chapters will then be brought together in chapter 7 to consider the intervention's strengths and weaknesses in promoting abstinence, partner reduction, fidelity, and condom use with young people.

Chapter Five

The *MEMA kwa Vijana*
School Program[1]

Schools and teaching staff provide an extraordinary opportunity to intervene with large numbers of young people at a fairly low cost, so many African countries have integrated HIV prevention education into their standard teaching curricula. School-based programs vary widely in terms of their objectives, structure, length, content, and implementation strategies (Gallant and Maticka-Tyndale, 2004; Paul-Ebhohimhen, Poobalan, and van Teijlingen, 2008; UNESCO, 2008; Harrison et al., 2010; Michielsen et al., 2010). They range, for example, from being very didactic to highly participatory in their approach. Generally, however, they can be categorized by whether they are led by adults or youth peers, and whether they are based on a curriculum or not. Curriculum-based programs often have an explicit theoretical basis and tend to be more extensively pilot-tested and sanctioned by authorities than other programs, as well as being more structured and intensive (Kirby, Obasi, and Laris, 2006).

Overall, reviews of school sexual health programs in sub-Saharan Africa have found that adult-led, curriculum-based programs improve participants' knowledge and reduce their reported risk behaviors (Gallant and Maticka-Tyndale, 2004; Kirby, Obasi, and Laris, 2006; Mavedzenge, Doyle, and Ross, 2011). However, reviews have found less evidence that peer-led and non-curriculum based programs have a desired impact, suggesting that they need more evaluation and evidence of positive effect before wider implementation (Kirby, Obasi, and Laris, 2006; Harrison et al., 2010; Mavedzenge, Doyle, and Ross, 2011).

As discussed in the last chapter, research generally suggests that good school-based HIV prevention curricula address facts and information, relationship and interpersonal skills, values, peer norms, attitudes, and intentions (UNESCO, 2008). Importantly, however, the quality of school programs can be negatively affected by implementation issues, such as poor teacher training, teachers being unconvinced of the program's importance and practicality, and/or insufficient time for program delivery (e.g., Dane and Schneider, 1998; Kinsman et al., 2001; Visser, Schoeman, and Perold, 2004; Harrison et al., 2010). Interventions also may be detrimentally affected by preexisting, problematic teacher-pupil relationships, unless these are adequately resolved during training and monitored during program implementation. For example, sexual abuse of school girls by male teachers has been found to be a problem in many countries in sub-Saharan Africa, and this is a particularly great concern within adolescent sexual health interventions (e.g., WHO, 1997; Mlemya, Justine, and Mgalla, 1997; Kinsman et al., 1999; Jewkes et al., 2002; O-saki and Agu, 2002; Panos Institute, 2003; Andersson and Ho-Foster, 2008).

Relatively few adolescent sexual health interventions involving peer education have been evaluated in sub-Saharan Africa (UNAIDS, 1999b; Brieger et al., 2001; Speizer, Tambashe, and Tegang, 2001; Macdowall and Mitchell, 2006; Bastien, Flisher et al., 2008; Kim and Free, 2008; Maticka-Tyndale and Barnett, 2010; Mason-Jones, Mathews, and Flisher, 2011). In addition, those which have been evaluated have often been small and intensive participatory programs which would be difficult to implement on a large scale, because they require in-depth, specialized training and supervision (e.g., Agha, 2002a; Campbell, 2003; Agha and Van Rossem, 2004; Onyango-Ouma, Aagaard-Hansen, and Jensen, 2005; Kafewo, 2008).

In a rare evaluation of a school-based peer education program in rural East Africa, Kenyan teachers trained Year 5 pupils in in-depth information about malaria and hygiene, with the goal that those pupils would each teach the same information to at least one Year 3 child and one adult in their home (Onyango-Ouma, Aagaard-Hansen, and Jensen, 2005). When the peer educators, adults, and Year 3 pupils were surveyed four and fourteen months after the training, each group demonstrated significantly improved and sustained knowledge. However, observations over the fourteen-month period found that pupils had difficulty implementing many of the recommended behaviors because of external constraints. For example, each pupil started the week with one clean school uniform, but these became unclean as the week progressed due to play and required manual work at school, and they were unable to clean them as recommended because they did not have enough soap at home.

Within peer education, a "peer" can be defined in diverse ways, including by age, sex, ethnicity, or shared interests. Peer education may address a diverse range of topics, and the educational activities may take a variety of forms depending on the goals, the context, and the target group, including counseling, lecturing, discussion facilitation, distribution of materials, and drama, music, or sport presentations (Harden, Oakley, and Oliver, 2001; Bastien, Flisher et al., 2008). Proponents of peer education believe that it has several advantages as a complement or an alternative to other intervention methods. They argue that peer education can: utilize already established means of sharing information; reinforce learning through ongoing contact; empower both the peer educators and the peers; engage hard-to-reach individuals; and provide trusted sources of information and role models for the targeted behavior (e.g., Turner and Shepard, 1999; Macdowall and Mitchell, 2006). To achieve this, peer educators need to be adequately trained and have a sound grasp of the concepts being taught, as well as the pedagogic tools to deliver them (Bastien, Flisher et al., 2008). The credibility of the peer educator and the message is also important, including the peer educator's personal characteristics (e.g., similar age, sex, or ethnicity to peers); his or her experience (e.g., training and/or personal background); and the credibility of the content and delivery of the message (Bastien, Flisher et al., 2008).

The previous chapter described the *MEMA kwa Vijana* school curriculum development and design, including pre-test, pilot test, modification during the trial, and final content. This chapter will now evaluate the school program as implemented during the trial. First, it will consider the teacher component of the school program, including teacher training, curriculum coverage, teaching practice, pupil understanding of curriculum content, and intervention teachers as role models. Then it will examine the peer education component of the school program, including peer educator training, peer education in the classroom and out of school, and peer educators as role models.

TEACHERS' ACTIVITIES

Teacher Training

In 1998, prior to the first year of formal intervention implementation, one-week *MEMA kwa Vijana* training courses were held for head teachers and two other teachers from each intervention school. Shorter refresher training courses were subsequently conducted annually for experienced *MEMA kwa Vijana* teachers as well as new ones who were replacing those who had transferred, retired, or moved. Teachers volunteered and/or were selected by head teachers to become *MEMA kwa Vijana* teachers. Concern about the potential for male teacher sexual abuse of female pupils led to preferential recruitment and training of female teachers. However, this was only partially successful because female teachers were in the minority in rural Mwanza, particularly in the most remote villages, and some primary schools had no female teachers.

Thus in the first year of the intervention only 35 percent of the *MEMA kwa Vijana* teachers were female.

All *MEMA kwa Vijana* teachers were trained to use the Swahili teacher's guides (Appendices 1–3), the teacher's resource book, and flipcharts. Many of the participatory teaching methods were unfamiliar to teachers, so the training focused heavily on modeling and practicing such methods. In addition, each method was broadly explained at the introduction of individual teacher's guides and then was described step-by-step when used for particular session tasks, including scripting of seemingly spontaneous discussion prompts. The *MEMA kwa Vijana* training strongly discouraged corporal punishment, although it was officially sanctioned within the school system and widely and routinely practiced in schools.

Observation of several teacher training courses by the author, external evaluators, and senior intervention staff found these courses were implemented with a high quality and consistency across the four project districts (e.g., Lugoe, 2001). Teachers' baseline levels of reproductive health knowledge were low, but in the first year the proportion responding correctly to reproductive health questions in pre- and post-training questionnaires tripled after the training course (Obasi, Chima, Mmassy, et al., 2002). Teacher's reported attitudes also improved significantly with initial training. For example, reports that there were circumstances in which a girl must have sex (such as after receiving money or gifts) fell from 36 percent before training to none afterwards. Prior to that training, 83 percent of teachers reported feeling "good" or "very good" about adolescent sexual health education, and this increased significantly to 93 percent afterward. In the second year, of those who had taught *MEMA kwa Vijana* classes the year before, 72 percent reported being very happy to continue being a *MEMA kwa Vijana* teacher, while 16 percent reported being moderately happy to do so.

Most teachers were enthusiastic about the new teaching methods and approach and showed progress in adopting them in the training courses. However, during training sessions some teachers lectured only and did not adopt participatory methods; some had difficulty teaching relatively complex sessions (e.g., explanation of the menstrual cycle, or leading games simulating disease transmission); some used patronizing terminology; and some made undesirable personal statements, such as judgmental comments about traditional medicine or abortion. In addition, in annual feedback meetings teachers frequently said they found it challenging and contradictory to advise pupils to be abstinent while also promoting monogamy and condom use if pupils were sexually active. Reported sexual behavior in the confidential training questionnaires also indicated challenges for some teachers to be role models. For example, of the 81 percent of teachers who were married, 27 percent reported that they had an extramarital sexual partner. Such high rates of extramarital sexual relationships were not unusual in rural areas, as discussed in chapter 3.

Curriculum Coverage

Some school sexual health programs in sub-Saharan Africa have not succeeded because they were optional curricula and few teachers ever implemented them (e.g., Kinsman et al., 2001). Knowing this, the *MEMA kwa Vijana* intervention team advocated with regional education authorities for two unusual and important conditions: first, that the program be assigned a timeslot within the broader school curriculum, and second, that it be formally examined alongside other subjects during the national examinations at the end of Year 7. The intervention team worked closely with the Mwanza Region Education Officer, and although he did not initially agree for condom use to be discussed in detail in classrooms, as described in chapter 4, he did fully support implementation of the *MEMA kwa Vijana* curriculum in the school timetables and its examination in Year 7. Indeed, he attended meetings with District Education Officers to stress his expectation that the curriculum would be implemented, and followed up with them in writing reaffirming his authorization of the program and giving guidance on its inclusion in the Year 5–7 timetables.

Teachers were thus expected to teach the *MEMA kwa Vijana* curriculum as part of their general workload, rather than as a voluntary or optional extracurricular activity. There were more sessions allocated for the program in the school year than the ten to thirteen sessions specified in the *MEMA kwa Vijana* teacher's guides (Appendices 1–3). This allowed repetition of difficult sessions, and ensured that the program could be completed despite high periods of teacher and pupil absenteeism, for example, during seasonal cultivation. In the final year of the trial, the AMREF intervention team arranged for curriculum content to also be included in a special examination that took place alongside the national Year 7 examination for other core subjects. This was intended to legitimize the topic and motivate teachers and pupils to fully engage with the material, and also to provide additional assessment of intervention impact.

During the school year, teachers were asked to complete brief report forms after teaching *MEMA kwa Vijana* sessions. In the first year of the intervention 1,416 (51 percent) of the total possible report forms were returned by 109 (89 percent) of the *MEMA kwa Vijana* teachers. For the majority of these sessions, teachers said that they did not skip or change any material specified in the curriculum (95 percent); that they themselves (92 percent) and their pupils (82 percent) enjoyed it; that they had enough time to teach it (78 percent); and that pupils were not embarrassed (68 percent). None of these findings varied significantly by class year. The most common responses to a free-text question about problems were that: pupils were embarrassed (8 percent), pupils did not participate (4 percent), and the content was too difficult (3 percent). In contrast, the most common free-text responses about good experiences were that pupils enjoyed the session (22 percent); pupils asked and answered questions (13 percent); the content was good (9 percent); the dramas were effective (5 percent); girls liked the session (5 percent); and pupils wanted to know more (4 percent). In the second year of the intervention the results were similar but somewhat improved, for example, 84 percent of teachers reported that they did not think their pupils were embarrassed by the sessions.

As another measure of teaching coverage, the AMREF intervention team systematically reviewed pupil exercise books and found that the vast majority of *MEMA kwa Vijana* sessions were taught during the January–December academic year. For pupils in Year 7, for example, 87 percent of sessions had been taught by November of the first year of the intervention (1999), 80 percent by August of the second year (2000), and 93 percent by August of the third year (2001) (Obasi et al., 2006). Participant observation and in-depth interviews suggest that the active monitoring of *MEMA kwa Vijana* teaching by district authorities and AMREF staff may have contributed to this high coverage, as occasionally respondents reported teachers taught sessions specifically in anticipation of a supervisor's visit. For example, a secondary school student recalled, "Sometimes when *MEMA kwa Vijana* teachers learned that their supervisors were coming, they would check whether there were past lessons which they had failed to teach and teach them in the morning before the supervisors arrived, which they then back-dated to tally with those days when they didn't teach" (PO-01-I-1-3m).

Nonetheless, participant observation and in-depth interviews with intervention participants from all ten intervention communities found that the vast majority had participated in *MEMA kwa Vijana* classes once per week for a large part of the school year. For example, of the thirty-three randomly selected intervention participants who participated in the second series of in-depth interviews at the end of the trial, only four reported little intervention experience. Two of these were young women who had not attended classes because of domestic responsibilities or pregnancy. One young man instead reported he intentionally did not attend *MEMA kwa Vijana* classes because he was embarrassed to discuss sex in the presence of female relatives in the same class. A fourth pupil reported that her teacher had not allowed her to participate in *MEMA kwa Vijana* classes because she could not read and write. Her lack of participation was evident in her comments about condom use, as she made unusually negative comments about them for an intervention participant. When asked if she would feel shy to buy condoms, she replied: "I would be ashamed . . . because they are for evil purposes. They are offensive/insulting . . . certainly, they are immoral" (II-02-I-272-f). This was the only time an intervention participant reported being excluded from *MEMA kwa Vijana* sessions.

At the third annual teacher's training only 8 percent of teachers reported having ever had a pupil withdraw from *MEMA kwa Vijana* classes due to parental concern about the subject matter. However, at the same training course 51 percent of teachers reported that, if they taught more about condoms in class, they believed parents would perceive them negatively as encouraging pupils to have sex.

Teacher turnover was a challenge in sustaining the intervention over the three years of the trial, and the annual training courses were introduced partly to ensure replacement of trained teachers who were transferred or moved for other reasons. For example, at the beginning of the second year of the intervention a teacher in a remote, participant observation village told a researcher she was planning to move:

> She said that when the intervention started, she and one other teacher from that school were trained to deliver the sessions. But after a short time the male teacher was transferred. When the project came again, she and a third teacher went for the training . . . so now when she goes away, he will be the only *MEMA kwa Vijana* teacher left in the school. (PO-00-I-4-1m)

It was not unusual for schools to lose trained *MEMA kwa Vijana* teachers within the three years of the trial, but the annual training courses helped ensure that the curriculum continued to be taught in those schools. There was also evidence that, occasionally, new teachers within schools had already been trained in their prior school, or teachers who did not move far away returned to their old schools to continue teaching *MEMA kwa Vijana* lessons. An example provided by a girl in Year 6:

> *R*: We were taught *MEMA kwa Vijana* lessons by a teacher from [another village].
>
> *I*: You don't have your own teacher?
>
> *R*: The *MEMA kwa Vijana* teachers were transferred there, so they come back now to teach those lessons. . . . That teacher taught us, "If you use condoms, you can't contract HIV or sexually transmitted infections, or become pregnant." (II-00-I-105-f)

Pupil Experience of the Taught Curriculum

In the sixty-two intervention schools, routine monitoring and supervision by intervention staff and district education officials found that the overall quality of *MEMA kwa Vijana* curriculum teaching was good. Teachers often

demonstrated mastery of curriculum content while teaching it, and also attempted to use participatory teaching methods in class, although their success in achieving the latter was quite variable.

Unlike the intervention supervisors, HALIRA researchers only occasionally observed teachers teaching *MEMA kwa Vijana* sessions in class, so
most HALIRA data collected on this intervention component were indirect,
such as intervention participants' descriptions of their *MEMA kwa Vijana*
lessons and what they had learned in them. When describing *MEMA kwa
Vijana* in their own words, for instance, pupils frequently said they had
been taught about sexual and reproductive biology, sexually transmitted
infections, and especially HIV/AIDS. Almost all of the randomly selected
in-depth interview respondents said they were very grateful to learn such
information, because they had little prior understanding of the topics and
believed them to be important. For example, a sixteen-year-old girl who had
recently completed Year 7:

> *R*: I liked when the teachers taught information about avoiding diseases, or that
> you should use a condom. . . . We were taught that we shouldn't feel shy. Not to
> turn our backs to the class, and to speak loudly if we wanted to say something.
> . . .
>
> *I*: Was there anything that you did not like about those classes?
>
> *R*: I liked everything . . . just everything. (II-00-I-94-f)

Some pupils were unconditionally positive about their *MEMA kwa Vijana*
classes, like this girl above. Most said they liked the drama, songs, and other
participatory methods that *MEMA kwa Vijana* teachers used. Many pupils
reported that teachers were more patient and respectful and less likely than
usual to use corporal punishment in *MEMA kwa Vijana* classes. Two examples from an in-depth interview and a group discussion:

> *I*: Earlier you said that you are beaten when you make mistakes in class. If you
> make mistakes during the HIV/AIDS lessons, are you also beaten?
>
> *R*: No. . . . When they are teaching us about that subject, they don't hit us. (II-99-
> I-46-m)
>
> *P*: No one was forced to step forward [to participate in role plays], because some
> felt shy. The experienced ones stepped forward and began to conduct plays
> without fear or trembling. (GD-99-I-15-m)

Occasionally, however, there were reports of teachers using corporal punishment to make children participate during their *MEMA kwa Vijana* lessons.
An example from a male peer educator discussion group:

P: Some pupils agreed [to participate in a *MEMA kwa Vijana* roleplay], but others refused. A boy and a girl were appointed. The teacher had to hit them . . . The girl agreed, the boy refused.

F: Until the teacher hit him?

P: He had to hit him before he agreed. (GD-99-I-14-m)

As noted above, almost all intervention participants said they appreciated the factual information they learned in their *MEMA kwa Vijana* classes. Sometimes respondents identified other aspects of the curriculum that they particularly liked. The following two examples were provided by a seventeen-year-old girl in Year 5, and a nineteen-year-old man in Year 7, respectively:

R: Too many men try to seduce me. . . . Like at the auction market one may tell you, "Come and take this sugarcane." The *MEMA kwa Vijana* teacher tells us we should not accept gifts. Sometimes a man might give you a skirt, or shoes, or socks. If you accept gifts, there will definitely be a day when he'll come and tell you that he always buys things for you . . . and you will have to pay for that [with sex]. So you shouldn't accept presents.

I: Were you pleased or not pleased when the teacher was teaching you that lesson?

R: I was really impressed with those lessons. . . . What I liked most was the lesson when the teacher teaches you not to have sex when you are still under age. I was really impressed by that. (II-99-I-68-f)

R: The teacher asked us to think about how our future life will be. . . . We were told not to answer the question right then, but just to remain with it, to reflect on it. . . . And, in fact, I found that issue to be very important. It's a question to think about a lot. (II-02-I-242-m)

Participant observation and in-depth interviews typically found that intervention participants had better reproductive and sexual health knowledge than their control counterparts or other villagers. Generally male intervention participants seemed to retain more accurate sexual health information than females. This may have reflected how parents and teachers encouraged and supported boys more than girls in their learning, and also how boys typically were more confident and dominated question-and-answer sessions and discussions in class. However, in their training courses *MEMA kwa Vijana* teachers were encouraged to engage girls more, and many small discussions were designed to be same-sex to reduce this gender imbalance. Participant observation found that female intervention participants sometimes described information taught within the *MEMA kwa Vijana* curriculum accurately. For example, in one village a sixteen-year-old girl "said she had been taught at school during *MEMA kwa Vijana* lessons that if they have [genital] itchiness, sores, or discharge, they should go to the dispensary for free treatment" (PO-01-I-1-2f). Another example from when a researcher passed school girls hauling materials to build a latrine:

> I asked about the number of the subjects they have in school and they listed all of them, including *MEMA kwa Vijana* lessons. They said in that lesson they are taught about the transmission and prevention of AIDS and other sexually transmitted infections, and unintended pregnancies. One of them [a peer educator] explained how pregnancy can occur. Three simultaneously said, "Millions of sperm are ejaculated, but only one fertilizes an egg." The whole group laughed while two others who were sitting to the side came closer and joined us. One of them was also a peer educator. They mentioned the sexually transmitted infections they have been taught about are gonorrhea, syphilis, and *Kabambalu* (a symptomatic form of chlamydia). (PO-01-I-7-5f)

The three young people quoted the same line above because it was a phrase that was repeated throughout the curriculum, both to explain the nature of reproduction and to emphasize the ease with which a girl could become pregnant. Participant observation researchers heard key intervention messages like this repeated verbatim many times in informal settings, sometimes in unexpected ways. In each of the participant observation intervention villages, for instance, researchers were present when intervention participants spontaneously used phrases in joking or mocking ways, including sometimes as a pick-up line during seduction.

In another example, in multiple villages researchers heard intervention participants criticize the intervention slogan "*hata mara moja*" ("even one time"), which was intended to emphasize that a person could cause a pregnancy or contract a sexually transmitted infection from just one sexual encounter. Instead, this was sometimes misinterpreted to mean that, if someone has vaginal intercourse once, they *will* (not *could*) cause a pregnancy or contract an infection. As many sexually active youth had not experienced such consequences, the statement was seen as invalid, raising questions about the validity of *MEMA kwa Vijana* more broadly. For example, a fifteen-year-old daughter of a Pentacostal pastor: "Some girls used to say that *MEMA kwa Vijana* is cheating them because it taught them that if a girl has sex once she'll get pregnant. But most of them have had sex several times and have never conceived" (PO-99-I-1-2f).

The degree to which condom use was taught and promoted in school seemed to vary greatly by teacher and school. A small minority of teachers independently decided to teach detailed information about condom use, including providing condom demonstrations. An example provided by an eighteen-year-old woman who had recently completed Year 7:

She said her teacher demonstrated condom use by putting it on a piece of wood shaped like a penis. She said the teacher explained the condom should be held at the tip to press out air so no air bubble is in it when it is put it on the penis. She said she plans to use condoms the next time she has sex, since they prevent sexually transmitted infections and pregnancy. She knows that condoms are supposed to be obtained at the [local] dispensary, but it is impossible for her to do this as she is too shy. (PO-99-I-1-2f)

In most schools, however, teachers did not seem to teach clear and accurate information about condom use in class. Many teachers were hesitant to teach detailed condom use information for several reasons, including the constrained and ambiguous guidelines from the Ministry of Education (and as a result, the *MEMA kwa Vijana* program); concern about what adult villagers would think of such material; and/or how they themselves found it challenging to promote abstinence and condom use simultaneously. As a result, most teachers only described condom use very superficially in class, but arranged for class visits to health facilities to provide pupils with an alternative source of information.

As had been found during the first pilot tests of the curriculum, some teachers reconciled the promotion of abstinence and condom use by telling pupils that they were too young to have sex, so they should abstain, but when they were sexually active adults it would be best to use condoms. The following example was provided by a sixteen-year-old boy in Year 7:

R: The teachers took us to the hospital to be taught how to use condoms. . . . In *MEMA kwa Vijana* they say . . . it is not good to use condoms at a young age. Yes, condoms are only good for adults. . . .

I: Do they say anything else to other youths, who might still have sex?

R: We are just told that we are children and we should completely abstain. . . .

I: Have the people from *MEMA kwa Vijana* told you there are adverse effects if you, a child, were to use condoms?

R: Actually we have never been told there are any adverse effects. But we have been forbidden to use condoms . . . because we are still young. (II-00-I-80-m)

In multiple villages, intervention participants referred to such statements to justify their unprotected sexual activity. For example, a report from a fifteen-year-old Year 7 pupil during participant observation:

He said that all the times he had sex he never used a condom. But he said he knows what condoms look like, how to use them, and where to get them at shops or the health facility. He said that he didn't use condoms when he had sex because they [primary school pupils] are not allowed to use them. He said that in *MEMA kwa Vijana* lessons they are taught that they are still young, thus they are not allowed to use condoms. He said during *MEMA kwa Vijana* lessons they are always told to abstain from having sex until they complete school or get married. However, he said that in normal circumstances it is difficult for a young man like himself to stop having sex when he has already started. (PO-01-I-7-3m)

Intervention participants were sometimes confused about condom use in other ways, particularly those who had not observed a condom demonstration at a health facility, as they often had difficulty visualizing condoms and understanding exactly how they were used. For example, a twenty-year-old, married HIV-positive woman who had not gone on a class visit to a health facility before she finished school two years earlier:

R: [*MEMA kwa Vijana* teachers] were teaching us those things, like that a condom protects against diseases like AIDS.

I: Is there anything that confuses you about condoms?

R: Yes. It is that I don't . . . I don't know what a condom is. . . . They only told us that condoms are a form of protection. But how . . . how to use it, how and when a person uses it, they didn't tell us. (II-02-I-293-f)

Other Teacher-Led Activities

In most villages, teachers facilitated intervention health worker visits to schools and class visits to health centers for a Youth Health Day. Given the constraints in teaching condom-related information as described above and in chapter 4, the teacher-health worker collaboration was very important in clarifying information about condom use and promoting pupils' appropriate use of health services. However, teachers and health workers occasionally collaborated in inappropriate ways which violated girls' privacy, for example, forcing school girls to undergo pregnancy examinations. Their collaborative work will be described in detail when the *MEMA kwa Vijana* health services component is evaluated in the next chapter.

In addition to the teacher-health worker collaboration, an annual *MEMA kwa Vijana* Youth Health Week was held in each community, during which pupils from intervention schools competed in performing dramas, *ngonjera* (traditional poetry recitation), songs, and dance with a sexual and reproductive health theme. This interschool competition was open to the local community and followed a similar format to preexistent interschool sports competitions. Pupils were asked to develop their own material for these performances, but in practice almost all such activities were developed and led by teachers, so they depended on the enthusiasm and skill of each school's *MEMA kwa*

Vijana teachers. In two participant observation villages, for example, teachers wrote *MEMA kwa Vijana* songs which they taught their pupils for Youth Health Week, and researchers occasionally came across pupils singing those songs independently while carrying out daily chores.

Participant observation generally found that pupils and parents were supportive of the Youth Health Week activities, although sometimes parents did not think they were important and instead kept their children home to do domestic or farm work. *MEMA kwa Vijana* provided prizes for the schools that won Youth Health Week competitions, such as a soccer ball, volleyball, or *MEMA kwa Vijana* T-shirts. As noted earlier, these were valued highly in a context where pupils might only have two or three sets of clothes and soccer balls often consisted of rags sewn together. In one example an informant explained, "It is true that some parents don't allow their children to go to school when there are *MEMA kwa Vijana* games. . . . [But eventually] some parents agree, as they can't buy their children those special T-shirts" (PO-01-I-4-5f). Indeed, new T-shirts were so valuable that participant observation researchers often observed peer educators' parents or older siblings wearing the *MEMA kwa Vijana* T-shirts the peer educators had received during training.

Teachers as Role Models

As noted in chapter 3, many teachers in rural Mwanza tried to teach children to the best of their abilities, despite tremendous resource constraints. This included *MEMA kwa Vijana* teachers who put many extra hours into teaching the intervention without compensation. Most pupils in intervention and control schools respected and appreciated their teachers, and they often liked one or two teachers in particular. In both intervention and control communities, the qualitative research also found that there were individual teachers who seemed to successfully discourage pupils from engaging in sexual risk behaviors by giving them appropriate guidance and intervening with nonpunitive concern, as shown in case studies 1.2, 1.3, and 3.2 later in this book.

During the trial, participant observation in four intervention villages suggests that adult and pupil attitudes toward the *MEMA kwa Vijana* intervention partly related to the reputations of the local school teachers. For example, in one multicultural fishing village (number 7), teachers generally seemed to have good reputations and were well respected by adults and children alike. In that village there were isolated incidents of adults criticizing the intervention program—most often reports that it promoted youth sexual activity—but overall adult villagers seemed to appreciate it and to view it favorably.

In contrast, in a remote inland village (number 4) several male school teachers had reputations for being drunkards and—to a lesser extent—womanizers. Fieldworkers themselves sometimes encountered the head teacher and other teachers when they were drunk during the day, suggesting there were grounds for those reputations. In that village some adults and children perceived the teachers as negligent and irresponsible, and attitudes toward the intervention seemed more mixed than in the fishing village mentioned above. Several adults in that village questioned whether the intervention had reduced pupils' risk behaviors, but few seemed concerned that it might increase them.

In a third example, in the inland intervention village near a mine (number 1), almost all male primary school teachers (including two of the three trained *MEMA kwa Vijana* teachers) were rumored to have sexual relationships with female school pupils. Numerous first- and third-hand pupil reports suggested that this was true both before and after the intervention began. Case study 1.1 describes one example. As noted in chapter 3, there was plausible evidence from multiple in-depth interviews and eight of the nine participant observation villages that one or more local teachers had pressured or forced school girls to have sex. However, this was particularly common in participant observation village number 1, where many pupils and adults also considered the intervention teachers to be hypocritical and poor intervention role models. A peer educator there described how a married *MEMA kwa Vijana* teacher even acknowledged his sexual relationship with a pupil during a *MEMA kwa Vijana* lesson:

> She said that the teacher who pressured her for sex also tried to seduce her friend, but her friend also refused. . . . She said when that teacher teaches them *MEMA kwa Vijana* lessons he asks each pupil, "Do you think you can control yourself?" If pupils respond that they can control their sexual desire, the teacher tells them that they cannot, that they are lying to themselves and it is better to just admit it and use condoms. She said that teacher tells them he himself cannot control his desire, and that is why he has [a certain school girl] as a sexual partner. (PO-01-I-1-2f)

In that village, the main strategy girls seemed to employ in resisting a teacher's sexual pressure was to avoid being isolated with the teacher, although this was not always possible. One pupil told a researcher that she resisted her *MEMA kwa Vijana* teacher's sexual pressure by referring to his own teachings:

> She said that the teacher has become a bother and when he meets her along a path, he keeps asking her for sex. . . . [The last time] she sang a song that he had taught them for *MEMA kwa Vijana* week competitions. The song had the theme, "Refuse by body and actions." (PO-01-I-1-2f)

Teacher-school girl sexual relationships were widely known amongst pupils in that school, and they were rumored and discussed to a lesser extent amongst adult villagers, but no public action seemed to be taken against the teachers involved. For example, the Village Chairman openly discussed the teachers' behavior during a formal interview with a participant observation researcher:

> He said that the *MEMA kwa Vijana* teachers have failed to be good role models for their pupils or other people in the community. He said they teach well but they also seduce pupils, a situation that he thinks has contributed to the failure of the *MEMA kwa Vijana* intervention, including the feelings amongst some parents that *MEMA kwa Vijana* lessons spoil their children by teaching them about sex. (PO-02-I-1-3m)

After the first round of participant observation, HALIRA researchers informed the AMREF intervention team of the findings of widespread sexual abuse within that village's school. The intervention team arranged for the abusive *MEMA kwa Vijana* teachers to be replaced, and confidentially reported the situation to the district and ward educational authorities. It is unclear, however, whether any further investigation or action was taken by those authorities.

PEER EDUCATORS' ACTIVITIES

Peer Educator Training and Drama Content

As discussed in chapter 4, preliminary research and a review of existing local programs during *MEMA kwa Vijana* intervention development suggested that rural primary school pupils lacked the cognitive and social skills necessary to independently teach sexual health information and risk reduction skills in reliably accurate ways. Within the *MEMA kwa Vijana* program it was thus decided that peer education would primarily consist of trained pupils assisting teachers in a structured way in class. Preliminary research found dramas to be both popular and feasible for pupils to perform well, so a series of carefully scripted short dramas were developed for pupils to perform in class to facilitate teacher-led discussions.

To select *MEMA kwa Vijana* peer educators, pupils in Years 5–7 in the sixty-two intervention schools nominated a shortlist, from which teachers and intervention staff selected eight per class to participate in the training, after which six per class were selected to be *waelimishaji wa rika* (peer educators). The qualitative research found that peer educators were often unusually confident, popular, bright, and/or respectful of authority, and it seems likely that many were selected because of one or more of those qualities. Because of these different criteria and the substantial age range within classes, peer educators within the same class sometimes represented very different age groups, such as twelve- to thirteen-year-olds who excelled academically and eighteen- to nineteen-year-olds who were admired for their experience and confidence.

Peer educators participated in a three-day training course that was led by AMREF intervention staff and sixty-three out-of-school youth—three males and three females per community—who had been elected by local advisory committees and who had participated in a two-week training-of-trainer course themselves. These young trainers-of-peers were the only non-AMREF staff to receive a regular allowance during the first two years of the trial, and their activities were devolved to teachers in the third year of the trial. In 1998, 1,124 peer educators were trained for the first year of the intervention, while in 1999 372 new Year 5 pupils (six per school who were not in the trial population) were trained for the intervention's second year. Thus peer educators made up approximately 12 percent of the trial population of 9,645, and that minority effectively participated in a more intensive sexual health intervention than their peers.

The first peer educator training focused on drama line memorization, acting skills, and character practice. Each drama episode lasted only a few minutes and was designed to be compelling, entertaining, and informative, so it could be used as a helpful discussion starter for teachers. The dramas acknowledged common local motivations for adolescents to have sex, such as peer pressure for boys and girls, and material desire for girls. In one of the drama series, three characters suffered different adverse consequences of unprotected intercourse and multiple partnerships, and three others gave advice and demonstrated the benefits of desired behavior (box 5.1). Peer educators were taught to speak loudly and clearly and to follow the script exactly, but to nonetheless perform their parts in a natural and animated way (figure 5.1). They were reminded to use the names of the characters frequently, so that the audience would not confuse the names and actions of the characters with those of the actors.

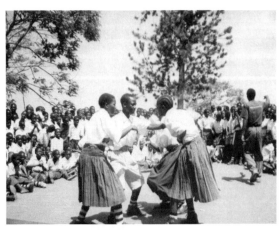

Figure 5.1. Pupils watching peer educators performing a drama at a *MEMA kwa Vijana* Youth Health Day event.

BOX 5.1. *MEMA KWA VIJANA* DRAMA, STORY, AND LETTER SERIAL[a]

This drama, story, and letter serial takes place over four sessions of the Year 5 curriculum (Appendix 1) and one session of the Year 6 curriculum (Appendix 2). It involves peer educators acting in two dramas, and the teacher reading two stories and one letter aloud. Each session begins with one of these activities to illustrate the session's themes and set the context for subsequent teacher-led discussions, personalization exercises, role plays, or small group competitions.

A. EXCERPT FROM "MISCONCEPTIONS ABOUT SEX" SESSION: JUMA, SAIDI, AND JOHN'S DRAMA

Juma meets Saidi when he is returning from school. Saidi is reading a letter from his lover. When Juma comes closer, Saidi hides the letter. He greets Juma and congratulates him on his excellent examination results. Then Saidi teases Juma about Rehema, who also did well in the exams. He says that now that Juma and Rehema both have excellent results, they must congratulate each other, meaning they should have sex.

Juma tells Saidi that Rehema is just a normal friend and that they are not having sex. Saidi does not believe him and finally tells Juma that, if he is not having sex with Rehema, then he is stupid (figure 5.2). Saidi says it is not easy for a boy and a girl to be friends without having sex with each other. Juma gets angry and tells Saidi that he is the one who is stupid because he thinks about sex all the time. Then Juma leaves.

Just as Saidi starts to read the letter again, John arrives. John asks Saidi if that letter is from his brother. Saidi laughs and says no. He explains that he has many lovers, and this letter is from the one he likes the most. Saidi starts to tease John because John has never had sex. Saidi warns John that if he does not have sex, he will become impotent and he may even die. John is surprised. He does not know what impotence is, and Saidi tells him that it means he will never be able to have sex or to have children, unless he has sex soon.

Saidi knows that John likes Sikujua, so he encourages John to have sex with her. John says he has heard that you can make a girl pregnant even if you only have sex one time, but he is not certain. Saidi tells him this is not true. He tells John that he will teach John a special way of

(continued)

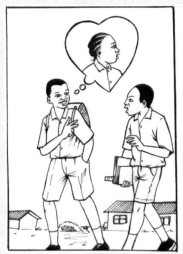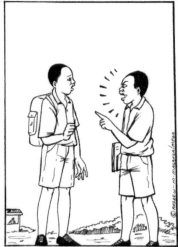

Figure 5.2.   Saidi pressuring Juma to have sex with Rehema, and Juma's angry response (a drama illustration).

having sex so Sikujua does not get pregnant. John hesitates and asks Saidi whether he should use a condom. Saidi tells him that condoms are dangerous, but that John will not make Sikujua pregnant if they have sex while standing up. Ultimately, John agrees and says he will ask Sikijua to have sex with him.

B. EXCERPT FROM "REFUSING TEMPTATIONS" SESSION: AMINA, REHEMA, AND SAIDI'S DRAMA

Rehema tells Amina that she has heard that Amina is having sex with Saidi. Rehema has heard bad things about Saidi's behavior, so she advises Amina to be careful. Amina replies that she has not done anything bad with Saidi. Rehema again cautions Amina to be careful, then she leaves.

Then Saidi appears looking very happy and energetic. He is happy to see Amina because his brother has traveled, and he thinks that he and Amina can be alone together at home. He tries to persuade Amina to go with him. However, Amina is anxious and demands to know what Saidi wants. Saidi does not say anything. Amina knows that Saidi wants her to go to his place to have sex, so she refuses right away, showing this both in her words and actions (figure 5.3).

(continued)

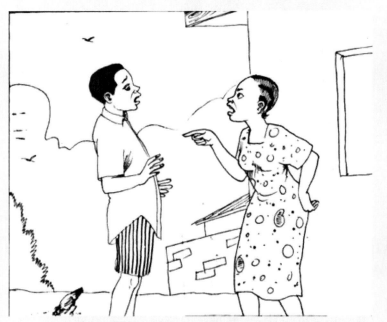

Figure 5.3. **Amina rejecting Saidi's sexual advances (a drama illustration).**

C. EXCERPT FROM "SAYING NO TO SEX" SESSION: JOHN, SIKUJUA, AND SAIDI'S STORY

After Saidi tells John that John will become impotent if he does not have sex, John asks Sikujua to have sex with him. Sikujua agrees and advises him to use a condom, but John refuses, because Saidi had told him that condoms are not safe. Instead, they try to prevent pregnancy by having sex while standing up, as Saidi recommended.

After a few months pass, Sikujua tells John that she is pregnant. She says that he is the father, because she has never had sex with anyone else. John realizes that this must be true. John is very surprised and quickly goes to tell Saidi. Saidi asks him, "What happened? How could Sikujua be pregnant? Didn't you do what I told you to do?" John replies regretfully, "I did exactly what you told me to do, so I am surprised that Sikujua is pregnant! I am sad that I have ruined her life, and mine as well."

(*continued*)

D. EXCERPT FROM "SEXUALLY TRANSMITTED INFECTIONS" SESSION: SAIDI AND JUMA'S STORY

Juma is working at home. He hears someone come to the door and is surprised to see Saidi. Saidi is in pain and clearly can not walk easily. Juma welcomes Saidi inside. Saidi is not able to sit comfortably. Saidi complains that for the past few days strange liquid has come out of his penis, and he has experienced severe pain when urinating. Yesterday he saw a sore on his penis, which is also very painful. He doesn't know what is happening and asks Juma to help him. Juma thinks that Saidi has at least one sexually transmitted infection, perhaps more. Saidi is surprised. He says, "How could I have a sexually transmitted infection?"

Juma reminds Saidi that he often boasts in class about having many lovers. But Saidi says that he was very careful and only had sex with each of them one time. Juma asks him if he used condoms. Saidi tells Juma that he never used them because he heard they are not safe. Juma tells him if he had used condoms, he probably would not have been infected. Saidi still does not believe Juma. But then the pain comes back and he asks Juma what he should do. Juma tells him that they must go to a health facility (figure 5.4).

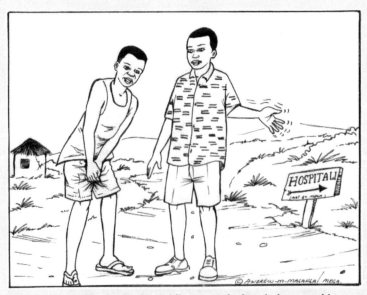

Figure 5.4.   Juma encouraging Saidi to go to the hospital to treat his sexually transmitted infection (a story illustration).

(*continued*)

Saidi says that he has relatives who live near the health facility. He doesn't want to go there because he is certain that his relatives will find out. Juma assures Saidi that the health workers are good at keeping secrets. He says there isn't any place at the health facility specifically for people with sexually transmitted infections, so no one will know why he is there. Saidi agrees to go to the health facility.

E. EXCERPT FROM "REVIEW OF LAST YEAR'S LEARNING" SESSION: SIKUJUA'S LETTER

In a letter to her classmates, Sikujua explains what has happened to her since she became pregnant. She tells them that she had to leave school, and her father kicked her out of his house, so she went to live with an aunt instead. She explains that she had difficulty delivering her child, because she is still young and her body had not fully matured. She says the delivery was painful, and she had to have an operation. She is grateful that she and her baby are both healthy. However, Sikujua works long hours and struggles to support herself and her daughter, and she has many regrets.

[a]Excerpted from the *MEMA kwa Vijana* teacher's guide for Year 5: a. Session 7 ("Misconceptions about Sex," 39–41); b. Session 8 ("Refusing temptations," 45–47); c. Session 9 ("Saying No to Sex," 50–51); and d. Session 10 ("Sexually Transmitted Infections: Going to the Hospital," 55–58) (Obasi, Chima, Cleophas-Frisch et al., 2002a). Also excerpted from the *MEMA kwa Vijana* teacher's guide for Year 6: e. Session 1 ("Review of Last Year's Learning, 3–4) (Obasi, Chima, Cleophas-Frisch et al., 2002c). Used with the authors' permission.

Observation of peer educator drama performances by the author, external evaluators, and the AMREF intervention team during the trial found that peer educators performed characters and dramas very consistently across the four project districts (e.g., Guyon et al., 2000). However, across the study area there were reports that girls who played characters with undesirable behaviors were sometimes teased or stigmatized by their peers. For example, a sixteen-year-old in Year 6 who played such a character:

. . . said she felt shy during her first appearance in the drama. She said after she was selected, the pupils who were not selected started telling her that *MEMA kwa Vijana* teaches prostitution and bad behavior, such as sexual activity. She said even her neighbors said that she was a prostitute. But then when they were given *MEMA kwa Vijana* T-shirts, the pupils who were jeering and insulting them were envious and said they also should have become peer educators to get such T-shirts. (PO-00-I-4-4f)

In contrast, process evaluation during the first years of the trial suggested that male drama characters whose storylines involved high-risk behaviors and negative consequences were sometimes admired, specifically because the roles were relatively complex and the best actors had been assigned to them. As a result, these characters and dramas were modified over the course of the trial. In the final version, female drama characters with disreputable behavior were replaced with stories about those characters, which were read aloud by teachers. In addition, male drama characters who practiced low-risk behaviors were made more interesting and complex, and teachers were encouraged to assign popular pupils and/or good actors to those roles.

During the first training course for peer educators, participants were only taught very basic information about sexual and reproductive health. Educational authorities limited the discussion of condom use in the training course to general statements that condoms prevent pregnancy and sexually transmitted infections, without visual depiction of condoms or explanation of correct condom use. HALIRA project and AMREF intervention team process evaluation during the first year of the program suggested that after their training some peer educators were confused about basic adolescent sexual and reproductive health information, and particularly condom use. To address this, intervention staff developed a simply worded information booklet for peer educators, which educational authorities allowed to be distributed at the end of the first year of the trial.

Additional training sessions were added to the second annual training course for peer educators, which included both new and old peer educators. These sessions included increased information about HIV/AIDS and other sexually transmitted infections, risk behaviors, and risk reduction, as well as exercises designed to improve peer educator personal risk assessment, self-efficacy, and communication skills. While the factual information was very well received by peer educators, observation by the author, external evaluators, and the AMREF intervention team found that the skills-building activities and exercises intended to develop pupil abilities as "agents of change" with their peers sometimes confused them, and in their subsequent work in the village the targeted skills were difficult for them to practice (e.g., Guyon et al., 2000).

To accommodate annual pupil turnover within the trial population, it was necessary to train 372 new Year 5 pupils as peer educators each year. This was difficult to sustain, so when the intervention was expanded ten-fold after the trial, *MEMA kwa Vijana* teachers were asked to select and train new Year 5 peer educators within their schools each year. A portion of the teacher training was modified to better prepare them for this additional task.

In-Class Peer Education

Peer educators generally had a detailed understanding of the dramas, and also better sexual health knowledge and stronger communication and assertiveness skills than other pupils (e.g., Makokha et al., 2002). Pupils almost universally reported that peer educators conducted in-class dramas and roleplays well, and in some schools said they also assisted teachers in answering pupils' questions in class or conducting special events. Most pupils and peer educators enjoyed and appreciated the dramas. The use of recurrent characters and realistic situations seemed to entertain pupils and keep their attention, while also helping them identify with the characters and reinforcing messages about the consequences of sexual decision-making. An example from a male peer educator group discussion:

> *P1*: *MEMA kwa Vijana* dramas teach us. If one didn't understand the lesson before, he/she will [see the drama] and know that I shouldn't do this thing. So the drama also carries a lesson. . . .
>
> *P2*: I think that they are good, because . . . if some pupils were about to fall asleep, they will become alert, and the lesson continues. (GD-99-I-13-m)

Two years after intervention participation, a small minority of in-depth interview respondents said they could not recall peer educator contributions in the classroom, or remembered very little about them. Many, however, could clearly recall specific aspects of the drama series. The following two examples were provided by a twenty-year-old woman and a twenty-one-year-old man, both of whom were farmers:

> *R*: Peer educators used to perform some plays. The plays were about diseases, and boys and girls.
>
> *I*: Can you tell me the message of those plays?
>
> *R*: Yes. Refuse to be seduced. Speak to him rudely and then leave, so you do not have sex with him. You shouldn't entertain him. If he tells you to have sex with him, you just refuse and leave that place. (II-02-I-322-f)

> *R*: Peer educators performed dramas, and then after performing the teacher came to give us a warning. . . . For example, there is the drama of Saidi and Juma. Saidi was a certain young man who was an *mhuni* (a badly behaved person). Now after his friend gave him a lot of advice to stop having sex, he [nonetheless] had sex, and later got a sexually transmitted infection. After he got it he went to his friend Juma, who advised him and took him to the hospital. After going there he was treated and was finally cured. . . . Also, if peer educators were just in a group, talking, if someone said things about having sex they advised them and told them, "If you can't completely stop sex and you want to have sex, use condoms." That was their activity. (II-02-I-298-m)

Peer educators often said they became more confident through their intervention training and experience. During participant observation, for example, a
female peer educator explained that she felt very shy when she first performed
the drama, but her shyness dissipated over time. Occasionally, peer educators
said it was difficult to portray drama characters who were sexually active. As
noted earlier, girls seemed especially vulnerable to teasing or stigma related
to a character's undesirable behavior, but boys sometimes also were targeted.
For example, an eighteen-year-old young man who worked in his family's bar
explained how he was ambivalent about performing the dramas:

I: Can you tell me anything you enjoyed about performing the dramas?

R: Maybe when [my character] got sexually transmitted infections. I was very
interested in showing how he went to the hospital and was examined and received an early treatment, before they got worse. Because the effects of sexually
transmitted infections usually are not seen so vividly.

I: And was there anything you did not like about performing the dramas?

R: What part I disliked? . . . Afterward, when some pupils joked that I had sexually transmitted infections [Laughter]. I was very annoyed. . . . And maybe when
you act the role of someone planning to have sex. I disliked that role. Some of
my classmates told me that I must be having sex, because I know how to do it
from my drama performance. But that was just acting. (II-02-I-249-m)

Pupil comments also revealed occasional misunderstanding or misuse of
drama content. For example, in two group discussions and several participant
observation villages, male respondents reported that *MEMA kwa Vijana* dramas demonstrated words or techniques that they or other boys subsequently
adopted to seduce girls or to deny responsibility for a pregnancy.

In addition to performing the scripted dramas, pupils said peer educators
sometimes led other activities in class, such as the unscripted roleplays if
other pupils were too shy to participate in them. There were also isolated
reports of peer educators teaching entire classes on their own when teachers were absent. An example from an in-depth interview with a randomly
selected sixteen-year-old boy in Year 7:

R: There were some days when the teacher did not come, in which case we had
to take the book and starting teaching our fellow pupils. . . .

I: Did they pay attention as if you were a teacher?

R: They paid great attention and understood me very well.

I: Did you feel comfortable or were you a bit shy?

R: I was not at all shy. Yes, I was very pleased. . . . They understood me very
well, and when I asked them questions they were able to answer me.

I: How many times have you taught like that?

R: Many times. Because whenever a teacher did not come, I just took the book and started teaching. . . . Some days when I was late the other pupils even came to find me to tell me to go teach. (II-99-I-42-m)

Informal Peer Education

Process evaluation by the AMREF intervention team, HALIRA researchers, and external evaluators found that many peer educators provided other pupils with basic sexual health information and advice, particularly when drawing on the peer educator workbook. Generally this took place in the classroom, but sometimes it also happened outside of school. The two following examples were provided by eighteen-year-old and seventeen-year-old males in Year 7:

R: After class one day, we were the only two left. [The peer educator] then told me we that we pupils should not have a lot of sex any more. It helped me to not have sex.

I: And was it easier to talk with a pupil about this than a teacher?

R: It was easier, because when you talk with the teacher you feel . . . somehow shy. With a pupil, you are not afraid of each other. (II-99-I-48-m)

I: Are peer educators liked by other pupils?

R: Yes. . . . Because they are inquisitive, they like to ask and to understand.

I: Have they ever talked with you about sex or AIDS outside the classroom?

R: Yes. It . . . it helped me, because . . . they educated me. They advised me to abstain from sex. They told me why. How AIDS . . . can be had by a person, and can spread to all people. They helped me understand.

I: Was it easier to talk with other pupils about this than to teachers?

R: Yes, because we have very close relationships with those pupils. We see each other very often. . . . When we go home after school, we leave the teacher there and walk home together. (II-00-I-98-m)

The most common reports of informal peer education outside of school took place in discussions between peer educators and their siblings, cousins, or close friends. Examples from a female peer educator group discussion and an in-depth interview with a randomly selected young man follow:

P1: We help [educate] our younger sisters, and our elder sisters. Even at the farm, when you and your sister are cultivating. . . .

P2: For example, at school, whatever time, and at any hour. Or on any day you want to tell family members, if parents are not present.

F: If parents are not present?

P2: Yes. . . .

F: Why can't you tell them in the presence of parents?

P2: Those are secret issues.

F: What do [other group discussion participants] say about what she has said?

P3: In my case, I tell them even if parents are present. (GD-99-I-16-f)

R: Occasionally we taught each other when we were resting after farming. . . . Those who came from the same school started telling stories or asking each other questions. . . . They would ask me, "With your *MEMA kwa Vijana* education, can you tell us how to wear condoms?" And I would tell them to do this and this. . . . The answers were still just in my head. . . . Some of them paid attention to what I said, but others didn't. . . . Some were argumentative. Some feel it is not acceptable to be taught by a young man of the same age, that we should be taught by a teacher instead. . . . Like if you tell him, "You are supposed to use condoms when you have a lover," he says, "I can't use condoms, I don't enjoy them." Then some argument ensues. But others listened to my words. (II-02-I-243-m)

Peer educator ability to communicate educational information beyond acting out dramas and answering pre-scripted questions seemed quite variable, with the examples above representing unusually active and independent peer educators. Most randomly selected in-depth interview respondents said that they had never talked with peer educators about *MEMA kwa Vijana* topics outside of class, or they had only done so briefly. In addition, in informal settings young people sometimes attached no more importance to peer educators' opinions than those of other youth, and sometimes peer educators' opinions were aggressively rejected. The following example was observed by a researcher, after a number of pupils accurately described *MEMA kwa Vijana* material:

Then they said that only adults are supposed to use condoms. One peer educator objected, saying, "Even we can use condoms, if we can't resist having sex." About eight others objected that pupils are not allowed to use condoms. One said, "We pupils are taught how to refuse seduction, 'verbally and physically— by saying "NO" in capital letters'" [a key intervention slogan]. They all laughed . . . and repeated that they were not advised to use condoms, as they are only for adults. (PO-01-I-7-5f)

A fourteen-year-old, Year 6 peer educator described a more hostile response:

She said they were never taught about [specific] sexually transmitted infections as a class. Only peer educators were taught and told to teach the rest. She said she tried to teach regular pupils about those sexually transmitted infections in their free time, but most resisted by telling her, "Hey! Take your *uhuni* away from here!" (PO-99-I-1-2f)

As described in chapters 3 and 4, the age range within Years 5–7 was substantial. In Year 7, for example, most children were fourteen- to eighteen-years-old, but it was not unusual to have children as young as twelve and as old as twenty-one in the same class. Peer educators on the young end of this age range may have been bright and enthusiastic, but their relative youth and inexperience may have been a detriment when trying to advise their older classmates.

The topic of condom use was particularly difficult for both male and female peer educators to discuss with their peers. In two of the four peer educator group discussions, participants were confused or frustrated by this topic. For example:

P1: A pupil asked me if a pupil is allowed to use condoms. I told him/her that a pupil is not allowed to use condoms, but an adult is allowed to use them. . . .

P2: If you begin counseling pupils to abstain from having sex, they begin murmuring, and some of them even leave the classroom. In our discussions outside . . . they say that abstinence requires too great a sacrifice, so we tell them to use condoms. And finally they ask us, "Should we use condoms?! Now where are the condoms?" We fail to tell them. (GD-99-I-13-m)

Condom distribution and access will be discussed in the next chapter. Despite the potential challenges involved, peer educators almost always reported gratitude for their training and experience as peer educators. Other pupils also often said that they would like to have such an opportunity, and sometimes said they envied it, as seen in case study 1.2.

In interviews conducted three months to two years after peer educators had left school, some said they still drew on their training in informal discussions with friends, and particularly that they continued to refer to their information booklets. For example, an eighteen-year-old young woman who had left school fifteen months earlier: "I remember [curriculum content] because they gave us information booklets. Now, even if I forget about family planning methods or how to protect against AIDS and sexually transmitted infections, I just go read it to remember" (II-02-I-285-f).

Finally, participant observation found that some intervention participants who were not peer educators shared or taught intervention material to their siblings, cousins, or close friends. The following examples were provided by a twenty-four-year-old male trader and a secondary school girl in her late teens, both of whom were visiting their families in the village:

He said his little brother [an intervention participant] gives him a lot of information about sexually transmitted infections, reproductive organs, and pregnancy.

He explained that most young villagers say they don't use condoms because condoms don't give pleasure. He said school children view this differently because they know the importance of condoms due to the education they receive from *MEMA kwa Vijana*, but nonetheless they still have sex without using condoms. (PO-00-I-4-4f)

She said she was never taught *Mema kwa Vijana* lessons because she left the year before they began, but she was eager to learn about them so she asked her younger sister and other pupils about them. Those pupils told her they were being taught seduction refusal techniques. She also said that *Mema kwa Vijana* is rumored to encourage pupils to have sex. She said that the messages to refuse men or, if unable to do that, to use condoms were somewhat misunderstood by pupils and parents. She said that even she found those messages confusing and contradictory. (PO-01-I-1-2f)

Peer Educators as Role Models

In group discussions and in-depth interviews, peer educators generally reported lower sexual risk behaviors than their peers. For example, in the group discussions held by HALIRA researchers and the AMREF intervention team with peer educators who were still in school, all reported that they had been abstinent since their training. In the second in-depth interview series, when respondents had left school three months to two years earlier, six male and two female randomly selected respondents said they had been peer educators. At that time, two of the males said they had never had sex, three males and two females said they had occasionally used condoms, and one male said he had used condoms many times. Specifically, the four sexually experienced young men said they had had one, two, three, or six lifetime sexual partners. The one who reported six partners was also the one who said he had used condoms many times, although his current sexual partner was pregnant. One of the young women was unmarried and reported three lifetime partners, while the other one was married and reported two. However, like several other women who had married between in-depth interviews, her reports were inconsistent, as she had reported several more lifetime sexual partners in her first interview two years earlier.

A minority of peer educators gave plausible, detailed, and consistent reports that they had actively tried to practice low-risk sexual behaviors, and particularly condom use, arguing for the validity of their reports. Case studies 3.1 and 3.2 provide two examples. While this is a promising finding, it is difficult to know if these young people were selected to be peer educators specifically because of unusual qualities that made them more risk averse, and/or they became more risk averse through their relatively intense *MEMA kwa Vijana* training. The characteristics of young people who actively tried to abstain, reduce partner number, practice fidelity, and/or use condoms will be examined more in chapters 8–10.

Overall, however, in-depth interviews and participant observation suggest that most peer educators engaged in sexual risk practices which were very similar to their peers. In one fishing village, for example, a female participant observation researcher got to know four fourteen- to eighteen-year-old Year 7 peer educator girls, all of whom seemed to be sexually active. Although these girls knew condoms protected against pregnancy and sexually transmitted infections, none had ever seen, let alone used, a condom. Two of them described their sexual relationships to the researcher, and the researcher witnessed the other two speaking closely and/or negotiating material exchange for sex with boys. In addition, one of the fourteen- to fifteen-year-old girls had unusually disreputable behavior in public. On one occasion the researcher saw that girl and a girlfriend laughingly remove their shirts, so that they were left only wearing their brassieres while walking down a path near some young men. Another time the researcher saw the same girl wearing a tight blouse and mascara, lipstick, and face powder at an afternoon soccer match, when very few others were similarly dressed and this might have been considered inappropriate.

In some villages, peer educators like the girl above had reputations for having unusually high-risk or disreputable behaviors. Some of these rumors seemed implausible (e.g., three female peer educators had sex with one man at the same time), but sometimes they clearly had some factual basis (e.g., in two villages female peer educators dropped out of school due to pregnancy). Female peer educators were especially vulnerable to rumors and criticism about their sexual activity. In interpreting such data it was difficult to determine if such peer educators had been nominated by their peers specifically because they were considered relatively sexually experienced, if they had increased their sexual activity after becoming peer educators, or if they had behavior typical of other youth but were simply subject to more scrutiny and false rumors because of their positions. Each of those possibilities probably had some validity in different peer educator experiences.

Generally, it seems likely that most peer educators had very similar sexual practices to their peers, with some perhaps briefly trying low-risk behaviors (e.g., condom use), but few intentionally and consistently doing so in an effective way long-term. This is reflected in comments made by a fourteen-year-old Year 6 peer educator:

> She said that other girls complained about [a certain girl] becoming a peer educator because she is an *mhuni*. She said that girl doesn't stay at home with

her aunt, but roams about in the village pretending to visit other girls until late in the evening. . . . She said that most girls and boys who are peer educators are just like any other pupils. The girls have boyfriends, and the boys have girlfriends. (PO-99-I-1-2f)

Similarly, when a participant observation researcher asked a male in his late teens what he thought of the *MEMA kwa Vijana* behavioral goals, he replied laughingly, "*MEMA kwa Vijana* peer educators themselves have sex without using condoms. So why shouldn't we?" (PO-01-I-4-5f).

DISCUSSION

A review of 162 preventative interventions with children found that high quality programs had carefully designed training manuals, well-conducted training courses, and reliable supervision of implementers (Dane and Schneider, 1998), all of which the *MEMA kwa Vijana* school program achieved. In addition, school programs may have disappointing outcomes if teachers or peer educators are unconvinced of the program's importance and practicality, and/or there is insufficient time for program delivery (e.g., Dane and Schneider, 1998; Visser, Schoeman, and Perold, 2004), but again the *MEMA kwa Vijana* school program did not experience such implementation problems. Strengths and limitations of the *MEMA kwa Vijana* school program will be considered more below.

The Role of Teachers

MEMA kwa Vijana teachers generally developed positive attitudes about teaching sexual and reproductive health topics and successfully imparted important information to pupils. The *MEMA kwa Vijana* curriculum (Appendices 1–3) was fairly simple and would not be considered unusual in North America or Europe. However, many aspects of it were exceptional within a Tanzanian primary school setting, including the participatory and entertaining teaching methods, and the discussion of HIV/AIDS, reproductive biology, and sexual behavior. Given teachers and pupils had little prior exposure to such techniques or information, they were eager to participate in training courses to improve their skills and understanding, even without financial compensation.

Almost all *MEMA kwa Vijana* teachers delivered the overwhelming majority of sessions and followed the detailed curriculum with remarkable quality and consistency. In addition, most intervention schools were visited by a health worker who addressed adolescent sexual health issues with pupils, and a large proportion of classes visited a health facility where they were introduced to adolescent sexual health services and saw a condom demonstration. It was helpful that the *MEMA kwa Vijana* curriculum was scheduled as a regular class within the broader school curriculum, and that related questions were included in the Year 7 examination, as this probably contributed to teachers and pupils taking *MEMA kwa Vijana* lessons seriously. The trial thus demonstrated that, despite great resource limitations, it is feasible to implement an intensive adolescent sexual health curriculum through existing government schools in a rural African setting. This is promising given that some other studies in sub-Saharan Africa have found problems with less formal implementation in school systems (e.g., Kinsman et al., 2001; Visser, Schoeman, and Perold, 2004).

Nonetheless, several important difficulties were encountered during the development and implementation of the *MEMA kwa Vijana* curriculum during the trial. From the onset, educational authorities required that the *MEMA kwa Vijana* curriculum focus on abstinence. This is not unusual in sub-Saharan Africa. In other school programs in Tanzania and neighboring Uganda, for example, official and/or community opposition to condom education in schools also led program implementers to remove condom-related material from their curricula, although such material was provided for teachers to use on an optional basis in the Tanzanian program (e.g., Klepp et al., 1994; Klepp et al., 1997; Shuey et al., 1999; Gallant and Maticka-Tyndale, 2004). For Years 5–7 of the initial *MEMA kwa Vijana* curriculum, the AMREF intervention team was able to negotiate permission to have very brief, positive messages about fidelity and condom use, and then in later versions of the curriculum they successfully advocated for more detailed information about condoms in Years 6 and 7. However, even this was very limited, as condoms could only be verbally described in class, and skills modeled in dramas and role plays focused on sexual refusal, not negotiation of premarital fidelity or condom use.

Preexisting teaching methodology and pupil-teacher dynamics also posed challenges for the *MEMA kwa Vijana* school program. Tanzanian primary school teachers typically used very didactic teaching methods, but *MEMA kwa Vijana* trained teachers to teach the curriculum using more interactive methods, as is widely recommended within global adolescent health education (e.g., WHO, 1997; WHO, 2003a; UNESCO, 2009a; UNESCO, 2009b). The *MEMA kwa Vijana* activities were fairly simple and neither as subtle nor as participatory as some active-learning and inquiry-based teaching techniques promoted within international "best practice" HIV prevention curricula. Nonetheless, *MEMA kwa Vijana* teachers often had difficulty adopting these new approaches, as has also been found in some other studies in sub-Saharan Africa (e.g., Kuhn, Steinberg, and Mathews, 1994; Shuey et al., 1999; Kinsman et al., 1999; Campbell, 2003; Ahmed et al., 2006; Mukoma et al., 2009; Njue et al., 2009).

In addition, although intervention teachers may have reduced some undesirable practices after *MEMA kwa Vijana* training (e.g., corporal punishment), it is less clear that they reduced others (e.g., sexual abuse of pupils). Male teachers who sexually abuse school girls can cause great harm to a sexual health program by modeling inappropriate behavior, by instilling fear and distrust of the curriculum associated with the teacher, and even by exploiting intervention classes as new opportunities to abuse pupils. In such settings, close supervision and appropriate responses are crucial for sexual health programs, and there is a broader need for national policies and norms that better prevent, monitor, and correct such abuses (WHO, 1997; Panos Institute, 2003). A recent campaign in Kenya shows promise in this area, as authorities there took advantage of the now widespread use of mobile telephones and sponsored a nationwide confidential helpline to identify teachers who sexually abused pupils. Their subsequent investigation led to the firing of over one thousand teachers, who were mostly teachers working in rural areas (British Broadcasting Corporation, 2010).

The Tanzanian primary school system was one of the most disadvantaged in the world at the time of the *MEMA kwa Vijana* trial. Some improvements have been made to it since then due to government efforts as well as nongovernmental programs working at a district level (United Republic of Tanzania, 2003; World Bank, 2004; Sedere, Mengele, and Kajela, 2008). For example, the national Primary Education Development Plan dramatically increased primary school enrollment, refurbished and built new classrooms, and developed stronger local management and financial systems (Benson, 2006). However, it has been far less successful in motivating teachers and improving teaching quality (Benson, 2006). Substantial long-term improvements of infrastructure, resources, and teacher capacity and supervision remain critical. Such efforts may be important in improving adolescent sexual health even in the absence of specific sexual health programs.

In addition, however, a more cost-effective and sustainable way of providing teachers with the knowledge, skills, and motivation to deliver high quality sexual education would be to incorporate a training course into their initial education in teacher training colleges. This could have other potential advantages. Being new to the profession, teacher trainees might be more open to adopting progressive styles of teaching. In addition, the participatory teaching skills they develop through such training could improve their generic teaching style, and thus benefit all pupils and courses they taught from the start of their career. Finally, it would increase the possibility that all teachers in a school were supportive of sexual health curricula and capable of teaching it, which can be particularly important in schools where there is frequent staff turnover, as was common in rural Mwanza during the study period.

The Role of Peer Educators

Limited and well monitored peer education within the *MEMA kwa Vijana* school program was useful. The vast majority of *MEMA kwa Vijana* peer educators seemed enthusiastic to participate in the training and very appreciative of the information they learned there. The dramas were also popular amongst intervention participants, as has also been found in other programs in sub-Saharan Africa (e.g., Bagamoyo College of Arts et al., 2002; Middelkoop et al., 2006; Kamo et al., 2008). Most peer educators acted out the dramas in a consistent and entertaining way; critically, this seemed to succeed on a large scale because the dramas were carefully scripted. Similarly, the other peer educator activities in the classroom seemed effective because they were structured and complemented and supported the teacher-led curriculum. The limited nature of those activities and their close monitoring seemed to help avoid unintended consequences, such as the provision of misinformation or other pupils stigmatizing peer educators.

The qualitative evaluation also suggests that many peer educators personally benefited from their relatively in-depth training and experience. Often the intervention seemed to have more of an impact on peer educator knowledge, attitudes, and—to a lesser extent—behaviors than those of their peers. Some other studies in Africa and elsewhere have also found that in-depth training for peer educators can be an effective intervention in itself, enhancing peer educator understanding, self-efficacy, and low-risk practices beyond those of their peers (e.g., Forrest, 2004; Bastien, Flisher et al., 2008). This will be discussed more in chapters 8–10, which describe young people who practiced low-risk behaviors.

Despite these positive findings, several challenges were also evident within the peer education component. Intervention participants sometimes misconstrued drama content or used it mockingly outside of class, and peer educators—especially girls—were sometimes stigmatized for performing "bad" characters, until the curriculum was revised to eliminate such roles. Peer educators' ability to informally educate their peers and to be role models for them seemed quite variable. Peer educators sometimes had difficulty understanding and independently conveying key concepts to peers in an accurate and clear way. Importantly, providing peer educators with detailed information books seemed to address this to a limited extent in the latter half of the trial. In addition, while many peer educators supported the intervention behavioral goals, they often did not perceive them as realistic and did not practice them themselves. The wide age range within many classes posed further challenges to peer educators, some of whom were at quite different cognitive, social, physical, and sexual life stages than many of their classmates.

These findings suggest that the brief *MEMA kwa Vijana* peer educator training was not enough to overcome several barriers to effective peer education, especially for a sensitive, controversial, and potentially stigmatizing topic such as sexual behavior. Barriers included pupils' low literacy and education levels; their subservience within a hierarchical, punitive, and didactic school setting; social norms discouraging young people from acting as experts with their peers or the general community; and powerful, contradictory sexual norms and expectations.

Similarly, in a process evaluation of peer education in one South African school, Campbell (2003) found that a tradition of authoritarian teaching and rote learning made it difficult for peer educators to work independently and to use participatory methods as intended. Despite being trained to use drama and roleplays, the peer educators in her study tended to use didactic teaching methods. Campbell (2003) further notes that, without explicit training in critical thinking skills, the peer educators lacked the skills and social insights to lead discussions about factors which place young people in vulnerable situations. Teacher-pupil dynamics also posed challenges, as teachers did not take a supportive and non-directive role within the program as intended, but instead took absolute control over it, insisting that peer educators emphasize abstinence over other low-risk behaviors, determining the timing of their work and their access to resources, and selecting new peer educators themselves.

Such findings suggest that, to maximize the potential of school-based peer education in sub-Saharan Africa, much more in-depth training is needed. Within the *MEMA kwa Vijana* intervention, however, a more intensive peer educator training course would have been difficult to achieve given the large scale of the program. It also would have been logistically challenging to sustain long-term, because of the need to train six new Year 5 peer educators per school per year. The practical difficulty of implementing large-scale and sustainable peer education has been recognized in other studies also. For example, to implement a peer education program in fifteen South African public high schools, different non-governmental organizations were tasked with training peer educators over a wide geographic area. In practice, this resulted in very different approaches to program implementation, for instance, trainers from faith-based organizations only promoted abstinence and did not speak openly about sex or condoms (Mason-Jones, Mathews, and Flisher, 2011). An evaluation of the overall program found no evidence of intervention impact on any reported sexual risk behaviors (Mason-Jones, Mathews, and Flisher, 2011).

In summary, the HALIRA study found that peer education can be a valuable, subsidiary component of a school-based sexual health intervention in rural Africa. However, the logistical challenges involved in maintaining a large-scale and sustainable peer education program means that training courses may need to be fairly simple. In addition, peer educator activities must be very carefully designed and monitored throughout intervention implementation to avoid unintended consequences, particularly in a context where adolescents have very low education and social status.

Scale-Up of the School Program

From 2004 to 2008, the *MEMA kwa Vijana* school program was scaled up from 62 to 649 rural Mwanza primary schools. A detailed description and evaluation of that scale-up is provided elsewhere, and those findings will only be summarized below (Renju, Andrew, Medard et al., 2010; Renju, Makokha et al., 2010). During the scale-up, the AMREF intervention team no longer had responsibility for teacher training and supervision; those tasks were instead carried out by government authorities. The scale-up began with twelve-day training courses for forty-four district and seventy-eight ward education officials, who together then led three-day training courses for 1,395 head teachers and support teachers, and twelve-day training courses for new *MEMA kwa Vijana* teachers (Renju, Andrew, Medard et al., 2010). For the scale-up, several modifications were made to intervention implementation and supervision, including: teachers were trained one time only (not annually); teachers selected and trained new peer educators themselves; the peer educator training was ad hoc and focused on drama performance only; school program supervision took place as part of routine district supervision visits (rather than special quarterly visits); and the dedicated annual Youth Health Week was eliminated or replaced by activities incorporated into existing commemorative events, such as the Day of the African Child, or World AIDS Day.

The *MEMA kwa Vijana* school program scale-up was impeded by delayed training courses, high teacher turnover, and limited incentives for teachers to teach *MEMA kwa Vijana* activities (Renju, Andrew, Medard et al., 2010). Process evaluation in eighteen representative schools found that teachers were enthusiastic and interacted well with pupils, pupils enjoyed the sessions, and the scripted drama serial continued to be a valuable participatory method. However, there was no uniformity in the number of peer educators teachers chose in each school (ranging from two to nine per class). In addition, although many teachers reported that they selected peer educators immediately after the teacher training, observation indicated that the majority of peer educators were only selected and taught the dramas after teachers were informed that evaluators would be visiting the school. These findings suggest that the devolution of the peer educator training to teachers is likely to have substantially diluted the quality and consistency of the peer education component.

Within the taught curriculum, coverage of biological topics, which were usually scheduled early in the school year, was better than coverage of the skills-oriented, psychosocial sessions. During the scale-up, there were relatively few reciprocal visits between the school and health facilities when compared to the trial. Scale-up evaluators recommended that any further expansion of the program should include: (1) more intensive training of teachers to teach complex, skills-related activities; and (2) strengthening of external factors to motivate teachers to fully implement the curriculum, that is, increased supervision, national directives, and inclusion of curriculum material in pupils' national examinations.

The next chapter will provide process evaluations of the two remaining *MEMA kwa Vijana* intervention components: youth-friendly health services and out-of-school youth condom distribution. Chapter 7 will return to the process evaluation findings presented here in examining the impact of the *MEMA kwa Vijana* intervention on abstinence, sexual partner number, fidelity, and condom use.

NOTE

1. Some material in this chapter was adapted from Plummer, Mary L., D. Wight, A. I. N. Obasi, J. Wamoyi, G. Mshana, J. Todd, B. C. Mazige, M. Makokha, R. J. Hayes, and D. A. Ross. 2007. A process evaluation of a school-based adolescent sexual health intervention in rural Tanzania: The *MEMA kwa Vijana* programme. *Health Education Research* 22(4): 500–12.

Chapter Six

MEMA kwa Vijana Health Services and Condom Distribution

HIV prevention experts increasingly recommend that interventions combine multiple, promising approaches to better promote low-risk sexual behaviors, as discussed in chapter 1 (Coates, Richter, and Caceres, 2008; Piot et al., 2008; Hankins and Zalduondo, 2010; Kurth et al., 2011). In keeping with that principle, the *MEMA kwa Vijana* health service and condom distribution components were developed to complement the main, school-based intervention component described in chapters 4 and 5. Both of these components will be described and evaluated in this chapter.

The chapter begins with a review of health services in rural Mwanza at the start of the study. That will be followed by a brief background of "youth-friendly" strategies to promote adolescent sexual health services in sub-Saharan Africa. Then the *MEMA kwa Vijana* health service component will be evaluated, including the training of health workers, the outreach they conducted in primary schools and health facilities, and the clinical sexual and reproductive health services they provided to young people within facilities. The second half of the chapter will then evaluate the *MEMA kwa Vijana* out-of-school youth condom distribution initiative. It will begin with a brief background on condom distribution in sub-Saharan Africa, and will then describe the availability of condoms in rural Mwanza at the beginning of the study. *MEMA kwa Vijana* condom distribution will then be evaluated, including public awareness of the initiative, outreach, sales, and the potential of condom distributors to be role models.

HEALTH SERVICES IN RURAL MWANZA
AT THE TIME OF THE STUDY

At the start of the *MEMA kwa Vijana* trial, the government supported six district hospitals, twenty-three health centers, and about 150 health dispensaries in rural Mwanza Region; in addition, there were three private missionary hospitals (Changalucha et al., 2002). A government health center was supposed to have eight to twelve trained personnel and to be managed by a clinical officer who had completed secondary school and received three additional years of medical training. A government dispensary instead was supposed to have two or three trained staff and was to be led by an assistant clinical officer who had some secondary school education and three additional years of medical training. However, shortages of health workers in all types of health facilities mean lower cadre staff often worked above the level for which they were qualified (Renju, Andrew, Nyalali et al., 2010). A health center typically had twenty to twenty-five beds for inpatients, while a dispensary had three for short-term observations which were usually used by women after childbirth (Changalucha et al., 2002). Sometimes a health center also had a laboratory technician and a microscope, but such equipment was often damaged and supplies of laboratory reagents were irregular (Changalucha et al., 2002).

The twenty *MEMA kwa Vijana* trial communities were served by thirty-nine health facilities (eighteen intervention, twenty-one control). A few facilities in each arm were health centers, but most were dispensaries. There were also a few private health facilities in the study area. The AMREF intervention team ensured that both intervention and control facilities met certain basic standards of service during the trial. First, each received quarterly supervision of their general sexually transmitted infection treatment services. Second, each was provided with an adequate supply of sexually transmitted infection medications, condoms, other contraceptives, and related medical supplies. Third, the intervention team tried to ensure that at least two prescribing health workers in each facility had received training in the prior two years to treat sexually transmitted infections syndromically. As noted in chapter 1, syndromic management of infection involves treating a patient for all infections that could cause his or her symptoms when laboratory tests are not available (Grosskurth et al., 1995; Johnson et al., 2011). However, ensuring this level of training throughout the trial proved difficult, because health worker turnover rates were high. In the three years between the 1998 *MEMA kwa Vijana* baseline survey and the 2001–2002 final trial survey, for example, 30 percent of intervention prescribing staff and 49 percent of those in control facilities were replaced (Larke et al., 2010).

None of the four intervention villages which were visited during HALIRA participant observation had a government health facility within the village. In one village, however, a private, Protestant health dispensary provided local people with medical services. In the remaining three villages, residents who needed health care typically first treated themselves with home remedies (e.g., traditional or over-the-counter medications). If symptoms did not resolve, then they usually sought treatment from a local traditional healer or private medical practitioner before traveling to another facility in another village or town. In the inland village near a mine, for example, two untrained men illegally practiced western medicine out of their homes. One was a former nursing assistant and the other was a health officer, whose official responsibilities were health education and monitoring public hygiene. These men prescribed villagers with medications, including giving them injections using needles and syringes which they said had been sterilized in boiling water. They also assisted pregnant women who were having difficult deliveries. In another inland participant observation village, residents expended a great deal of time and effort trying to build their own dispensary, including raising funds from each family and slowly amassing almost one thousand cement bricks. At the end of the study, however, that project seemed to have stalled.

"YOUTH-FRIENDLY" SEXUAL HEALTH INTERVENTIONS IN SUB-SAHARAN AFRICA

Medical services were extremely limited in rural Mwanza at the time of the study, as described above and in chapter 3, but sexual health services for adolescents were particularly weak. In Mwanza, as elsewhere in sub-Saharan Africa, such services were often constrained by limited resources and staff training, low levels of efficiency, poor privacy and confidentiality, and negative health worker attitudes (e.g., Langhaug et al., 2003; Wood and Jewkes, 2006; Kipp et al., 2007; Arube-Wani, Jitta, and Ssengooba, 2008; Mathews et al., 2009).

"Youth-friendly" health service interventions attempt to address many of these challenges through specialized staff training courses and facility improvement. These interventions generally intend to provide young people with: information about HIV and other sexual health issues; condoms and other contraceptive services; diagnosis and treatment for sexually transmitted infections; confidentiality, privacy, respect, and lack of judgment during health care visits; reduced fees or subsidized commodities; convenient working hours and locations; and/or community outreach (WHO, 2002). They may also provide male circumcision and HIV testing and counseling services.

Most youth-friendly service interventions in sub-Saharan Africa have attempted to improve existing public services (e.g., Kim et al., 2001; Mmari and Magnani, 2003; Okonofua et al., 2003; Dickson, Ashton, and Smith, 2007; Mathews et al., 2009; Cowan et al., 2010). A few, however, have created new health facilities or clinical services integrated within multi-purpose youth centers (e.g., Neukom and Ashford, 2003). Reviews of youth-friendly programs in sub-Saharan Africa have found that they can increase young people's use of services, particularly if health worker training is accompanied by outreach and other activities to make the services more accessible to young people (Dick et al., 2006; Tylee et al., 2007; Mavedzenge, Doyle, and Ross, 2011).

MEMA KWA VIJANA HEALTH SERVICES

Health Worker Training and Supervision

The youth-friendly health services component of the *MEMA kwa Vijana* intervention involved training two to four health workers per facility with the goal of promoting privacy, confidentiality, and empathy in adolescent sexual and reproductive health services. First, the six-day training course sought to improve health worker understanding of reproductive biology, adolescent sexuality, and the importance of free and confidential contraceptive advice and sexually transmitted infection treatment for adolescents. Second, it sought to develop health worker ability to discuss young people's sexual health concerns in a private and non-judgmental way. Third, the training engaged with health workers about how they could feasibly conduct outreach to promote their services with young people in their communities. By the end of the training course, health workers typically planned three types of outreach service: health worker visits to *MEMA kwa Vijana* intervention schools to encourage appropriate health facility attendance; health worker hosting of class visits at their facilities to provide condom demonstrations and an overview of services ("Youth Health Day"); and health worker participation during Youth Health Week activities.

In questionnaires completed before the first (1998) *MEMA kwa Vijana* health worker training course, the vast majority of health workers reported positive attitudes toward teaching young people about condom use. A comparison of health worker and head teacher attitudes prior to training found that health workers were less likely to believe that condom discussion or distribution would encourage youth sexual activity (1 percent versus 18 percent, respectively), and more likely to report use of condoms themselves (69 percent versus 47 percent, respectively) (Obasi et al., 2000). However, many were concerned that community members would perceive condom promotion for young people as promotion of adolescent sexual activity in general

(Obasi et al., 2000). Overall health workers responded quickly and favorably to the training courses, particularly as many had seen evidence of the high prevalence of sexually transmitted infections in rural areas first-hand. In post-training questionnaires, health worker attitudes toward adolescent confidentiality and access to contraceptives other than condoms improved significantly.

A three-day refresher training course was conducted with new and experienced intervention health workers approximately eighteen months after that first one. In addition to quarterly supervision of general sexually transmitted infection services, intervention health facilities also received quarterly supervision of the quality of their sexual health services for young people.

Health Worker Outreach

At the end of the first year of the intervention (1999), 89 percent of intervention teachers reported that health workers had visited their school class to discuss *MEMA kwa Vijana* topics, and 92 percent said they had taken a *MEMA kwa Vijana* class to visit the local health facility (Obasi et al., 2006). This was supported by the 1999 process evaluation survey, in which teacher reports of health worker visits to schools differed considerably between randomly selected intervention and control schools, including the number of schools visited by health workers (10/11 versus 3/10, respectively); discussion of sexual and reproductive health with pupils during such visits (9/11 versus 2/10); and health worker invitations to pupils to visit health facilities (5/11 versus 1/10).

Surveyed pupils and health workers reported similar patterns. At the 2001–2002 trial *MEMA kwa Vijana* survey, for example, 65 percent of intervention participants reported that a health worker had visited their class, compared to only 34 percent of control participants. In addition, 44 percent of intervention participants reported that their class had visited a health facility, compared to only 10 percent of control participants (Larke et al., 2010). In addition, in all four participant observation intervention villages, intervention participants reported that their classes had visited the nearest government health facility for Youth Health Day activities once or twice, and a large majority of in-depth interview respondents reported this as well. Those few respondents who said they had not attended a health facility with their class said their class never went, or they missed school that day due to other responsibilities (i.e., domestic responsibilities for several girls, and school prefect responsibilities for one boy).

Qualitative research found that the collaboration between schools and health facilities generally worked very well, particularly in the critical areas of increasing young people's familiarity with health facilities and improving their understanding of condom use. During class visits to health facilities, intervention participants almost always observed a condom demonstration and often also were given a brief tour of the facility and were told about family planning methods and treatment services for sexually transmitted infections. For example, during participant observation a twelve-year-old girl in Year 5 told a researcher:

> One day her class went to a health center, where they were taught how to use condoms. She explained that when the health workers teach this they roll a condom on to something made in the form of a penis. . . . She said those who wanted to take condoms and contraceptive pills were allowed to take whatever quantity they wanted. (PO-01-I-4-5f)

Many young people lived far from health facilities and had never previously attended one, so class visits were memorable ways to introduce them to health workers and the services. These experiences seemed to be quite salient for young people, as months or years later most in-depth interview respondents could describe such visits in some detail. The following examples were from in-depth interviews at the end of the trial, one to two years after respondents had participated in the intervention:

> *R*: A condom is a soft tube specifically made for prevention of pregnancies during sexual intercourse. . . . Let's say it's as long as this bottle. Now it's a bit round, and it's very soft. It's used when you want to perform a sexual act. You put it on your penis to prevent pregnancies or HIV and other diseases during sexual intercourse.
>
> *I*: Is there any person that showed you a condom?
>
> *R*: Yes, at the health center. . . . We [pupils] were told to go to the health center to see a condom and how to use it. . . . The doctor showed us.
>
> *I*: Did he/she explain how a condom works?
>
> *R*: Yes, he/she said during sex it prevents vaginal fluid from penetrating the penis, in case that vaginal fluid is mixed with a disease that the girl may have. If that vaginal fluid enters you, you too will suffer from that disease. (II-02-I-280-m)

> *R*: Health workers say, "Please come and get treated, the services are free. No one will demand money." And they also say, "We are doctors and we have taken an oath, we cannot tell patients' secrets. So don't fear to come and get treated." So they help people in that way.
>
> *I*: Did they come to your school?
>
> *R*: Yes, they came to school to talk with us twice. Teachers also took us to the hospital twice. . . . [The health workers] told us, "Here is where we treat sexu-

ally transmitted infections. So if you feel that you have a disease, come here, the services are free, don't hesitate." (II-02-I-298-m)

Teacher and health worker initiative and collaboration were encouraged by the *MEMA kwa Vijana* program. Their success in this is noteworthy, particularly as it involved extra effort on the part of both health workers and teachers without compensation, as well as visits to schools or health facilities which usually required traveling many kilometers on foot or bicycle. Despite these achievements, however, there were occasions when health workers and teachers worked together in ways that were undesirable and inappropriate. Occasionally, for instance, intervention participants reported that boys were shown and offered condoms at health facilities but girls were not. One example: "The boys were told, 'If you want condoms, you should follow me.' That they should follow those [male] teachers and hospital workers. . . . And the girls instead should follow the women [female health workers]. . . . Girls never went for condoms, girls only went for oral contraceptives" (II-02-I-290-f).

School girls' privacy was also sometimes violated when teachers and health workers collaborated together. In one extreme incident reported during an in-depth interview, teachers and health workers instructed several girls to show their genitals to other girls at school, including one who had gone to a health facility for treatment of a sexually transmitted infection. An eighteen-year-old woman explained:

R: We saw a girl at school whose private parts were infected. . . . People came from [the government health facility]. I think she had gone there to be treated. Then the teachers called her into their office. They made her spread her legs apart, and beside her they made some younger girls [with no visible symptoms] do so also. Then we were called, just a few of us, to go see . . . her private parts . . . which had become white. . . . They asked, "Between this one and those ones, who is healthy?" The younger girls said, "We are healthy." (II-02-I-333-f)

This incident violated the privacy and dignity of all of the girls who were made to expose their genitals, and it also stigmatized and violated the confidentiality of the girl who had sought treatment at the health facility. There were no other reports of an incident like this, suggesting that it was an isolated event. However, there was one inappropriate practice that was widespread before the trial and which continued in both intervention and control communities during the trial, that is, the practice of teachers taking groups of school girls for mandatory pregnancy examinations at the nearest health facility. Data from all research methods suggest that this practice continued in many schools after the intervention began, even sometimes taking place within a Youth Health Day visit to a health facility. One example was provided by a married and pregnant eighteen-year-old who had completed school fifteen months earlier:

> *I*: Has anyone ever shown you a condom? . . .
>
> *R*: I have seen them . . . we went there to [the hospital] . . . to see examples of how men put on condoms. . . . We were told, "Go to the hospital to be examined for pregnancy. Go now, and you will also see what the environment is like there at the hospital." (II-02-I-290-f)

Some school girls seemed to take such pregnancy examinations for granted and did not consider them a problem, but others feared and/or disliked them. While some teachers and health workers may have had good intentions in carrying out this practice— trying, for example, to ensure that a girl who was pregnant received adequate prenatal care—its forced and often punitive nature undermined intervention goals. Some teachers and health workers incidentally mentioned this practice during *MEMA kwa Vijana* training courses early in the trial, when they clearly did not see it as problematic. In subsequent training courses it was systematically addressed and discouraged by trainers, and it was reported less frequently in later training courses and group discussions.

Extent of Clinical Services

Despite the high rates of sexually transmitted infections among young people in rural Mwanza prior to the *MEMA kwa Vijana* trial (Obasi et al., 2001; Changalucha et al., 2002), very few young people went to health facilities to seek treatment for them. At the onset of the trial, only one fifteen- to twenty-four-year-old woman sought such treatment in each health facility per month, and for fifteen- to twenty-four-year-old men this was even less frequent, that is, one man every two months (Larke et al., 2010). Treatment rates may have been higher for women because many attended health facilities for prenatal and pediatric care, so those services may have been more familiar and accessible to them.

By the end of the trial, there was weak evidence that the intervention had increased fifteen- to twenty-four-year-old women's attendance at health facilities for treatment of sexually transmitted infections, but this was not significant (p = 0.087). In contrast, fifteen- to twenty-four-year-old men's attendance for this reason increased significantly in intervention health facilities, although this was only a very modest increase in absolute terms (i.e., an increase to one male patient per month) (p = 0.005) (Larke et al., 2010). This probably reflected changes in health-seeking behavior rather than a higher incidence of sexually transmitted infections, because there were no significant differences in rates of infection between young men in intervention and control communities at the end of the trial (Ross et al., 2007).

In the late 1990s, the Tanzanian Ministry of Health supplied government health facilities across the country with condoms which were to be distributed to patients for free; in 1999 alone, for example, health facilities were sent forty million condoms (Brent, 2010). However, all of the *MEMA kwa Vijana* intervention and control health facility records indicated that they had not distributed any condoms prior to the trial. During the trial, the number of condoms distributed increased in both intervention and control facilities, and the increase was significantly greater for fifteen- to twenty-four-year-olds in intervention communities ($p = 0.008$) (Larke et al., 2010). Again, however, the absolute numbers of condoms distributed remained extremely low, peaking at five condoms per facility per month in intervention health facilities in 2000.

By the end of the trial most intervention participants knew that condoms and other contraception were available to them free-of-charge at health facilities, as well as treatment of sexually transmitted infections. However, it is likely that young people with sexual and reproductive health needs did not seek clinical services for several reasons. These include having no symptoms or only minor symptoms of infection; not feeling comfortable attending a health facility without their parents' awareness (and not wanting to tell their parents about their health concern); and/or being embarrassed or worried about poor confidentiality and stigma, particularly girls. In addition, the distance between most villages and their closest health facility remained prohibitive, as this could make a visit to a health facility an all-day undertaking. Although such a distance was a barrier in and of itself, in combination with class visits to health facilities it sometimes reassured youth of the confidential nature of health services, because they came to believe health workers would not recognize them or know their families. The following in-depth interview excerpts were typical:

R: Health workers will keep [patient information] secret . . . because it is not easy for them to go and tell somebody else, like maybe a neighbor in the village. It is not easy, unless he/she is very close to that patient. (II-02-I-331-f)

R: It is the custom of a doctor is to keep a patient's secrets. . . . Because there are many people that go to get services there. Given how many patients there are, the doctor doesn't say about each one, "He/she is ill in such-and-such a way." (II-02-I-295-m)

However, the relatively few young people who lived in a village close to a health facility and who knew health workers personally tended to be less confident of patients' privacy and confidentiality:

R: It is possible . . . that health workers will tell others patients' information. Because I have heard about it . . . I have heard a certain health worker telling people such a thing, saying, "We have diagnosed so-and-so and we have seen that he/she has a certain disease . . . a sexually transmitted disease." (II-02-I-287-f)

Quality of Clinical Services

In both intervention and control communities, villagers usually were appreciative of government health services, because most individuals or a family member had been treated for a common condition (e.g., fever or diarrhea) at a health facility at some point. The following comment by a twenty-year-old woman was typical: "People with diseases go to the health facility and are given medicine to swallow. I think the services are good because they make people recover and no longer feel pain" (II-02-I-314-f). When a respondent did criticize the clinical services at a particular health facility, it was usually because they or a family member had had difficulty obtaining treatment (e.g., due to equipment failure or medication shortages), or they perceived the treatment they received to be ineffective (e.g., because symptoms reoccurred).

The few in-depth interview respondents and young participant observation informants who said they had sought treatment for sexually transmitted infections at health facilities said they only did so after experiencing severe symptoms over an extended period. Those who were treated successfully were usually very grateful for those services, as seen in case study 3.3.

The simulated patient exercises suggest that the provision of such services or contraceptive services were of a somewhat higher quality and consistency in intervention facilities than in control facilities. That research suggested that intervention health workers were relatively matter-of-fact and non-judgmental in responding to adolescent sexual health requests. Control health workers instead sometimes initially voiced shock, uncertainty, and disapproval before, usually, providing the young person with the requested services.

Specifically, based on simulated patient transcripts alone, five out of six of the intervention health workers and five out of ten of those in control facilities were fairly responsive and non-judgmental, and provided patients with basic to good information. Of the three simulated patient scenarios, this included four of the six about sexually transmitted infection concerns, and five of the six condom requests, but only one of the four (female only) family planning requests. It is not clear why the results for family planning requests had generally poorer results than the other simulated patient scenarios. It may be due to chance, greater judgment of sexually active girls than boys, and/or the relatively complex nature of that visit, which could involve a description of diverse family planning methods and a physical examination.

The following excerpt is taken from the one family planning visit that was ranked highly amongst the simulated patient exercises. It involved an intervention health worker who provided one of the most patient, respectful, and informative responses in any of the simulated patient exercises:

HW: Mm, now . . . there are several types of family planning methods. . . . There are oral pills, to be swallowed daily. Then there is the loop [intra-uterine device]. It is placed in the uterus. It stays there and normally lasts eight years before it becomes ineffective.

SP: Fine.

HW: Then there is the injection [Depo Provera]. Each injection is given after this many months [holds up three fingers and awaits response] . . .

SP: Three.

HW: Three. Then you are injected again. And then there are condoms. This condom is used during sexual intercourse. Yes, you should put it on [words unclear]. . . . Mm, I think there at school, you have already been taught about condoms, have you not?

SP: Yes.

HW: Yes, therefore, when he ejaculates, his sperm remain inside what?

SP: Inside the condom.

HW: Inside the condom, so it is difficult to impregnate you, and even to become infected. A condom has this number of benefits [holds up two fingers].

SP: Two.

HW: Preventing disease and preventing pregnancy. Those are the benefits of a condom. . . . Now, for you, I don't know which of these methods you have chosen? (SP-00-I-14-7f)

Health workers who were ranked highly, such as the one above, generally corrected myths volunteered by a simulated patient. For example, during one condom demonstration, a female simulated patient asked whether it is true that new condoms have holes, and an intervention health worker replied, "People who tell you that are lying to you. Condoms have been checked by the International Bureau of Standards specifically to ensure that they are safe" (SP-00-I-28-10f).

Simulated patients who requested condoms at health facilities were all given condoms if condoms were available, regardless of intervention status. Even in the one instance when condoms were not available, the intervention health worker was responsive and encouraged the girl to abstain until they were available, saying, "Now, just try to exercise self-control, just for this week, because then condoms will be brought here, right? So even if you come, say, on Friday, you can get them then" (SP-00-I-29-10f).

Male simulated patients requesting condoms were only given a condom demonstration in intervention facilities, although females were given demonstrations irrespective of the health facility intervention status. For example, an intervention health worker gave the following description as he provided a condom demonstration for an adolescent boy, pausing to wait for affirmation after each question:

> *HW*: First, it's a matter of opening [the package] right? . . . Mm. Now you're erec-erect . . . you hold this nipple, you press it first. You put your iron bar [slang for penis] inside of it. It will roll downwards, right? Until it reaches its end. Then you will start work [intercourse]. After one ejaculation, you do what? Remove the condom while the penis is still erect. . . . It's weak then, so it will be easy to get out, right? Now . . . the sperm will have dropped into [the condom]. Therefore, you should tie it up, tie it up completely, right? And put it aside. If you want to continue, you take another one. Every . . . let's say, every time you "work," you will use a new condom, right? . . . Now, do you have any other questions you want to ask?

> *SP*: Yes! I have heard some people say that condoms have holes. Others say they have AIDS.

> *HW*: No. Those are false beliefs, because condoms are absolutely approved. Right, sir? So you should neither worry nor allow anybody to tell you lies, like condoms have AIDS or condoms have holes, okay? You should go and use them as best you know how. (SP-00-I-26-9m)

Simulated patient exercises suggested that intervention health workers were more comprehensive than control health workers in the information they provided about condoms. Two of the three intervention health workers gave condom demonstrations to simulated patients who expressed concern about a sexually transmitted infection but did not specifically request condoms. None of the control health workers did so. Similarly, some intervention health workers gave condoms as well as oral contraceptives to girls who requested oral contraceptives. Again, none of the control health workers did this. However, enthusiasm to promote condoms may have sometimes contributed to the perpetuation of misinformation. For example, one intervention health worker initially encouraged a simulated patient to adopt condoms rather than another method of contraception by saying that Depo Provera can "mess up your [future] childbearing" (SP-00-I-21-7f). This health worker later correctly explained that a woman may not be able to become pregnant for several months after stopping her Depo Provera injections, but the initially extreme phrasing was misleading.

In a minority of control health facilities—but none of the intervention facilities—health workers were very rude or judgmental and did not provide adequate information to simulated patients. For example, in one control facility the health worker refused to see a boy who voiced concern about a sexually transmitted infection, because the boy did not bring payment. Although the service should have been provided free-of-charge, when the boy said he could not pay the health worker replied, "Nonsense! Get out of here!" (SP-00-C-11-8m).

Despite this evidence of higher quality youth-friendly services in intervention health facilities, the simulated patient exercises indicated several problems which were common to both intervention and control health facilities during the trial, including late opening times, poor privacy, and inappropriate personal questions. In almost all facilities, health workers arrived two to three hours after the scheduled opening time each morning. Less than half of simulated patients were able to discuss their problems with a health care worker in a private and confidential setting, and this did not differ by intervention or control status. Patients were typically expected to discuss their problems in an open room with staff members walking in and out during the consultation and with other patients able to overhear. For example, the consultation room in one intervention health facility was separated from the waiting area by a half-built wall, so that conversations on either side could easily be overheard.

In addition, almost every health worker asked simulated patients unnecessary questions about their identity during their conversation, such as the names of their parents and local relatives. The timing, intensity, and tone of these questions varied, ranging from brief and curious to disapproving and interrogatory, but no intervention or control health workers seemed to feel such questions were inappropriate. Similarly, when a physical examination was expected, as was the case in two intervention and two control facilities where oral contraceptives were requested, health workers provided very little or no explanations of the purpose or nature of the examination before attempting to proceed with it.

Health Workers as Role Models

Adult villagers usually had relatively little contact with health workers and that contact usually took place within a professional setting, so they knew relatively little about health workers' personal lives. Thus unlike *MEMA kwa Vijana* teachers and condom distributors, villagers rarely seemed to criticize particular health workers for being hypocritical and not practicing the low-risk sexual behaviors they recommended. Similarly, intervention participants usually had little personal experience with health workers beyond *MEMA kwa Vijana* class visits. In in-depth interviews they thus usually said they had no opinion of health workers as behavioral role models, other than to assume that they practiced the low-risk behaviors they promoted.

CONDOM PROMOTION AND DISTRIBUTION
IN SUB-SAHARAN AFRICA

Condom distribution in sub-Saharan Africa has often taken place through social marketing initiatives. These programs adapt commercial marketing and sales techniques to promote condom use. Socially marketed condoms are sold at a fraction of their actual cost in order to make them affordable to poor populations. These subsidized condoms are not given away for free, however, because free distribution has been found to contribute to waste and misuse. In 1999, for example, over half of the condoms distributed and/or sold in Tanzania are believed to have been used for unintended purposes, such as to carry or store water (Brent, 2010).

Condom social marketing typically involves private-sector distribution of condoms through a variety of formal and informal venues, such as health facilities, shops, kiosks, pharmacies, bars, discos, hotels, and guesthouses (Knerr, 2011). In many African countries, the organization Population Services International has coordinated national distribution of free and subsidized condoms (e.g., Neukom and Ashford, 2003; Pfeiffer, 2004; Agha and Meekers, 2004; Papo et al., 2011). Their efforts have typically focused on urban areas because of the relatively high HIV prevalence in those areas and the great logistical difficulties involved in supplying rural regions. For example, an affiliate of Population Services International conducted a multimedia condom social marketing campaign for urban fifteen- to twenty-four-year-olds in Cameroon that consisted of peer education; a monthly magazine; an eighteen-episode radio drama; integrated television, radio, and billboard campaigns; and youth-friendly condom outlets (Meekers, Agha, and Klein, 2005; Plautz and Meekers, 2007). Such condom distribution campaigns for youth have been rare in sub-Saharan Africa, because of adult concerns that condom promotion may promote youth sexual activity in general. The limited condom distribution that has targeted adolescents has typically been integrated within larger, complex adolescent sexual health interventions (e.g., Agha, 2002b; Campbell, 2003; Molassiotis et al., 2004; Meekers, Agha, and Klein, 2005; Plautz and Meekers, 2007).

CONDOM AVAILABILITY IN RURAL MWANZA
AT THE TIME OF THE STUDY

In 1993, Population Services International began social marketing the *Salama* brand of condoms in Tanzania with an intensive, national, multimedia campaign. In its first few years this included over two thousand messages through radio, TV, billboards, and newspaper; training 3,100 community-based agents to sell condoms; and hundreds of mobile video presentations that were estimated to reach well over a million people (Eloundou-Enyegue, Meekers, and Calvès, 2005). In 1999 they sold eighteen million condoms at approximately one-third their actual cost; this was half of the number of the free condoms distributed to government health facilities during the same year (Brent, 2010).

These efforts were largely limited to urban areas, however. In 1998, for example, when the *MEMA kwa Vijana* intervention was being developed, Population Services International only supplied condoms to three shops in all of the four *MEMA kwa Vijana* districts, an area that encompassed 475 villages and a population of 1.5 million people (United Republic of Tanzania, 1997). From those three shops, condoms were informally distributed to other villages by bus, bicycle, or on foot. Many villages did not have a condom supply. For example, a 1999 needs assessment conducted by the AMREF intervention team in three central and three peripheral intervention villages found that condoms were completely unavailable in the peripheral villages, and they only were available in a few outlets in larger villages, at twice the recommended retail price (Cleophas-Frisch, Obasi, Rwakatare et al., 2000).

During participant observation, shopkeepers reported that they mainly sold condoms to men in their twenties and thirties. In a village with a large, mobile population of fishermen, two shopkeepers independently estimated that they sold three to five packs of three condoms on a normal day, and as many as eight packs per day on market days or video show days. Reports of condom sales were substantially lower in other villages. Cost was rarely mentioned when people discussed reasons why they did not use condoms, and a number of young men specifically noted that the cost of condoms was not a problem.

MEMA KWA VIJANA CONDOM DISTRIBUTION

Condom Distributor Recruitment and Training

Intervention and HALIRA research findings about the very low availability of condoms in intervention villages in the first year of the trial led the AMREF intervention team to design and test a condom distribution initiative with the assistance of Population Services International in the second year of the trial. In this intervention component, out-of-school youth were trained in basic condom social marketing with the primary goal of increasing rural young people's access to condoms in a private and confidential way. These young people were called *mawakala wa usambazaji kondom*, which literally means "condom distribution agents." Specific objectives of this component were to assist young people by selling condoms at an affordable price, to teach accurate condom use, to discuss beliefs and mis-conceptions about condoms, to promote condom use among those who were sexually active, and to keep accurate records of condom sales. It was also hoped that condom distributors might model low-risk sexual behavior and help shift youth norms related to condom use.

To select condom distributors, AMREF intervention staff first hosted a video show and discussion for the general public in each village before facili-tating a public meeting the next day for young adults. Both young men and women were invited to those meetings, but they were primarily attended by young men, probably for several reasons, including that young women had more domestic and farming commitments, and that condoms were perceived as sexual, male, and/or disreputable for young women to discuss. At each of those meetings, young people were asked to nominate eight young people (ideally four males and four females) to be local condom distributors. Any youth living in the community could be nominated, but AMREF staff recom-mended young people between sixteen to twenty-five years of age who were approachable by both in-school and out-of-school youth, and who ideally had an existing economic activity in the village, such as a shopkeeper, food kiosk worker, carpenter, or barber. Candidates also were required to purchase twelve packs of three condoms and thirty-six individual condoms for half the price recommended for retail, that is, Tshs 50 ($0.06) per packet and Tshs 10 ($0.01) per condom. Once eight young people had been nominated and consented, four were elected to become distributors.

This condom distribution design was pilot tested in six villages to assess its acceptability and feasibility (Cleophas-Frisch, Obasi, Manchester et al., 2000). Over forty young people attended each of the pilot meetings to elect condom distributors. Despite encouragement, young women were much less likely to volunteer than young men, and only four of the twenty-three youths who were trained during the pilot study were female. Half of the condom dis-tributors required re-stocking within one month, and the majority of their cli-ents were males aged between twenty and thirty years. The pilot study found that packs of three condoms with illustrated instructions were as popular with customers as the cheaper, loose condoms, suggesting that people were eager to have clear, detailed information about condom use, and/or they might be willing to pay more for condoms which they perceive to be of higher quality.

Minor modifications were made to the condom distribution initiative after the pilot test, and then 228 distributors (twenty-four of whom were female) were recruited and trained in a two-day course on HIV/AIDS, condom use, record-keeping, and marketing. Condom distributors were to replenish their stock from twenty-eight individuals who were selected from all of the condom distributors and intervention health workers to be central distributors. AMREF intervention staff supervised condom distributor activities during prearranged, quarterly visits which included a review of their sales records.

Condom Distributor Outreach

Participant observation found that, early in their work, some *MEMA kwa Vijana* condom distributors used public meetings to educate people about condoms and their availability. For example, in one remote inland village:

> We passed by the Village Executive Officer's house and he mentioned that he went to a sub-village meeting yesterday accompanied by *MEMA kwa Vijana* condom distributors, who explained condom use to the villagers there. He said the distributors were asked several questions and they answered them well. [The twenty-year-old woman accompanying the researcher] said that the condom distributors are trying very hard to explain their work whenever they are asked about it. (PO-01-I-4-5f)

In addition to such formal meetings, a minority of condom distributors reported that they attempted informal peer education as a public service and/or to promote business. For example, a twenty-three-year-old married minister (Thobias):

> He said that sometimes when he wants to motivate the trawl net fishermen, he follows them to places where they fish or prepare nets, whereas the *dagaa* fishermen are usually available during the day when they are resting. . . . Thobias also said that sometimes when he is preaching in the church he tries to educate people about AIDS and how to protect themselves. (PO-01-I-7-3m)

In an example from a village near a mine, an unmarried condom distributor (Gabriel) explained how he tried to convince his peers of the value of condoms in informal discussions:

> Gabriel said there are some people who don't use condoms and who would like to influence others not to use them. . . . He said, "There are provocateurs who say, 'I might as well buy chewing gum and chew it in its wrapper,' and I tell them, 'If the gum had a disease, then we would chew it in its wrapper.'" (PO-01-I-1-2f)

There was no formal collaboration between the school and the condom distribution components of the intervention, and there generally seemed to be little contact between them. However, two of the in-depth interview respondents who were peer educators reported that condom distributors had taught them helpful information about condom use. Similarly, there were isolated reports in other interviews that condom distributors educated specific individuals about condoms. For example:

> R: The condom distributors have never taught me. . . . But I think they teach people individually, people who have a problem and go to them to be advised about condom use. I have heard that. He/she could even be walking on the road and others start asking him/her questions, so they have to answer. (II-02-I-296-m)

Public Awareness and Attitudes toward the Condom Distribution Initiative

Although there was evidence of limited outreach such as that described above, most *MEMA kwa Vijana* condom distributors did not seem to attempt broader outreach and instead established fairly small clienteles to whom they discreetly sold condoms. Participant observation suggests that most villagers did not know about the *MEMA kwa Vijana* condom distribution initiative. For example, a male bar worker in his early twenties in a fishing village:

> . . . said that most villagers don't know what *MEMA kwa Vijana* does, but some know that it teaches how to use condoms. Regarding condom distributors, he said he personally doesn't know anything about them and he has never heard anyone mention them. (PO-01-I-7-3m)

Similarly, at the end of the trial almost all intervention participants knew that condoms could be obtained at kiosks or health facilities, but in in-depth interviews and participant observation only a small minority said they had heard of *MEMA kwa Vijana* condom distributors.

When adult villagers did know about this initiative, it did not seem to be the focus of as much controversy as the in-school program, most probably because condom distributors and their customers were usually young men, and young men were expected to be sexually active. Nonetheless, one female intervention participant whose brothers were condom distributors said they sometimes had to address villagers' concerns about their work:

> R: Probably there are some who think badly about them, that they sell shameful things . . . things that are not supposed to be shown to people.
>
> I: Do such people hinder them and ask, "Why do you sell those condoms?"
>
> R: Yes. There are some who say that. . . . But my brothers just reply, "The person who has a lover should come and I will sell it to him/her so that they are safe . . . because they should not get illnesses." (II-02-I-325-f)

Young women who were elected and agreed to be condom distributors were almost invariably single mothers who already had somewhat tarnished reputations. These young women were more likely than men to be judged negatively for working as condom distributors, and they tended to be even more discreet than the men in their condom promotion and distribution efforts.

The minority of intervention participants who knew about the condom distribution initiative viewed it positively. For example, an eighteen-year-old secondary school student reported that he had never had sex, but he had a good understanding of condom use and was aware of this intervention component:

> R: When one decides to have sex, he should first give a girl some money, which will make her agree to have sex with him. Perhaps if he has some money left, he will have enough to buy that prevention method [condoms]. . . . Some youths buy them from shops. . . . There are also some villagers who were appointed by *Mema kwa Vijana* to sell those condoms . . . so that everyone who wants to use a prevention method can get it easily. (II-02-I-280-m)

Similarly, the young woman whose brothers were condom distributors viewed the initiative positively. A twenty-one-year-old single mother herself, she had never seen condoms while in school, but she knew what they looked like and was open to using them because of what she had learned through her brothers:

> I: Has anyone ever shown you a condom?
>
> R: No, but I saw them at home . . . after *MEMA kwa Vijana* gave them to my brothers to sell.
>
> I: Have you ever seen a condom?
>
> R: Yes. . . . It is like a . . . like a gourd. It has a whitish color. You find that there is something like milk on it . . . I don't know, like sweat. . . . One puts it on like a sock, on the man's private parts.
>
> I: Mm. Have you ever used a condom?
>
> R: No . . .
>
> I: If you agreed to have sex with a boy and he wanted to use a condom, how would you feel?
>
> R: I would just feel good. . . . I would think, "It is possible this one is healthy, that he has no infections." Yes, or he doesn't want to get illnesses, the illnesses you might have.
>
> I: Would you feel embarrassed to get a condom yourself?
>
> R: Yes. . . . Because when you buy the condom, the person selling it to you suspects, "This one probably is going to have sex." (II-02-I-325-f)

Condom Distribution and Sales

Participant observation found that most condom distributors—including the females—mainly sold condoms to a small number of twenty- to thirty-year-old male acquaintances and friends. They also occasionally sold condoms to single women and rarely to school pupils. Similarly, broader condom distributor sales records indicated that 15 percent of customers were pupils, 23 percent were other youth under twenty years of age, 40 percent were twenty- to twenty-nine years old, and 22 percent were thirty years old or older (Cleophas-Frisch et al., 2002). In total, 15 percent of customers were female. By the end of the *MEMA kwa Vijana* trial, the 228 condom distributors had sold 57,610 condoms, averaging eleven condoms sold per distributor per month (Terris-Prestholt et al., 2006).

Condom sales varied widely based on the particular distributor's efforts, the characteristics of the village, and seasonal activities. For example, in one remote inland village where no kiosks sold condoms, a twenty-five-year-old farmer and small businessman named Mabina estimated he sold about forty condoms per month, a relatively high rate of sales. The researcher noted: "Mabina says he sells more condoms on market days and during *ngoma* gatherings for the *Saba saba* holiday. He said that his stock of condoms ran out during *Saba saba*, because people have sex more frequently then than on other days" (PO-02-I-4-1m). Despite this relative success, Mabina was doubtful about the impact his work would have on a broader level:

> Mabina said a young man could have sex as many as three times during a week. And [during one sexual rendezvous], a young man could even ejaculate three times. So he estimated such a person could use nine condoms in a week. So even if Mabina sells forty condoms in one month, he thinks many young men have sex without using condoms. (PO-02-I-4-1m)

Mabina reported that he had a regular clientele of twelve male and two female twenty- to thirty-five-year-old clients. He explained that his female clients bought condoms infrequently but in large amounts, to minimize the chance that they might run out of condoms or be seen buying them. A female condom distributor in the same village told a researcher she also mainly sold condoms to twenty- to thirty-year-old men, but she had also sold condoms to five unmarried young women and two school pupils. On average, however, she only sold six condoms per month.

Thobias, the minister in a fishing village, reported that his condom customers mainly were young fishermen, but on occasion he also had sold condoms to Year 4 and Year 5 pupils. Thobias explained that people were often uncomfortable when they sought condoms from him:

He said that many people are afraid of going to his home to buy condoms. Thobias thinks they fear his wife. Those who come to his house ask him to give them condoms without his wife's knowledge, so when they leave the house he escorts them and carries condoms in his pocket to give to them once they are further away. (PO-01-I-7-5f)

Condom distributors reported that it was difficult to teach people about condoms while making a sale. They believed some of their customers were curious and had questions about condom use, but they also often were shy and pretended that they were purchasing condoms for friends. As had been found in the pilot study, some condom distributors believed their customers preferred to purchase a manufacturer's pack of three condoms, rather than the cheaper alternative of three individual condoms, specifically because the pack came with illustrated instructions that explained condom use.

Participant observation suggests that condom distributors usually sold condoms at the prices recommended by the project. During training the distributors had been asked not to sell any of their stock to local shops. However, some distributors owned kiosks and told participant observation researchers that they primarily sold their condoms through those kiosks. In addition, two of the condom distributors who were interviewed during participant observation reported sometimes selling their stock to other people's shops and then falsifying their *MEMA kwa Vijana* records as if they had sold them directly to customers. For example, the minister Thobias:

> Thobias said he is given condoms that he sells for Tshs 50 ($0.06), but this work is hard . . . so he sometimes gives his condoms to shopkeepers, who sell them at Tshs 100 ($0.12) and keep the profit. . . . He said, "It is impossible to only devote your time to *MEMA kwa Vijana*'s work, but you have to keep their things [records], so when they arrive suddenly you just show them and they will know that you are working." (PO-01-I-7-5f)

Other condom distributors also said that it took substantial effort to sell condoms. For example, Gabriel, the unmarried distributor from the village near a mine:

> Gabriel said he has talked to other condom distributors and they say a distributor has to actively mobilize people to use condoms to succeed in selling them. He said those condom distributors who sat and waited for people to go to them rarely sold a single condom. (PO-01-I-1-2f)

The HALIRA research suggests that the school pupils who were the most likely to know and obtain condoms from condom distributors had a familial connection to them. In the second series of in-depth interviews, for example, only three of the thirty-three randomly selected intervention participants had, on rare occasions, obtained condoms from a condom distributor. They included a man whose brother was a condom distributor, and a woman whose husband was one. None of the eleven intervention participants in the third interview series said they had received condoms from a condom distributor.

While *MEMA kwa Vijana* condom distributors generally seemed to be discreet in their services, it is unclear how consistently they protected their customers' privacy. During a conversation with a researcher about his work as a condom distributor, for example, Thobias named individuals who bought condoms from him, and she also heard him mentioning customers' names in conversations with others.

Condom Distributors as Role Models

In HALIRA research, most *MEMA kwa Vijana* condom distributors were rumored not to use condoms themselves, or only rarely to do so, and this was generally confirmed by their own reports and those of their sexual partners. For example, the twenty-year-old wife of a condom distributor:

I: Have you ever used any prevention method against pregnancy during sex?

R: Yes, condoms. . . . That is to say, the man used it, I didn't use it myself.

I: And have you often used a condom, or rarely?

R: Rarely. . . . We just get them from the kiosk we have at my husband's homestead, because he sells them there for *MEMA kwa Vijana*. (II-02-I-314-f)

In contrast, the young man whose older brother was a condom distributor believed his brother used condoms consistently: "We always talk together, and he told me that—if he gets a girl—it is important that he use condoms" (II-02-I-298-m).

None of the six condom distributors who participated in in-depth interviews during participant observation reported consistent condom use. All of the men reported trying to use condoms but giving up after a short time due to reduced pleasure or delayed orgasm. None used them with their wives, but some used them with partners who they perceived to be high risk. For example:

Gabriel said, "The first time using condoms truly does not bring pleasure. It is necessary to get used to using them. Also, condoms delay ejaculation, so you are delayed in finishing [reaching orgasm]." . . . He said that although he can now have complete intercourse with a woman without removing a condom halfway through, he rarely uses one. . . . He said that he knows all the girls and women in the village and he knows those with multiple partners, like some *wasimbe*, so he only uses condoms with them. (PO-01-I-1-2f)

A male researcher lived in Mabina's family's household over three participant observation visits. During the first visit, Mabina had not yet been recruited and trained as a condom distributor. At that time the researcher frequently witnessed Mabina negotiating sexual liaisons with girls or young women, and he was also present when Mabina prepared himself to meet partners for sex at night, or returned after meeting them. The researcher's observations suggested that Mabina had several concurrent sexual partners, including a school girl, an out-of-school adolescent girl who lived next door, and two single and/or divorced young women. During that first participant observation visit Mabina did not seem to be concerned about his personal risk of contracting a sexually transmitted infection, although he actively attempted to protect himself against other perceived harms. For example, he applied traditional medicine to his armpits and face before leaving home at night in order to protect himself from witches. Mabina knew that condoms were promoted for protection against sexually transmitted infections, but at that time he said he had never used one and he believed that few other villagers had either.

Ten months later, Mabina was elected to be a *MEMA kwa Vijana* condom distributor. During the second participant observation visit two months after that, he told the researcher he had tried using condoms but he disliked that it took him longer to have an orgasm when he wore one. Around the time Mabina became a condom distributor he decided to marry the young neighbor with whom he had an ongoing sexual relationship. They married informally, in that she snuck into his room one night and then simply did not return to her parents' household the next day. Eventually the two families negotiated an elopement fine of Tshs 20,000 ($24) and a bicycle, which Mabina and his family paid to his wife's family. During that participant observation visit and the subsequent visit one year later, Mabina said he did not use condoms with his wife, who he assumed to be faithful. However, his general comments suggested he might use them if he had sex with extramarital partners who he perceived to be high risk.

As discussed in chapter 5, in one of the participant observation villages (number 1) some of the teachers were widely known for very disreputable sexual behavior, and in that village some of the condom distributors also had bad reputations. Several single women there reported having had sex without condoms with two of the *MEMA kwa Vijana* condom distributors, both of whom were married. This included one man with a particularly bad reputation who was widely rumored to have impregnated five local girls and women. In addition, two women independently told researchers detailed and plausible accounts of having been sexually assaulted by him when they were fifteen years old, and several others independently reported that he had moved to the village only after being arrested for raping a young girl in another village. At least some of these incidents occurred prior to the man becoming a condom distributor, and it is unclear why other youth nonetheless perceived him as a suitable candidate and elected him for that role. A twenty-one-year-old bicycle taxi driver commented that such condom distributors had a negative impact on the broader *MEMA kwa Vijana* program:

> He said that the condom distributors are not fit to conduct education in the vil-
> lage because they are the chief seducers and tempters of girls. He went on to say
> that the condom distributors don't use condoms, and that if *MEMA kwa Vijana*
> wants success in their education, they should change the condom distributors.
> (PO-01-I-1-3m)

Discontinuation of the Condom Distribution Initiative

Most condom distributors were disappointed by the income-generating aspect of the initiative, as they found it challenging to sell even a small number of condoms and their profit margins were narrow (Cleophas-Frisch et al., 2002). Many also reported substantial difficulty managing money, keeping sales records, and accessing new condoms on foot or by bicycle from the central suppliers who were usually located ten or more kilometers away from their homes. Finally, many reported that community misconceptions and negative attitudes toward condoms were powerful and difficult to overcome.

Eighteen months after the initial training, 30 percent of condom distributors had stopped participating in the initiative due to relocation or other changes in their circumstances (Cleophas-Frisch et al., 2002). In addition, even with health facility staff and other central distributors to assist in supplying rural areas, this intervention component took up a disproportionate amount of AMREF staff time. It also was not cost-effective, so it would have been very costly to sustain on a large scale. For example, even though the *Salama* condoms used by the *MEMA kwa Vijana* intervention were already subsidized by Population Services International, the cost for each condom distributed by the condom distributor initiative was $1.54 (Terris-Prestholt et al., 2006). Due to the extremely low demand for condoms, difficulty monitoring and supplying condom distributors, and the costly nature of this intervention component, it was discontinued at the end of the *MEMA kwa Vijana* trial in 2001.

DISCUSSION

Youth-Friendly Health Services

Several aspects of the *MEMA kwa Vijana* youth-friendly health services initiative were successful. At baseline, health workers usually perceived adolescent sexual health education as important and were fairly comfortable with the idea of teaching young people such information. Moreover, health workers' professional role made it more socially acceptable for them to teach adolescents potentially controversial information, such as condom use, than was the case for teachers in schools. Most intervention health workers conducted outreach that was positive and salient for school pupils, both visiting schools and hosting class visits to health facilities. This is particularly notable as it took place above and beyond their regular duties and without compensation. Few interventions have explored the potential to utilize local health workers in school and community HIV prevention programs, but those which have done so also have found this to be an unusually acceptable and cost-effective approach (e.g., Agbemenu and Schlenk, 2011; Kaponda et al., 2011). Simulated patient exercises further suggest that the quality of *MEMA kwa Vijana* health workers' clinical interactions with adolescents improved modestly, as intervention health workers generally seemed more respectful and less judgmental with adolescents than their control counterparts. They also were more likely to promote condoms and to provide simulated patients with detailed information.

Despite these achievements, by the end of the trial very few young people had attended intervention health facilities for sexually transmitted disease treatment or to obtain condoms or other contraceptives, except for some young mothers who already were attending facilities for other services. This intervention component thus was unable to overcome some important barriers to service, such as distance from homes and fear of stigma. In addition, some problems within adolescent sexual health services which preceded the trial continued in intervention facilities during it, including poor privacy, inappropriate personal questions, and health worker participation in forced pregnancy examination of school girls.

After the trial, the *MEMA kwa Vijana* health services component was scaled up from 18 to all 177 health facilities within the four project districts. A detailed description and evaluation of that scale-up is provided elsewhere (Renju, Andrew, Nyalali et al., 2010; Renju, Makokha et al., 2010). In brief, a cascade approach to training was used during the scale-up, with a small number of AMREF staff first training local government officials and those officials then training 429 health workers. During the scale-up, health workers only participated in one training course, unlike those who participated in annual refresher courses during the earlier trial.

Evaluation found that the scaled-up training courses had a high coverage, were well conducted, and significantly improved health worker knowledge of HIV/AIDS and puberty, as well as their attitudes toward young people's confidentiality, right to treatment, and use of condoms (Renju, Andrew, Nyalali et al., 2010). In simulated patient exercises conducted during the scale-up, intervention facilities scored higher than control facilities in accommodating adolescent contraceptive and/or condom requests, but lower in response to adolescent concerns about sexually transmitted infections. Importantly, only 40 percent of the health workers who met with simulated patients in intervention facilities had actually participated in the *MEMA kwa Vijana* training course. Finally, as noted in chapter 5, during this scale-up relatively few reciprocal visits took place between school classes and health workers, and the dedicated annual Youth Health Week was eliminated or replaced by activities incorporated into existing commemorative dates (Renju, Andrew, Medard et al., 2010). The evaluation suggested that the scale-up was moderately successful, but the quality of training, outreach, and clinical services was diluted during scale-up (Renju, Andrew, Nyalali et al., 2010). In addition, this intervention component was hampered by the small number of trained health workers per facility and a high rate of staff turnover, suggesting a need to train more clinical and non-clinical staff in each facility. Ideally, intensive youth-friendly training would be incorporated into pre-service health worker training courses, to ensure large-scale consistency of services and to reduce the impact of high staff turnover.

Condom Promotion and Distribution

The *MEMA kwa Vijana* condom distribution initiative achieved some of its objectives, but ultimately these were not sufficient to warrant continuing it after the trial. This initiative was introduced into areas which were very difficult to access, where prior to the intervention there had been very little or no distribution of condoms, and where misinformation and negative attitudes toward condoms were powerful and widespread. In such contexts, the intervention succeeded in recruiting and training four young condom distributors per village, and those young people generally succeeded in establishing small clienteles of customers. However, negative attitudes toward condoms persisted, making it difficult for most distributors to sell more than a small number of condoms. In addition, the profit margin for condom sales was so low that most of these young people did not want to continue working as condom distributors long-term. These findings suggest that much more intensive, multimedia condom promotion is necessary to create enough demand among both adults and young people to drive condom sales in rural areas.

In addition, condom distribution in rural areas is likely to be more sustainable logistically if it is integrated within existing distribution networks, whether specific to condom social marketing, large-scale businesses for manufactured goods (such as soda companies), and/or other small-scale business (such as traveling petty traders). Reviews of other community-based HIV prevention work with young Africans have similarly found that programs which are not integrated within existing services may focus limited resources and capacity on creating infrastructure rather than developing and delivering intervention content (Maticka-Tyndale and Brouillard-Coyle, 2006; Mavedzenge, Doyle, and Ross, 2011).

This chapter has built upon chapters 4 and 5 to complete the process evaluation of the different components of the *MEMA kwa Vijana* intervention. Chapter 7 will now draw on the findings of all three of these chapters in examining the intervention's impact, and particularly its strengths and weaknesses in promoting abstinence, low partner number, fidelity, and condom use.

Chapter Seven

Impact of the
MEMA kwa Vijana Intervention

Within the *MEMA kwa Vijana* trial, multiple research methods were used to assess intervention impact, including biomedical surveys, face-to-face questionnaire interviews, assisted self-completion questionnaire interviews, semi-structured in-depth interviews, group discussions, simulated patient exercises, and participant observation. The general strengths and weaknesses of these methods and the particular ways they were employed within the trial are detailed in chapters 1 and 2.

This chapter will draw on all of the *MEMA kwa Vijana* research methods to assess the impact of the intervention on theoretical determinants of sexual behavior, on actual sexual practices, and on pregnancy and sexually transmitted infections. It will begin by examining the consistency and validity of trial participants' self-reported sexual behavior, because most intervention impact evaluations are based on such self-reported information. It will then describe the preliminary qualitative evaluation of intervention impact, which was completed prior to analysis of the trial's quantitative data. That section will be followed by a summary of trial findings of intervention impact on participant knowledge, attitudes, behavior, and biological markers. The next sections then will detail findings from the in-depth qualitative data analysis that took place after the trial results were known, particularly examining intervention impact on the theoretical determinants of abstinence, low partner number, fidelity, and condom use. The chapter then continues with an introduction to "positive deviants" in intervention communities, that is, unusual young people who actively tried to practice low-risk sexual behaviors, partly due to their intervention experience. The chapter will conclude with a comparison of the *MEMA kwa Vijana* intervention process and impact findings with those of the Stepping Stones randomized controlled trial in South Africa, which to date is the only sexual health intervention trial for young people in Africa to have found a statistically significant impact on a biological outcome (Jewkes et al., 2008).

THE VALIDITY OF SELF-REPORTED DATA
IN THE *MEMA KWA VIJANA* TRIAL

As noted in chapter 1, self-reported sexual behavior can be inaccurate due to a number of reasons, including poor recall, misunderstanding, or intentionally false statements made to avoid anticipated criticism or embarrassment (Catania et al., 1993; Huygens et al., 1996; Brewer, Garrett, and Kulasingam, 1999; Gersovitz et al., 1998; Stycos, 2000; Fenton et al., 2001; Hewett, Mensch, and Erulkar, 2004; Gersovitz, 2007; Palen et al., 2008; Beguy et al., 2009; Turner et al., 2009; Koffi et al., 2012). The latter issue is a particular concern within intervention evaluations, as participants are aware of promoted behaviors and may be biased toward falsely reporting them. Within the *MEMA kwa Vijana* trial, the validity of self-reported information was scrutinized in two ways using data collected during the first half of the trial (Plummer, Ross et al., 2004; Plummer, Wight, et al., 2004). First, the consistency of self-reported sexual behavior was assessed by comparing the logic of individuals' reports within and between surveys and in-depth interviews. Second, reported experience of sex was examined for those young people who tested positive for pregnancy or sexually transmitted infection.

In the 1998 *MEMA kwa Vijana* trial survey, for example, 9,283 trial members participated in a face-to-face questionnaire survey, and a sub-set of 4,958 boys (average age sixteen) and girls (average age fifteen) also completed an assisted self-completion questionnaire survey on the same day (table 1.1). For that sub-set, overall reports of sexual experience appeared very similar in both surveys. In the face-to-face and assisted self-completion questionnaire interviews, for instance, 52 percent and 56 percent of males reported having had sex, respectively, while 23 percent and 22 percent of females reported the same (Plummer, Wight et al., 2004). However, when these data were analyzed at an individual level, 40 percent of the males and 59 percent of the females who had reported sex only did so in one of the questionnaires, and not the other questionnaire. In addition, 1 percent (twelve males, forty-nine females) of the sub-set of 4,958 trial participants tested positive for one or more biological markers, but only 58 percent of those boys and 29 percent of those girls reported ever having had sex in both interviews (Plummer, Ross et al., 2004). Most of the remaining youth with biological markers denied having ever had sex in both surveys.

The in-depth interview respondents provided the greatest opportunity for comparison of data validity across several research methods. From 1998 to 2000, seventy-three trial participants participated in as many as five interviews, that is, in 1998 and 2000 face-to-face questionnaire and assisted self-completion questionnaire interviews, as well as in 1999–2000 in-depth interviews (table 1.1). For those individuals, responses to questions about whether they had ever had sex were considered "consistent" if they were consistently affirmative or consistently negative over time, or if they were first consistently negative and then became consistently positive. Thirty-two percent of these respondents provided inconsistent responses, while an additional 8 percent provided consistent but invalid responses, because they consistently denied ever having had sex but they were pregnant or had a sexually transmitted infection during the first survey (Plummer, Ross et al., 2004). It is possible that some of the HIV-positive adolescents contracted HIV from their mothers during pregnancy or soon after birth, and indeed had never had sex. However, only one of the six female in-depth interview respondents with HIV or another sexually transmitted infection reported sex in any of the four surveys, while five reported it in in-depth interviews which took place contemporaneously or prior to some of their survey interviews.

The findings above raise concerns about the accuracy of self-reported sexual behavior in general and particularly in surveys. The few other studies which have scrutinized the consistency and validity of adolescent sexual behavior reports in surveys in sub-Saharan Africa have identified similar problems (e.g., Palen et al., 2008; Beguy et al., 2009; Cremin et al., 2009). This poses challenges for evaluations of intervention impact. Nonetheless, the vast majority of evaluations of adolescent sexual health interventions assess program effectiveness based on such self-reported information (Gallant and Maticka-Tyndale, 2004; Michielsen et al., 2010).

PRELIMINARY QUALITATIVE IMPACT EVALUATION

At the end of the *MEMA kwa Vijana* trial and HALIRA fieldwork in mid-2002, the *MEMA kwa Vijana* trial director (David Ross) requested that the HALIRA research team draft a report describing their impressions of intervention content, delivery, and impact, based on preliminary qualitative data analysis. This was done in advance of quantitative analysis of intervention impact on knowledge, attitudes, behavior, and biomedical markers to avoid the possibility that awareness of trial results would bias the qualitative analyses (Oakley et al., 2006). To create this report, this book's author requested that the lead principal investigator (Daniel Wight) and each of the HALIRA field researchers at the time (Neema Busali, Gerry Mshana, Joyce Wamoyi, and Zachayo Salamba Shigongo) independently write responses to a series of questions related to intervention process and impact, without discussing them with other team members until they had finished. At the same time the author independently drafted a more detailed and lengthy report addressing the same questions. All of the HALIRA researchers then reviewed and gave feedback on one another's responses, and the author integrated all responses into a final 8,600 word report. There were few discrepancies of opinion between the HALIRA researchers, and they were noted in the final report. In 2002, this report was only read by the HALIRA team and the *MEMA kwa Vijana* trial director. It was otherwise kept confidential until early 2003, when preliminary analysis of the trial impact data had been completed. This confidentiality was maintained to reduce the possibility that preliminary qualitative findings might unduly influence the formal quantitative analyses.

The preliminary HALIRA findings were largely confirmed by subsequent in-depth qualitative analyses. For example, the preliminary process evaluation of each intervention component identified many of the same strengths and weaknesses described in detail in chapters 4–6 after more in-depth analyses. The preliminary HALIRA report also identified participants' knowledge as the most likely area where the intervention had had substantial impact. An excerpt from the preliminary report:

> Sexual and reproductive health knowledge seems to have greatly improved in the intervention side of the *MEMA kwa Vijana* cohort in the course of the trial. The dearth of basic information prior to the trial meant there was potential for a very high learning curve. Indeed, the simple presentation of key concepts, and their frequent reinforcement over the years of the intervention, seems to have succeeded in educating cohort members about basic reproductive biology, the nature of AIDS and other sexually transmitted infections, and the value of abstinence, reduction of partners, and condom use. (HALIRA, 2002, 13)

However, the preliminary HALIRA report noted that there was less evidence of substantial, genuine change to participants' attitudes and skills in the areas targeted by the intervention. Another excerpt from the preliminary report:

> It seems quite possible that reported knowledge, attitude, and behavior measures will show statistically significant improvement amongst intervention cohort members relative to control cohort members over the course of the trial. A challenge will then be to distinguish between those attitude and behavior results which are valid, and those which are biased self-reporting, given intervention participants are aware of the desired responses. . . .
>
> For example, attitudes toward gender rights and roles have a strong cultural and social basis and seem unlikely to change. . . . Girls' assertiveness is generally disapproved of within the predominant local ethnic group, the Sukuma, because girls are considered to be of low status in terms of both age and sex.

Girls are particularly discouraged from looking males directly in the eye, so intervention messages stressing assertive, direct eye contact during sexual refusal may be culturally inappropriate and misconstrued. Thus while there is evidence from participant observation that some girls have adopted and used the assertive behaviors taught in *MEMA kwa Vijana* classes, [many] do not seem comfortable with them.

Other attitudes, such as the fatalistic belief that disease avoidance is out of a person's control (for young people) or that sexually active young people should be chastised (for health care workers) may have been improved by the intervention to a moderate extent. A few attitudes seem to have improved substantially, such as young people's comfort and openness in talking about sexual and reproductive issues. For example, participant observation research and in-depth interviews with eighty-eight young people in 2002 found that intervention participants were much more inquisitive and comfortable using sexual vocabulary than their control counterparts. (HALIRA, 2002, 13–14)

The preliminary HALIRA report found that significant positive intervention impact on youth sexual behavior was unlikely. First, the issue of abstinence:

Abstinence until marriage was one of the strongest intervention messages, and it was undoubtedly the most socially acceptable amongst parents, teachers and the broader community. However, it does not seem to be a realistic option for more than a very small minority of young people. Just as young people already widely disobey the orders of their parents and teachers not to have sex, it is likely they will treat the *MEMA kwa Vijana* advice in the same way: as an injunction from adults that does not fit with young people's reality . . .

[By the end of the trial] the vast majority of cohort members appear to be sexually active, many having reportedly started sex at ages as young as ten or twelve years. Sexually active young people commonly report that it is extremely difficult to stop having sex once they have started, for financial (female), prestige (male), and biological (male, and to a lesser extent, female) reasons. Most youth see their elder brothers and sisters, friends, relatives, and parents engaged in sexual activities, and it becomes difficult to perceive or choose a different path. Thus while a few individuals who have already had sex may have decided to abstain until marriage after participating in the intervention, it seems highly unlikely that this represents a general trend. (HALIRA, 2002, 11)

The preliminary HALIRA report also addressed the likelihood that significantly higher proportions of intervention participants than control participants might practice monogamy, partner reduction, or partner selectivity:

There is evidence to suggest that both multiple, concurrent partnerships and serial monogamy with frequent partner change are fairly common among adolescents in rural Mwanza, particularly as opportunistic or casual sexual partnerships may be fairly common. Frequent partner change and serial monogamy is a particular concern because the long-term danger is relatively abstract, and the target population may have difficulty conceptualizing it, particularly as they are adolescents and may be focused on immediate, short-term goals. Similarly, some respondents report multiple, concurrent relationships are necessary for sexual satisfaction (male and female), financial need/desire (female) and/or prestige (male), although some male respondents instead report that they cannot afford to have multiple partners, as it is too expensive to provide money or gifts to more than one partner. . . .

[Nonetheless], some respondents reported having reduced partners as a result of the intervention, and many reported that this was the most feasible and realistic of the targeted behavior changes, because it is culturally sanctioned, it allows for reproduction and sexual satisfaction, and/or it does not involve learning an alien practice like condom use. This message may have been especially effective in combination with risk information that makes young people select their partners more carefully. The curriculum repeatedly stressed that a person with HIV can appear healthy, and that adults are more likely to be infected with HIV and other sexually transmitted infections than a young person. However, the curriculum did not address some other potentially high-risk partners, e.g., travelers and urban dwellers, and this is unfortunate given such individuals are often perceived as desirable partners in villages due to relative wealth or modern appearance. (HALIRA, 2002, 11–12)

Finally, the preliminary HALIRA report addressed the likelihood of significant intervention impact on condom use:

For sexually active youth, the intervention strongly encouraged condom use . . . but this message was necessarily limited due to national and local regulation. Nonetheless, the general condom use message appears to have been repeatedly reinforced within and across school years, and it is likely that the vast majority of intervention cohort members know that condoms prevent pregnancy as well as HIV and other sexually transmitted infections. However, the limited nature of in-school condom information may have led some pupils to pick up patchy and ultimately incorrect information.

Some intervention participants report having used condoms, and some of these reports seem plausible (e.g., school girls reporting occasional condom use to avoid pregnancy). However, it seems unlikely that more than a very small proportion of intervention participants have ever truly used condoms, and of those only a much smaller proportion is likely to have used them consistently. This is not to say that the condom use intervention message failed. The environment into which condoms were introduced was confused and hostile, and access was very limited; given those obstacles, the intervention may have achieved an important, long-term step in raising condom awareness and availability in general. (HALIRA, 2002, 12–13)

The preliminary HALIRA report concluded by saying that there did not seem to have been much intervention impact on sexual behavior in the course of the trial, so significant impact on pregnancy or sexually transmitted infections seemed unlikely. These findings were largely borne out in subsequent trial analyses, as will be described in the next section.

QUANTITATIVE IMPACT EVALUATION

The impact of the *MEMA kwa Vijana* intervention was primarily evaluated through the trial, in which twenty communities were randomly assigned to either the intervention or a control group (Hayes et al., 2005). During the trial, three surveys were conducted with 9,645 young people between 1998 and 2002, as described in chapter 1 (table 1.1). The 2001–2002 survey found that intervention participants had significantly better sexual health knowledge and were significantly more likely to report some desirable attitudes and behaviors than control participants (table 7.1) (Ross et al., 2007). However, there was no statistically significant and positive intervention impact on pregnancy, HIV, or other sexually transmitted infections.

The *MEMA kwa Vijana* intervention was continued and expanded in the same districts after the trial ended in 2002 (Renju, Andrew, Medard et al., 2010; Renju, Andrew, Nyalali et al., 2010; Renju, Makokha et al., 2010). From 2007 to 2008, a follow-up cross-sectional survey evaluated possible long-term intervention impact in a cohort of 13,804 young people aged fifteen to thirty years, all of whom had attended intervention or control schools during the trial but were not necessarily members of the original trial cohort (Doyle et al., 2010). That survey was conducted to evaluate whether greater time and broader population exposure had a greater impact on knowledge, attitudes, behavior, and biological outcomes. It found that, at an average of five years after school program participation, intervention participants still had significantly improved sexual health knowledge and were significantly more likely to report some desirable behaviors than control participants. However, the survey found that the intervention neither had a significant long-term impact on reported sexual attitudes nor on the prevalence of HIV or other sexually transmitted infections.

To describe these findings in more detail, the following sections summarize the results documented in the several publications for the 2001–2002 survey (Ross et al., 2007) and the 2007–2008 survey (Doyle et al., 2010; Doyle, Weiss et al., 2011). These and other results are also detailed in table 7.1.

Table 7.1. Impact of the *MEMA kwa Vijana* Intervention on Select Outcomes by Sex in the 2001–2002 and 2007–2008 Surveys

| | Males | | | | | | | | | | | | Females | | | | | | | | | | | |
| | 2001–2002 | | | 2007–2008 | | | | | | | | | 2001–2002 | | | 2007–2008 | | |
Outcome	I (%)	C (%)	aRR[a] (CI)	I (%)	C (%)	aPR[a] (CI)	I (%)	C (%)	aRR[a] (CI)	I (%)	C (%)	aPR[a] (CI)
Knowledge[b]												
HIV acquisition	65	45	1.44 (1.25, 1.67)	73	66	1.11 (0.99, 1.23)	58	40	1.41 (1.14, 1.75)	68	61	1.11 (1.00, 1.24)
STI acquisition	52	40	1.28 (1.07, 1.54)	54	46	1.18 (1.04, 1.34)	36	25	1.41 (1.06, 1.88)	38	30	1.24 (0.97, 1.58)
Pregnancy prevention	84	50	1.66 (1.55, 1.78)	83	69	1.19 (1.12, 1.26)	72	46	1.58 (1.26, 1.99)	71	60	1.17 (1.06, 1.30)
Attitudes[b]												
Attitudes towards a girl's right to refuse sex	22	12	1.77 (1.42, 2.22)	28	22	1.31 (0.97, 1.77)	27	19	1.42 (1.11, 1.81)	11	10	1.09 (0.67, 1.77)
Abstinence												
Sexual debut during the trial[c]	60	72	0.84 (0.71, 1.01)			—	68	67	1.03 (0.91, 1.16)			—
Age at first sex <16 years			—	25	28	0.91 (0.80, 1.05)			—	28	27	1.01 (0.80, 1.28)
Partner Number Limitation												
>1 partner in last 12 months	19	28	0.69 (0.49, 0.95)	41	45	0.92 (0.79, 1.08)	9	8	1.04 (0.58, 1.89)	10	10	0.97 (0.76, 1.23)
>2 (female) or >4 (male) lifetime partners			—	37	44	0.87 (0.78, 0.97)			—	34	37	0.89 (0.75, 1.05)
>1 partner in same time period in past 12 months			—	29	32	0.90 (0.76, 1.06)			—	6	7	0.87 (0.63, 1.20)
>1 partner in past 4 weeks			—	11	13	0.87 (0.65, 1.15)			—	2	2	1.04 (0.66, 1.66)

Condom Use												
First used condom during the trial[d]	39	28	1.41 (1.15, 1.73)	—	—	—	38	28	1.30 (1.03, 1.63)	—	—	—
Used condom at last sex[d]	29	20	1.47 (1.12, 1.93)	—	—	—	27	22	1.12 (0.85, 1.48)	—	—	—
Used condom at last sex in past 12 months[e]	—	—	—	34	29	1.19 (0.91, 1.54)	—	—	—	19	15	1.27 (0.97, 1.67)
Used condom at last sex in past 12 months with non-regular partner[f]	—	—	—	50	44	1.15 (0.97, 1.36)	—	—	—	45	31	1.34 (1.07, 1.69)
Treatment Seeking												
Went to health facility for most recent STI symptoms within past 12 months[g]	29	35	0.84 (0.50, 1.41)	48	43	1.19 (0.91, 1.56)	36	34	1.02 (0.62, 1.70)	47	47	1.02 (0.77, 1.37)
Biological Outcomes												
HIV incidence (/1,000 person years)	0.4	0.3	NA	—			3.2	4.7	0.75 (0.34, 1.66)	—		
HIV prevalence	11.3	12.5	0.92 (0.69, 1.22)	2.0	1.7	0.91 (0.50, 1.65)	—			3.9	4.2	1.07 (0.68, 1.67)
Herpes prevalence				25.0	26.7	0.94 (0.77, 1.15)	21.3	20.8	1.05 (0.83, 1.32)	40.3	42.5	0.96 (0.87, 1.06)
Syphilis prevalence	1.4	1.8	0.78 (0.46, 1.30)	5.8	5.3	1.06 (0.74, 1.52)	3.3	3.6	0.99 (0.67, 1.46)	6.3	7.5	0.86 (0.62, 1.21)
Chlamydia prevalence	0.5	0.5	1.14 (0.53, 2.43)	2.1	2.1	1.24 (0.66, 2.33)	4.9	3.6	1.37 (0.98, 1.91)	2.6	2.1	1.27 (0.87, 1.86)

Table 7.1. (continued)

| | Males | | | | | | Females | | | | | |
| | 2001–2002 | | | 2007–2008 | | | 2001–2002 | | | 2007–2008 | | |
Outcome	I (%)	C (%)	aRR[a] (CI)	I (%)	C (%)	aPR[a] (CI)	I (%)	C (%)	aRR[a] (CI)	I (%)	C (%)	aPR[a] (CI)
Biological Outcomes (continued)												
Gonorrhea prevalence	0.4	0.1	NA	0.3	0.4	0.71 (0.21, 2.41)	2.4	1.2	1.93 (1.01, 3.71)	0.3	0.4	0.73 (0.20, 2.63)
Trichomonas prevalence[h]			—			—	28.6	25.8	1.13 (0.92, 1.37)			—
Pregnancy (test) prevalence[h]			—			—	19.2	18.0	1.09 (0.85, 1.40)			—
Reported pregnancy during trial[h,i]			—			—	46.9	45.5	1.03 (0.89, 1.20)			—

aPR = adjusted prevalence ratio; aRR = adjusted relative risk; C = control; CI = confidence interval; I = intervention; NA = Not applicable as number of cases too small to justify comparison (<10 in each group); STI = sexually transmitted infection; — = not measured.

[a]Adjusted for: age group (2001–2002: ≤17, 18, ≥19 years old at survey; 2007-2008: <21, 21-22, 23-24, ≥25 years old at survey), ethnic group (Sukuma vs. non-Sukuma), and trial stratum (low, medium, or high HIV risk). Community categorization within trial strata was based on HIV prevalence in 15–19 year olds in a 1997-1998 survey (Obasi et al. 2001), and geographical characteristics of the communities, e.g., whether villages were remote or close to towns, major roads, or gold mining areas (Hayes et al. 2005). 2001–2002 data are also adjusted for number of lifetime partners at baseline in 1998 (0, 1, 2, ≥3).

[b]Proportion who answered all three variables for each category correctly or desirably.

[c]Among those who reported never having had sex at the 1998 baseline survey.

[d]Among those who reported having had sex.

[e]Among those who reported having had sex in the past 12 months.

[f]Among those who reported having had sex with a non-regular partner in the past 12 months.

[g]Among those who reported having sexually transmitted infection symptoms (genital discharge or genital ulcer) within the past 12 months.

[h]Females only.

[i]Among those who reported never having been pregnant at the 1998 baseline survey.

Adapted with permission from Ross et al., 2007 and Doyle et al., 2010.

Knowledge

The 2001–2002 *MEMA kwa Vijana* trial survey assessed participants' knowledge of pregnancy prevention, HIV acquisition, and the acquisition of other sexually transmitted infections by asking three questions about each topic, and then determining the proportion of participants who answered all three questions correctly for each topic. These questions were very basic, such as, "Can a person who looks strong and healthy have the AIDS virus?" and, "Is it possible for a person to prevent pregnancy by using a condom while having sex?" For each of the topics, significantly higher proportions of intervention participants than control participants answered all three questions correctly; this was true for both males and females (table 7.1).

In 2002 the intervention's impact on knowledge was independently confirmed by responses to the sexual health questions placed within the national Year 7 examination in trial schools, as described in chapter 5. Those questions were answered by 4,707 intervention and control participants in the school year below the trial cohort, so they had not participated in trial research. However, all of those in intervention schools had participated in three years of the *MEMA kwa Vijana* school program. Tests were administered under examination conditions and were supervised by a teacher from a different school. In that examination, 88 percent of male and 80 percent of female intervention participants answered half or more of the sexual health questions correctly, compared to only 59 percent and 41 percent of male and female control participants, respectively. In addition, 32 percent of male and 20 percent of female intervention participants answered 80 percent or more of the sexual health questions correctly, compared to less than 1 percent of both male and female control participants. For both males and females all of these differences were statistically significant by intervention status.

The 2007–2008 long-term cross-sectional survey assessed participant knowledge about pregnancy prevention, HIV acquisition, and the acquisition of other sexually transmitted infections by asking the same questions that had been asked in the 2001–2002 trial survey. For almost all of the knowledge questions, higher proportions of both intervention and control participants gave correct answers than had been the case in 2001–2002. For several of these, significantly higher proportions of intervention participants than control participants answered correctly, namely for HIV acquisition (females), sexually transmitted infection acquisition (males), and pregnancy prevention (males and females) (table 7.1).

In both the 2001–2002 and the 2007–2008 surveys, males and females who had participated in two or three years of the intervention, rather than one only, were more likely to answer knowledge questions about pregnancy prevention correctly. In 2001–2002, this was also true for male responses to questions about HIV acquisition.

The consistent finding of significant and long-term intervention impact on knowledge is important, given improved understanding of sexual and reproductive health is considered to be a crucial step in risk reduction, and substantial knowledge gaps still exist in sub-Saharan Africa even thirty years into the AIDS epidemic (e.g., Uiso et al., 2006; Bastien, Sango et al., 2008; Dixon-Mueller, 2009; Ezekiel et al., 2009; Robins, 2009; Mkumbo, 2010; UNAIDS, 2010; Dimbuene and Defo, 2011). Critically, the trial demonstrated that a low-cost, large-scale participatory school program could achieve this impact despite great resource limitations. However, the surveys only assessed very basic knowledge about HIV, AIDS, and other sexual health issues. They thus did not reveal much about the depth, complexity, or extent of intervention participants' improved knowledge.

Attitudes

In both the 2001–2002 and the 2007–2008 *MEMA kwa Vijana* surveys, participant attitudes were assessed by asking whether they agreed, disagreed, or did not know how to respond to each of three statements. Intervention impact was then determined by comparing the proportions of intervention and control participants who responded to all three statements in the way desired by the intervention. Those statements addressed a girl's right or ability to refuse sex if a boy or man is older than her, if he is her lover, or if she has already accepted a gift from him. In the 2001–2002 survey, the overall proportion of trial members who gave the desired responses to all three of the statements was low. Nonetheless, significantly higher proportions of intervention participants than control participants gave the desired responses to all three statements, and this was true for both males and females (table 7.1). In addition, males who had participated in two or three years of the intervention were more likely to report the desired attitudes than males who had only participated in one year of it.

For males in the 2007–2008 survey, slightly higher proportions of both intervention and control participants consistently gave the desired responses to these statements, and there were no significant differences by intervention status. For females, in contrast, the proportion of intervention participants who consistently reported the desired attitudes decreased from 27 percent in 2001–2002 to 11 percent in 2007–2008, and similarly for control participants decreased from 19 percent to 10 percent; there were no significant differences by intervention status (table 7.1). It is striking that, with increased age and experience, markedly lower proportions of female intervention and control participants believed a girl has the right or ability to refuse sex in all of the three circumstances specified. Nonetheless, there was some evidence of intervention impact on women's attitudes based on the extent of their participation in the *MEMA kwa Vijana* program. Specifically, women who had participated in two or three years of the intervention were more likely to report the desired attitudes than women who had only participated in only one year of it.

Behavior

In the 1998 *MEMA kwa Vijana* baseline survey, 49 percent of males (average age sixteen) and 79 percent of females (average age fifteen) reported they had never had sex (Todd et al., 2004). As discussed earlier in the chapter, however, triangulation of different data sources suggests that this variable was underreported, particularly for females (Plummer, Ross et al., 2004; Plummer, Wight et al., 2004). Of those trial participants who reported they had never had sex at the beginning of the trial, approximately two-thirds said they had become sexually active by the 2001–2002 survey at the end of the trial (table 7.1). For this and other abstinence variables measured in the 2001–2002 and 2007–2008 surveys, there were no significant differences by intervention status.

The *MEMA kwa Vijana* intervention did, however, have a limited impact on male participants' reported partner number (table 7.1). In 2001–2002, a significantly lower proportion of male intervention participants (19 percent) than control participants (28 percent) reported they had had more than one sexual partner in the last twelve months. In addition, males who had participated in two or three years of the intervention were significantly less likely to report more than one partner in the last twelve months than males who had only participated in one year of the program. For females there was no significant difference by intervention status for this variable (9 percent and 8 percent, respectively), and also no significant difference by years of program participation amongst intervention participants.

In 2007–2008, there was no significant difference for this variable for either males (41 percent intervention, 45 percent control) or females (both 10 percent) (table 7.1). However, at that time a significantly lower proportion of male intervention participants (37 percent) than control participants (44 percent) reported more than four partners in their lifetimes. No similar difference was observed by intervention status for females for a similar variable, that is, more than two lifetime partners (34 percent and 37 percent, respectively). In addition, no significant difference by intervention status was observed for either males or females for another partner number variable (i.e., more than one partner in the last four weeks) or a concurrency variable (i.e., more than one partner during the same time period in the last twelve months).

The *MEMA kwa Vijana* intervention also had limited impact on some condom use variables reported by males and females (table 7.1). In 2001–2002, significantly higher proportions of both male and female intervention participants (39 percent and 38 percent, respectively) than control participants (both

28 percent) reported first use of condoms during the trial. In addition, significantly higher proportions of male intervention participants (29 percent) than control participants (20 percent) reported condom use at last sex. For females there was no significant difference by intervention status for this variable (27 percent and 22 percent, respectively). In contrast, in 2007–2008 there was no significant difference in reported condom use for males by intervention status, either for condom use at last sex in the past twelve months, or specifically for condom use at last sex in the past twelve months with a non-regular partner. Females did not show a significant difference by intervention status for the former variable, but female intervention participants (45 percent) were significantly more likely than their control counterparts (31 percent) to report condom use at last sex in the past twelve months with a non-regular partner.

Biological Markers

In the 2001–2002 survey, 14 percent of males (average age nineteen) and 45 percent of females (average age eighteen) tested positive for trichomonas, herpes, syphilis, chlamydia, gonorrhea, and/or HIV (Helen Weiss, personal communication). The incidence and/or prevalence of each of these infections is shown by sex and intervention status in table 7.1. Intervention status was not significantly associated with any infection or with pregnancy, except that gonorrhea was slightly higher among female intervention participants. This association was only of borderline statistical significance, and it was only seen in the school year that had had the least exposure to the intervention, suggesting that it was due to chance rather than intervention participation. Similarly, there were no significant differences in either direction by intervention status for any of the five sexually transmitted infections tested in the 2007–2008 survey (table 7.1).

In both the 2001–2002 and the 2007–2008 surveys, the proportions of male and female respondents who reported experience of abnormal genital discharge during the past year was lower in intervention communities than in control communities, sometimes significantly so. For males and females reporting symptoms of sexually transmitted infection, however, there were no significant differences by intervention status in the proportions who reported seeking care at a health facility for their most recent outbreak during the past year.

IN-DEPTH QUALITATIVE IMPACT EVALUATION

As discussed in chapter 4, the *MEMA kwa Vijana* school curriculum (Appendices 1–3) and other intervention components were based on two behavioral theories, the Social Cognitive Theory and the Theory of Reasoned Action. Those theories identify largely overlapping sets of factors which are believed to determine behavior, including knowledge of the risks and benefits of behaviors, perception of personal risk, anticipated outcomes, intentions or goals, sense of self-efficacy or control, observational learning or modeling, and contextual facilitators and impediments (Bandura, 2004; Michie et al., 2005; Aarø, Schaalma, and Åstrøm, 2008). Overall, the qualitative evaluation suggests that the intervention *did* have an impact on many of those determinants, but that this was only to a mild extent for most intervention participants, and/or to a great extent for a few, and this was insufficient to result in a significant and sustained impact on the trial population's behavior, unintended pregnancy, or sexually transmitted infections. The next three sections will examine these findings in more depth by considering the intervention's impact on each of the theoretically defined behavioral determinants of abstinence, low partner number, and condom use.

Theoretical Determinants of Abstinence

Knowledge of the Risks and Benefits of Abstinence

In the course of participating in the *MEMA kwa Vijana* school program, the vast majority of intervention participants' knowledge of the risks and benefits of abstinence improved. Almost all understood that unprotected vaginal intercourse could result in pregnancy, infection, and other reproductive health problems, and that abstinence was the only certain way to avoid such consequences. Male pupils generally seemed to understand and retain this information in greater detail than female pupils, which may reflect how boys were typically favored and encouraged more in their learning. In addition, the approximately 12 percent of the trial population who were peer educators had a particularly good understanding of these issues, which reflected their participation in the special training course as well as the school program.

Abstinence-Related Risk Perception

While almost all pupils' abstract understanding of sexual risk improved with intervention participation, this usually did not result in more accurate personal risk perception related to abstinence. Many intervention participants abstractly associated sexually transmitted infections with substantially older people, urban residents, and/or people with obvious symptoms, all of whom were indeed more likely to be infected with sexually transmitted diseases. However, in practice pupils rarely avoided older men and urban visitors as sexual partners, and on the contrary often considered them to be particularly desirable partners because of their perceived wealth, modernity, and/or style. In addition, although the biological surveys revealed that sexually transmitted infections were fairly common, many infected youth probably did not experience symptoms. Even if they did experience symptoms, however, they might not have recognized the condition as a sexually transmitted infection, or if they did they might not have revealed it in order to avoid stigma. Negative consequences related to unintended pregnancies were more visible in rural Mwanza, and female pupils were more likely to fear this than infection. Nonetheless, many girls felt pregnancy was a low risk—especially if they had already had sex without becoming pregnant—and some were ambivalent about potential pregnancy because they expected to leave school, marry, and have children soon regardless.

In the qualitative research it was very rare for pupils to give plausible reports of intentionally abstaining after sexual debut (i.e., secondary abstinence) in order to avoid infection or pregnancy. When they did, this almost always resulted from a frightening personal experience of negative consequences of sexual activity, as seen in examples provided by both intervention and control participants in case studies 1.3, 1.4, and 3.3.

Outcomes Expected from Abstinence

Intervention participants' limited ability to accurately assess their personal risk influenced their abstinence-related outcome expectations. For most, the immediate benefits of sex outweighed the possibility of pregnancy or other consequences later. Importantly, adolescents may have a limited ability to anticipate long-term behavioral outcomes, and their exploratory behaviors also may have had an impulsive component (Johnson et al., 2003; Breinbauer and Maddaleno, 2005). In addition, however, the *MEMA kwa Vijana* program only superficially addressed intervention participants' overriding motivations to have sex, that is, sexual desire for boys and material gain for girls. If participants' main incentives to have sex are not addressed in depth, they may mistrust the intervention and feel its goals are unrealistic.

It is not unusual for adolescent sexual health programs in Africa or elsewhere to avoid discussion of sexual pleasure, and also not to acknowledge masturbation as a safe way to satisfy sexual desire, because these are potentially controversial topics (Pattman and Chege, 2003; Mkumbo, 2009). However, in a context where masturbation may be perceived as more harmful than unprotected intercourse (e.g., where it may be believed to reduce a man's virility or his potential to reproduce), it is important to acknowledge it is a safe way to manage sexual desire. This acknowledgement may not only be relevant to primary and secondary abstinence but also to monogamy and condom use, as masturbation can also be a safe way to satisfy sexual desire when a monogamous person is separated from a partner, or a condom user does not have access to a condom.

Unlike sexual pleasure for boys, during the trial the *MEMA kwa Vijana* intervention increasingly addressed girls' expectation that they would receive money or materials in exchange for sex. As discussed in chapter 4, the school curriculum initially addressed material exchange for sex by encouraging girls to reject male offers of gifts and money, and providing them with opportunities to practice their refusal skills. The final version of the curriculum additionally acknowledged that girls might be motivated to have sex due to material gain, and might encourage one another to do so. However, the curriculum was not able to address the centrality of transactional sex in adolescent girls' lives and the frequent, fundamental dilemmas they faced in having few other ways to obtain basic necessities, such as underwear and soap. In addition, the final curriculum only superficially engaged with some deeply imbedded cultural beliefs about material exchange, reciprocity, and self-esteem, for example, beliefs that a girl who received a gift from a boy or man was indeed obliged to have sex with him, and that a sexually active girl who did *not* receive something in exchange for sex had little self-respect.

Abstinence Goals

Within the school program, pupils were encouraged to make goals to be abstinent while schooling and/or until marriage. Reflective exercises were intended to help participants focus on their short-term and long-term goals to guide them in their behaviors. The qualitative research suggests that sexual health intervention participation influenced a small minority of adolescents to actively set abstinence as a personal goal, particularly those who were highly motivated to go far in school and/or to establish financial independence before starting a family. This can be seen in the description of the *MEMA kwa Vijana* intervention participant in case study 1.2, as well as the two young people in case studies 1.3 and 2.2 who—unusually for pupils in trial control communities—had also participated in sexual health education while in school. These young people believed abstinence would help them achieve their ambitions, because they would not be distracted by sex and/or they would not have to leave school due to pregnancy. Some girls also had a goal to be abstinent to maintain their good reputations, as this had implications for their self-esteem, community regard, and future marriage prospects, as can be seen in case study 2.1. However, the qualitative research found that most intervention participants did not consider abstinence to be a realistic or feasible goal in either the short-term or the long-term. The following examples from an in-depth interview with an eighteen-year-old married woman and a participant observation group discussion with young men were typical:

R: Some people can reduce partners, some can use condoms. To abstain completely, I have never seen someone who has abstained completely. Very few abstain completely. . . .

I: Why do you think they don't abstain completely?

R: Maybe *tamaa* (literally "desire," "longing," "greed," or "lust"; colloquially often used to describe male sexual desire and female desire for nice commodities). (I-02-I-290-f)

P: As I see it, it is better that they stop shouting at people and telling a person not to have sex when his organ is fine and he is physically fit. I would suggest that they leave that and think of another plan, like teaching and convincing them to just reduce their partner number, and perhaps to be faithful to one lover. . . . It would even be better if you told a person to try to use condoms, to do it with condoms, but not to stop completely. That is impossible. (GD-02-I-1-1m)

Self-Efficacy to Be Abstinent

Almost all of the skills-building exercises in the school curriculum focused on abstinence, and particularly on girls' abilities to resist sexual advances from boys and men, and boys' abilities to resist peer pressure to have sex. The intervention participants who had the greatest perceived self-efficacy to be abstinent—that is, those who believed they could control themselves and successfully abstain—were almost always those who had never had sex. For some of these young people, strong intervention emphasis on abstinence and sexual refusal skills may have reinforced their sense of control and helped delay their sexual debut. However, the qualitative research found that widespread and persistent pressures and temptations for young people to have sex typically wore down the resistance of all but those most highly motivated to abstain. Notably, adolescent girls who abstained were often considered the most "hard-to-get" and desirable partners, so boys and men intensively targeted them with sexual propositions.

Adolescents who had already become sexually active rarely believed they had sufficient self-control to become abstinent again. Young men typically believed they had a natural, biological drive that they could not overcome once they had experienced sex. In contrast, once adolescent girls had had sex, it quickly became the main way for them to obtain basic needs and small luxuries and very few perceived abstinence as a feasible option any longer. In practice, many pupils who had already experienced sex, particularly school boys, *did* go through abstinent periods of weeks or months in length. However, for boys this typically was not voluntary or intentional and when they again had the opportunity to have sex—as most often happened around special events, such as a sports competition or *ngoma* celebrations—then they felt they could not abstain.

Modeling Abstinence

Within the school curriculum, abstinence was modeled in stories and dramas in which abstinent characters remained in school and healthy while some pupils who had sex became pregnant, contracted an infection, and/or dropped out of school (e.g., box 5.1). However, the intervention did not have much success in modeling abstinence in real life, that is, in providing new opportunities for pupils to learn how to abstain by observing others. In addition to talking about their abstinence goals and life priorities, for example, male role models might demonstrate abstinence skills by declining to participate in sexual pursuit of young women with their peers, while female role models might refuse to engage in sexual negotiation when approached by men and boys at special events or festivals. Peer educators were intended to be such role models, but the qualitative research suggests only a small minority of peer educators seemed to practice lower risk behaviors than other pupils, including abstinence. Abstinence also was not a behavior that adults modeled for adolescents, as abstinence was only perceived as a goal for unmarried youth. Virtually all adults of reproductive age were sexually active in rural Mwanza, whether they were married or not.

Contextual Impediments of Abstinence

Many of the social, economic, and cultural influences on young people's sexual behavior described in chapter 3 and this book's companion volume (Plummer and Wight, 2011) were contextual impediments of abstinence, and the intervention had very little impact on them. This included girls' low and subservient social status, which made it difficult for them to resist sexual pressure from men who approached them for sex and from female intermediaries who were authority figures. As already noted, girls' economic dependence on boys and men was also a great impediment to abstinence, because it contributed to sex being an important economic resource for them. For boys, contextual impediments to abstinence included the widespread beliefs that sexual activity was central to masculine identity and that continued sexual activity was inevitable once a boy had experienced sex.

Contextual Facilitators of Abstinence

The intervention's promotion of abstinence was in line with some contextual facilitators of abstinence, such as the common adult ideal that school pupils should be abstinent, especially pupils who hoped to go further in formal education. However, the intervention was not able to strengthen or reinforce such beliefs by making them more feasible to achieve. This was largely due to structural impediments such as poverty and gender inequality. For example, although intervention teachers repeatedly encouraged pupils to abstain so they could pursue further schooling, intervention participants knew that only a minority of Year 7 pupils ever won a place in secondary school, and that few girls who achieved this were supported by their parents to pursue secondary education.

Theoretical Determinants of Low Partner Number and/or Fidelity

Knowledge of the Risks and Benefits of Having Few Partners and/or Being Faithful

Young people's knowledge of the risks and benefits of having few partners and/or being faithful improved with *MEMA kwa Vijana* intervention participation. School sessions focused on reproductive anatomy, the local prevalence of sexually transmitted infections, disease transmission simulation exercises (box 4.1), dramas, and stories conveyed the basic principle that unprotected sex with multiple partners was associated with increased risk of infection.

However, the relationship between sexual partner number and infection transmission is complex and depends on many factors, such as the frequency of sexual encounters, the type of sexual activity, the rate of partner change, the overlap of partnerships, and the type of infection (Caldwell, Caldwell, and Quiggin, 1989; Halperin and Epstein, 2004; Buvé, 2006; Harrison and O'Sullivan, 2010). Given the low education levels of both teachers and pupils in rural Mwanza, the school program did not attempt to convey such concepts in their complexity. Instead, it noted that the protective potential of monogamy is difficult to assess, particularly as a sexual partner might begin a relationship already infected with a sexually transmitted disease, or might contract it from unacknowledged partners during the relationship. The curriculum also repeatedly stressed that HIV-positive people usually appear healthy for many years before developing symptoms. Intervention participants were thus encouraged to be abstinent until marriage, but if they could not be, they were encouraged to be monogamous and to use condoms. Mutual HIV testing prior to starting a sexual relationship was not addressed, because such services were hardly available in rural Mwanza at the time of the trial. Even if they had been more available for the general population, however, it may still have been very difficult for unmarried adolescents to access such services, given their sexual activity was very hidden.

Risk Perception Related to Having Few Partners and/or Being Faithful

While pupils' abstract understanding of the risk of multiple partnerships improved with intervention participation, their personal risk perception related to this often remained limited, for several reasons. First, very few villagers had ever had any biology education, and it was commonly believed that illnesses were cured once symptoms were gone. Although intervention participants developed a basic understanding that some infections can be asymptomatic for a long period, this was difficult for them to fully conceptualize and apply. Most still felt they were not at risk if a sexual partner appeared healthy and they had agreed to be faithful to one another. Second, concurrent sexual partnerships were fairly common but well hidden, so it was difficult to know when a partner had other partners. Third, while adolescents typically expected their partners to be faithful—and ended relationships if a partner's infidelity was discovered—they often did not hold themselves to the same standard and were not as concerned by the risk posed by their *own* infidelity. Fourth, many young people considered themselves to be safely monogamous, even if they had a series of monogamous relationships with only short gaps in between them over a period of months or years.

Despite these limitations, the intervention did seem to influence a small minority of pupils—particularly males—to become concerned about risk related to their multiple partnerships, or those of a partner. The few individuals who intentionally tried to reduce such risk usually tried to be mutually monogamous in their premarital relationships and then to marry and have a long-term, mutually faithful relationship. Some of these individuals also tried to be selective in who they chose as sexual partners, studying potential partners before choosing one who they believed had had few prior partners and who they believed would be faithful to them. Case study 3.3 provides one example. This attempt to reduce risk depends on subjective impressions and imperfect risk assessment, but nonetheless sometimes may have been protective.

Outcomes Expected from Having Few Partners and/or Being Faithful

The qualitative research found that some young people perceived immediate, positive benefits to having multiple partners, and the intervention did not have much impact on those expectations. Many young men sought new partners to maximize their sexual pleasure. Some young women instead took new sexual partners to maximize what they received in exchange for sex, because men typically offered the most money or gifts for sexual encounters early in a relationship. Such outcome expectations contributed to opportunistic sexual relationships (particularly when traveling or attending special events), serial monogamy, and concurrency.

Nonetheless, of the three low-risk sexual behaviors promoted by *MEMA kwa Vijana*, intervention participants typically perceived partner reduction and monogamy as involving the least sacrifice and thus being the most feasible and desirable. Unlike abstinence and condom use, these behaviors could still satisfy young people's main motivations to have sex, that is, the pleasure of unprotected intercourse for boys and the receipt of money or gifts for girls. Both also allowed for pregnancy, if desired. Fidelity was also a social ideal in rural Mwanza, and as such it was positively reinforced by sexual partners and the broader community, especially for girls. Thus, intervention participants often expected some positive personal, physical, and social outcomes related to partner reduction and monogamy.

Goals to Have Few Partners and/or Be Faithful

As noted above, the school program primarily promoted low partner number and fidelity for sexually active youth by stressing the increased risk involved in multiple partnerships. Most curriculum exercises focused on building skills and setting goals for abstinence, not reducing partner number and/or being faithful. For example, there were no exercises addressing how to discuss risk or how to negotiate mutual fidelity with a sexual partner. Critically, however, safe practice of monogamy does not rely solely on an individual's decision to be monogamous and his or her ability to follow through on that decision, but also on a partner's intention and restraint.

When the *MEMA kwa Vijana* intervention was developed in 1998, very few HIV prevention interventions in sub-Saharan Africa focused on fidelity and related interpersonal skills in depth. Even today few such interventions exist, and they mostly target married couples (e.g., Parikh, 2007). This evaluation suggests that intensive promotion of low partner number and/or fidelity with unmarried young people has promising potential, because those practices are social ideals shared by many youth and adults in rural Africa, and adolescents reported they were more feasible than either abstinence or condom use. Nonetheless, such intervention work is likely to be very challenging, for several reasons. First, if local authorities and adult community members require that an intervention primarily promotes abstinence, as was the case for *MEMA kwa Vijana*, it can become very difficult to have in-depth and complex discussions about pupil sexual relationships, which are typically hidden. Indeed, as noted in chapter 5, *MEMA kwa Vijana* teachers frequently said they found it challenging and contradictory to advise pupils to be abstinent while also promoting monogamy and condom use if pupils were sexually active. Other school-based interventions have had similar findings (e.g., Helleve et al., 2009; Njue et al., 2009).

Second, it may be difficult to promote fidelity and/or low partner number with adolescents because adolescence can be a time of personal exploration and transitory sexual relationships. Many youth in rural Mwanza entered into new sexual relationships with few specific goals for how the relationships would develop beyond the first encounter, but they were open to multiple possibilities and eventually hoped to find a suitable spouse. It was thus not unusual for young people to have overlapping, open-ended relationships in which partners did not necessarily plan to continue the relationship, but they had sex when circumstances were conducive and the opportunity arose. During such a life stage, it is unclear how to effectively promote mutual and long-term monogamy.

Third, it is not possible to unequivocally promote partner reduction and monogamy as behavioral goals because it is difficult to assess the extent to which these practices are protective in the absence of condom use. Practicing these behaviors in a safe way can be a complex, challenging, and ongoing process. If a couple does not use condoms, for example, fidelity is only protective against disease if both are uninfected and monogamous. Their relationship could instead be high risk if one or both individuals enters the relationship infected or is not faithful during the relationship. So while the *MEMA kwa Vijana* intervention stressed the risks involved in multiple partnerships, it could not unequivocally promote monogamy as low risk, particularly in a context where HIV testing was largely unavailable.

Self-Efficacy to Have Few Partners and/or Be Faithful

It is unclear whether the *MEMA kwa Vijana* intervention had much impact on participants' self-efficacy to have few partners and/or be faithful, for several of the reasons already discussed. On the one hand, intervention participants typically perceived these options as more realistic and feasible than abstinence or condom use. On the other hand, they may have felt little control over critical factors which made these practices safe, such as whether a partner entered a relationship with an infection, whether a partner was faithful during the relationship, and whether condoms were used. This may have reinforced a broader cultural belief that risk is inevitable and unavoidable, justifying high-risk practices. Importantly, the increased availability of HIV testing in Mwanza and elsewhere in sub-Saharan Africa today could partially address such fatalism and reduce the risk involved in monogamous relationships, if couples were to test themselves for HIV before having unprotected intercourse and then test again at routine intervals afterward.

Modeling Low Partner Number and/or Fidelity

In dramas and stories within the school program, characters with many partners developed sexually transmitted infections, while those who only had one partner long-term usually remained healthy. Those few monogamous individuals who did contract infections either had a series of monogamous relationships or had a partner who was not faithful, and their storylines were used to illustrate the importance of condom use even within monogamous relationships. These dramas were entertaining and popular among intervention participants, and many youth remembered details about them a few years later, suggesting that they were useful in modeling the practices of having few partners and/or being faithful. However, as noted earlier, the qualitative research found that only a small minority of the peer educators who performed the dramas actively reduced their sexual partner number and/or were faithful due to their intervention participation, suggesting they were not able to model those new behaviors for their peers in real life. For example, a sexually active male peer educator could have modeled these skills and behaviors if he made a personal commitment to have only one mutually faithful sexual relationship, if he explained his intention to his friends, and if he then did not succumb to pressure or temptation to have new partners when such opportunities arose.

Contextual Impediments to Having Few Partners and/or Being Faithful

As was the case with abstinence, some of the social, economic, and cultural norms and expectations described in chapter 3 and this book's companion volume (Plummer and Wight, 2011) were barriers to low-risk practices such as having few partners and being faithful, and the intervention did not seem to have an impact on them. Many intervention participants continued to manage contradictory social norms and expectations by hiding their sexual relationships from adults. This practice often also concealed an individual's partners from one another, helping to maintain concurrency and inhibiting realistic risk perception. The intervention also was not able to enhance adolescent girls' limited alternatives to sex to obtain basic supplies, and this economic dependence sometimes contributed to girls seeking new serial or concurrent sexual partners. Finally, the intervention only superficially addressed a common belief amongst young men that seducing new and/ or multiple partners demonstrated masculinity. It also did not promote alternative ways to establish masculinity, such as through sports, disciplined employment, or entrepreneurship.

Contextual Facilitators of Low Partner Number and/or Fidelity

In rural Mwanza, several contextual facilitators encouraged low partner number, particularly for women, but they mainly related to adulthood and marriage. By primarily promoting abstinence until marriage and fidelity after marriage, the *MEMA kwa Vijana* intervention was broadly in line with social ideals related to marriage. However, such ideals may not have seemed immediately relevant to school pupils who were at an exploratory stage of their sexual lives and whose premarital sexual relationships were hidden. Only a small number of intervention participants reported that the program influenced them to have one low-risk, long-term premarital partner with whom they had unprotected sex, as seen in case study 3.3.

Most intervention participants left school during the trial and about one-third of female participants were married by the end of it (Lutz, 2005). Young people chose to marry for many reasons, including a desire for offspring, economic security, adult status, or legitimate sexual access to a partner. Some also married to ensure a partner's sexual fidelity and/or to reduce their sexual risk related to multiple sexual partnerships. Marriage was considered protective because it involved an overt commitment of mutual fidelity, even if this was not always fully achieved in practice. In addition, marriage was perceived as protective because young people typically chose spouses who they believed were low risk, as opposed to partners who they believed had many prior or current partners, with whom they might enjoy sex but not want a more serious commitment. These issues will be discussed in more depth in chapter 9.

Theoretical Determinants of Condom Use

Knowledge of the Risks and Benefits of Condom Use

At the end of the trial, the vast majority of intervention participants had better knowledge of the risks and benefits of condom use than their control counterparts. Most knew that condoms protect against pregnancy and sexually transmitted infections, and most rejected common false beliefs, such as beliefs that new condoms have HIV or have holes in them. Health workers played an important role in teaching pupils correct information about condom use, for several reasons. Their prior training and experience made them unusually aware of youth sexual health needs and confident in teaching about condom use; other adult community members were usually comfortable with them in that role; and institutionally they were not constrained from engaging in explicit sexual discussion in the way that teachers were. Among pupils, intensive peer educator training helped peer educators have a relatively good understanding of the value and practice of condom use, even though this was still limited as they were not shown condoms during their training courses.

Educational authorities did not allow condoms to be shown within the school curriculum either, and proper condom use was not explained in detail until the last session of Year 7 (box 4.2), if teachers and schools elected that option. In addition, while class visits to health facilities were strategic in enabling many pupils to see condoms and a condom demonstration, most pupils only participated in such a visit once or twice. If teachers did not organize such a visit or pupils missed school that day, those pupils typically only had a vague idea of what condoms looked like and how they were used. Intervention participants' understanding of condom use thus varied greatly, with many having a positive but somewhat confused and incomplete understanding of it. Notably, an international review of adolescent HIV prevention interventions found that the more time programs devoted to condom instruction and training, including skills to negotiate and use condoms, the more likely participants were to later report condom use (Johnson et al., 2003). Similarly, in a study of four African countries Bankole, Ahmed, and colleagues (2007) found that adolescents who had seen a condom demonstration were two to five times more likely than others to know correct condom use.

During the *MEMA kwa Vijana* trial, educational authorities' increasing willingness to provide primary school pupils with detailed information about condom use illustrates the value of ongoing advocacy to support and improve adolescent sexual health programs. The final 2002 *MEMA kwa Vijana* curriculum had more condom-related information than the early trial versions, but it still had less than intervention implementers ideally would have included from the onset had they not been constrained by local and national policies. Recent research suggests that Tanzanian adults have become more open to the idea of teaching adolescents about condoms. For example, the 2004–2005 Tanzanian Demographic and Health Survey found that 65 percent of women and 72 percent of men aged eighteen to forty-nine years agreed that twelve- to fourteen-year-old children should be taught about using a condom to avoid AIDS (National Bureau of Statistics and ORC Macro, 2005). The proportions were even higher (80 percent and 82 percent respectively) in the Lake Zone, which includes Mwanza Region.

Similarly, a 2007 study of 86 parents of ten- to thirteen-year-olds in one of the *MEMA kwa Vijana* districts found that 73 percent supported the idea of sex and relationships education in primary schools (Mkumbo and Ingham, 2010). When compared to parents from an urban area who had participated in a different primary school sexual health program, the parents in the *MEMA kwa Vijana* district categorized far more topics as "very important" to address within a curriculum, and were more likely to identify potentially controversial issues as "important" or "very important," such as condom use (Mkumbo and Ingham, 2010). Parental preferences did not differ significantly by sex, education level, employment status, or religion, but younger parents were significantly more supportive of school programs than those forty-five years old or older. Over time, local attitudes and guidelines may become more permissive of previously controversial material, which highlights the need to routinely review and improve the content of school curricula in Tanzania and elsewhere in sub-Saharan Africa.

Risk Perception Related to Condom Use

As noted earlier, at the end of the *MEMA kwa Vijana* trial many intervention participants abstractly associated sexually transmitted infections with substantially older people, urban residents, and/or people with obvious, severe symptoms, but often in practice both older men and urban visitors were sought-after sexual partners. Condom-related personal risk perception skills remained limited and very few sexually active intervention participants were concerned enough about their risk of infection or pregnancy to use condoms. Those young people who did use condoms were extraordinarily fearful of infection (typically out-of-school young men) or pregnancy (typically school girls), such as male youths who had already experienced symptoms of sexually transmitted infection, or girls who were unusually determined to go to secondary school.

After leaving school, some male intervention participants said they sometimes used condoms with women who they considered to be high risk, such as bar maids, guesthouse staff, and other women who were reputed to have many partners. Case study 3.3 provides an example of this. Such selective condom use suggests there was some intervention impact on young men's personal risk assessment skills. This subjective approach to risk reduction is problematic, given someone can falsely conclude a healthy-looking HIV-positive person is low risk. Nonetheless, young men who tried to reduce their risk in this way considered it a feasible and practical strategy, and when compared to no condom use at all, it may indeed have reduced exposure to HIV sometimes. However, even this intervention impact was quite limited, as youths rarely continued to use condoms beyond a few sexual encounters with a new partner, even if the man had initially been concerned about the woman being unfaithful or having an infection from a prior relationship. Typically, when individuals began to trust a partner's current fidelity they also began to perceive the partner's risk as low, or as an acceptable trade-off for the emotional intimacy and physical pleasure of unprotected intercourse, as has also been found in other research with African youth (e.g., Hattori, Richter, and Greene, 2010).

Outcomes Expected from Condom Use

The *MEMA kwa Vijana* intervention had some influence on participants' condom use outcome expectations. At the end of the trial, most intervention participants expected condom use to be safe and that it would protect them against pregnancy and sexually transmitted infection. In addition, most female intervention participants seemed to perceive the potential physical experience of condom use neutrally, expecting that it would not affect their comfort or pleasure either negatively or positively. Most male intervention participants instead continued to expect that—as widely rumored—condom use would somewhat reduce their sexual pleasure. This was reported by male intervention participants in general as well as those few who had tried to use condoms. In contrast, control participants were more likely to expect condom use to be very unpleasant, harmful, and/or inadequate protection against pregnancy or disease.

As noted earlier, sexual pleasure was hardly discussed within the school program, even though this was the main motivation for male youth to have sex. In the first versions of the curriculum, the possibility of reduced pleasure during condom use was not addressed, although this was an oft cited reason why boys and men rejected condoms in rural Mwanza. Based on HALIRA feedback on this issue, the final version of the curriculum briefly acknowledged condoms might somewhat affect pleasure for some people, but stressed that the value of condom use in preventing pregnancy and infection made this an acceptable trade-off or compromise.

By only marginally addressing boys' and men's central concern about the possibility of reduced pleasure during condom use, some male participants may have felt the intervention was out of touch with their reality and their concerns. However, intervention teachers' feedback suggests that it would have been very difficult for them to engage with young people about ways to make condom use more pleasurable. Given health workers were generally more comfortable and accepted by the community when speaking frankly about youth sexuality, they may have been better placed to take on such a responsibility.

Condom Use Goals

While many pupils became neutral or positive toward condoms through their intervention exposure, few seemed to perceive condom use as realistic enough to plan to use them, even with high-risk partners. This related to multiple factors, including a limited sense of personal risk, low self-efficacy (especially for girls), and poor condom access. The *MEMA kwa Vijana* curriculum repeatedly recommended that sexually active young people use condoms, but personalization and reflective exercises within the curriculum did not focus on pupils actively setting a goal of condom use. Just as some teachers felt a conflict between the promotion of abstinence and premarital fidelity with school pupils, some felt a conflict between the primary promotion of abstinence and intensive promotion of condom use for sexually active pupils. It was not unusual for teachers to manage this by insisting that pupils abstain but also telling them that—once they left school and became sexually active adults—they could use condoms to protect themselves. Some other school-based HIV prevention programs in sub-Saharan African have encountered similar conflicts (e.g., Brouillard-Coyle et al., 2005; UNESCO, 2008; Ahmed et al., 2009). Within the *MEMA kwa Vijana* intervention, such statements seemed to confuse some sexually active pupils, and/or they used them to justify having unprotected sex, claiming that their teachers told them they were not allowed to use condoms until they had left school.

Self-Efficacy to Use Condoms

It is difficult to assess the impact of the *MEMA kwa Vijana* intervention on male participants' self-efficacy to use condoms, that is, on the belief that they had enough control over their behavior to use condoms. Even in optimal circumstances, when teachers taught the detailed condom session at the end of Year 7, practical instruction and exercises related to condom use only addressed how to obtain, put on, and dispose of condoms, not broader behavioral issues, such as negotiation with a partner, or strategies to use condoms consistently and long-term. It was not unusual for male intervention participants to say that they knew how to use condoms and where to buy them, and that they had enough money to purchase them and would not be inhibited in doing so. Many reported they would be able to use condoms if they wanted to do so, but they said they simply did not want to use them. Some said it would be very difficult to convince a girl to let them use a condom, and a few said they could not use condoms because, once aroused, they did not have the self-control to pause to put a condom on. Those few who did report condom use typically had enough control over their behavior to use them occasionally, but very few demonstrated self-efficacy to use them consistently with all partners, or with one partner beyond the first few encounters.

The *MEMA kwa Vijana* intervention seemed to have almost no impact on female participants' self-efficacy to use male condoms, that is, their belief that they could persuade and assist their partners to use them. Female intervention participants were more likely than female control participants to say they would agree to use condoms if a new sexual partner suggested it. However, very few young women ever reported initiating or insisting upon condom use, and even those who did report this said they had not obtained the condoms themselves, because it would have been embarrassing or inappropriate for them to do so. Case study 3.2 provides one example. Many intervention participants also reported that material exchange reduced a woman's ability to negotiate condom use, because a boy or man would demand his money or gift back if a partner insisted on condom use.

Modeling Condom Use

Intervention developers hoped that *MEMA kwa Vijana* peer educators and condom distributors would not only broadly promote condom use for sexually active youth, but also use condoms themselves and acknowledge this openly and positively with their peers, in this way becoming role models of condom use. It seems likely that most, if not the vast majority, of condom distributors tried using condoms after receiving their brief intervention training. However, many of them found that condom use reduced their pleasure to an unacceptable extent, so they soon stopped completely or only used condoms in certain circumstances, such as when they considered a sexual partner to be high risk. While most condom distributors continued to promote condom use as a way for their peers to reduce their sexual risk, their own ambivalence was likely evident.

As school pupils, peer educators had far less access to condoms than condom distributors. Some had never seen a condom or a condom demonstration
themselves, and their peers knew that their attempts to promote condoms
usually were not based on personal experience. Most peer educators' sexual
behavior seemed similar to those of their peers, as discussed in chapter 5, but
after their intervention training a minority actively tried to reduce their risk by
using condoms, at least for a short period. For example, the few school girls
who initiated and insisted upon condom use were disproportionately peer
educators; case study 3.2 provides one example. However, even when a female peer educator negotiated condom use with a partner she was unlikely to
discuss it widely, and in that way be a role model of condom use, as acknowledgement of any sexual activity could damage a girl's reputation, and condom use was particularly stigmatized in the broader community. Similarly,
the qualitative research suggests that a small minority of male peer educators
tried condom use while still in school. Case study 3.1 describes an example
of an unusually old (twenty-two-year-old) pupil who seemed to use condoms
consistently. However, most male peer educators who used condoms used
them inconsistently, depending on several factors, such as their sense of risk
at the time, their access to condoms, and a partner's agreement. Chapter 10
will describe their motivations and experiences in more detail, within the
broader description of atypical trial participants who used condoms.

Contextual Impediments and Facilitators of Condom Use

The *MEMA kwa Vijana* intervention only had a very limited influence on
contextual facilitators and impediments of condom use. The most obvious
impediment was the difficulty intervention participants had in accessing condoms. Prior to the intervention, condoms were entirely unavailable in some
villages, and in others they were only available in very small numbers in a
few village kiosks. The *MEMA kwa Vijana* condom distribution initiative was
intended to improve condom access for sexually active pupils, but in practice
most condom distributors established very small clienteles which mainly
consisted of out-of-school male youths and adults. By the end of the trial few
intervention participants knew a condom distributor and very few had ever
obtained condoms from one.

Similarly, the intervention team ensured condoms were available in both
intervention and control health facilities during the trial, and intervention
health workers were more likely than control health workers to promote and
distribute condoms to unmarried young people. This probably contributed
to the significantly higher distribution of condoms recorded in intervention
health facilities during the trial, but the absolute numbers of condoms distributed remained extremely low (Larke et al., 2010).

An international review of adolescent HIV prevention programs found that intervention participants who received condoms did not later report more sexual risk behaviors, such as earlier sexual debut or higher numbers of partners (Johnson et al., 2003). However, at a later date they were more likely to report condom use. Nonetheless, improving adolescent access to condoms continues to be a challenge for school-based sexual health programs in sub-Saharan Africa (e.g., Njue et al., 2009). In South Africa, for example, where the Children's Act provides youth with the right to access condoms, government policies and public pronouncements regarding condom provision in schools have been confusing and contradictory, so few schools have taken the option to provide youth with condoms (Han and Bennish, 2009).

In addition to the logistical issue of condom access, there were other important contextual impediments to condom use in rural Mwanza which the *MEMA kwa Vijana* intervention was not able to address effectively. Many intervention participants came to perceive condoms as potentially valuable protection, but in the broader community negative attitudes toward condoms continued to be powerful and widespread. Adolescents—particularly adolescent girls—had such low social status relative to adults that even if condoms had been accessible to them it is unlikely that large numbers would have begun to use them consistently, given their out-of-school peers, sexual partners, and family members would not understand or support such a practice.

"Positive Deviants": Intervention Participants Who Reported Behavior Change

Despite the discouraging findings described above, there was some evidence of *MEMA kwa Vijana* intervention impact on sexual behavior at the individual level. Some intervention participants reported that the *MEMA kwa Vijana* program was useful for certain types of pupils, even if not for most pupils. A former peer educator and secondary school student explained: "*MEMA kwa Vijana* education helps people with good behavior. Pupils with good behavior are those who sit down and contemplate the importance of what they are being taught, even in other lessons" (PO-01-I-4-5f).

In in-depth interviews at the end of the trial, many intervention participants initially reported that the intervention had motivated them to reduce their sexual risk behavior, at least for a short period. Very few intervention participants in participant observation villages reported the same thing. Most of the in-depth interview respondents who reported this said that the intervention convinced them to abstain until marriage and to be monogamous after marriage. However, such reports of abstinence were sometimes contradicted by what respondents said later in an interview, or by positive biological test results. For example, a seventeen-year-old secondary school

student (Debora) said she had never had sex and attributed this to her
MEMA kwa Vijana participation:

> *I*: When do you think you will begin to have sex?
>
> *R*: [Laughter] I have not thought of that. . . . I don't even want to have sex. . . .
> I am afraid of getting pregnant. And sexually transmitted infections and AIDS.
>
> *I*: Was there a person who taught you about that?
>
> *R*: Yes, I was taught by *MEMA kwa Vijana*. . . . Different stories were read to
> us. . . . Like there was a girl who was in Year 5, she had sex and got pregnant,
> and she was expelled from school. . . . And another story, there was also a girl
> who had sex, she contracted AIDS. . . .
>
> *I*: Do young people usually use the methods you mentioned earlier [abstinence
> and condom use] to avoid getting sexually transmitted infections?
>
> *R*: There are some who use them, but I don't know about others. . . . I use them
> myself. I use that method of abstaining from sex. (II-02-I-300-f)

Despite Debora's convincing reports of never having had sex, four days
prior to her in-depth interview she had provided a survey sample that subsequently tested positive for pregnancy and gonorrhea.

At the end of the trial, some in-depth interview respondents instead reported that the intervention had influenced them to be monogamous. For
example, a twenty-two-year-old farmer named Nyamhanga:

> *I*: Do you think that education has helped you?
>
> *R*: Me? Of course it has helped me. . . . I have learned not to have many women.
> That you must remain with one only. Yes, because some people always have sex
> with different women. (II-02-I-297-m)

Nyamhanga may have been sincere in his intention to be monogamous,
and his intervention experience may have helped him have fewer partners
than he might otherwise have had. Nonetheless, when he participated in another interview seven years later, he was in a polygynous marriage with two
wives. At that time, Nyamhanga explained that he had had two extramarital
sexual relationships after he married his first wife. When his first wife did
not become pregnant in the first years of their marriage, he then decided to
marry one of his extramarital partners also (Wamoyi and Mshana, 2010).
Importantly, although polygynous marriages consist of concurrent sexual relationships, polygyny is not necessarily high risk. Indeed, it may be lower risk
for the individuals involved than other forms of concurrency, if no spouses
have sexually transmitted infections and their sexual network is closed, that
is, none of them have extramarital relationships. Nonetheless, Nyamhanga

initially aspired to be monogamous, and his subsequent extramarital relationships and polygynous marriage indicates he did not succeed in that goal.

Finally, at the end of the trial some sexually active in-depth interview respondents said that the intervention had convinced them to use condoms. For example, several months after completing the intervention, a sixteen-year-old farmer and former peer educator (Kashindye) provided a confident, detailed description of his use of condoms. He explained that he had witnessed a condom demonstration during a class visit to a health facility and he subsequently used condoms twice, with two of his three sexual partners. Kashindye described the school program and its influence on him:

> R: They used to teach through dramas. People used to act out plays and then were asked questions about the actors. How you saw them and the words you heard, and the topic itself. . . . We were taught things about AIDS . . . how it is passed from person to person. . . . The most important thing we were taught is to use protection or to abstain from sex completely. That was the important thing for me. . . . It helps me not to enter into the danger of being infected. . . . It has helped me personally to use protection [condoms], so that I don't get diseases, or else I should abstain completely. (II-02-I-295-m)

Each of the individuals described above was articulate in discussing the positive ways that the *MEMA kwa Vijana* intervention had influenced them. Similar testimony is the main evidence used in determining intervention effectiveness all over the world. What the *MEMA kwa Vijana* trial made clear, however, is that such reports should not be taken at face value. To ensure intervention effectiveness, it is critical to also examine the extent to which such reports represent genuine and consistent long-term behavior change, as well as significant and positive impact on sexual health.

DISCUSSION

When a carefully designed and implemented intervention does not have its intended impact, there is a critical need to learn from and build upon what worked well within it, and to improve upon what did not. As DiClemente and Wingood (2003, 319) comment in their editorial on HIV prevention with adolescents:

> [There is] a growing body of evidence indicating that HIV prevention interventions can effectively enhance the acquisition of preventive skills and behaviors. . . . It is unclear, however, whether the changes observed, particularly for HIV-preventive behaviors, are of sufficient magnitude to substantially affect the HIV epidemic among adolescents from a public health perspective. . . . As the lessons of history have shown, there are unfortunately no magic bullets or easy answers.

To date, few randomized controlled trials other than the *MEMA kwa Vijana* trial have evaluated the impact of a behavioral intervention on adolescent sexual health in sub-Saharan Africa (e.g., Cowan et al., 2002; Jewkes et al., 2006; Jewkes et al., 2008; Cowan et al., 2010). Of those, only the 2002–2006 Stepping Stones intervention trial in South Africa found a statistically significant impact on a biological outcome (Jewkes et al., 2008). That intervention did not have an impact on its primary outcome, HIV incidence, but it did have a significant positive impact on its secondary outcome, herpes incidence. In examining the limited impact of the *MEMA kwa Vijana* program here, it is thus worth exploring how its context, content, and impact contrasted those of the Stepping Stones intervention. The description of the Stepping Stones trial and context below draws on multiple sources (Jewkes et al., 2006; Jewkes et al., 2008; Jewkes, Nduna, and Jama, 2010; Jewkes, Wood, and Duvvury, 2010).

Comparison with the Stepping Stones Intervention Context and Process

The goal of the Stepping Stones intervention is to "improve sexual health through building stronger, more gender-equitable relationships with better communication between partners" (Jewkes et al., 2006, 5). Both Stepping Stones and *MEMA kwa Vijana* targeted rural African youth with an intensive, large-scale intervention that was well implemented and evaluated. However, unlike *MEMA kwa Vijana*, which was developed and tested over one year before the trial began, the Stepping Stones intervention was tested and modified over seven years before its evaluation in a trial. Specifically, it was developed in Uganda in 1995, adapted in South Africa in the Xhosa language in 1998, and then implemented for four years there before being revised for a second South African edition, which is the version that was implemented and evaluated in the trial.

The *MEMA kwa Vijana* trial took place in a generalized epidemic, where nationally 9 percent of fifteen- to forty-nine-year-old adults were estimated to be HIV-positive at the end of the trial in 2001 (UNAIDS, 2004). In that setting, AIDS was relatively uncommon and was further obscured because it often went undiagnosed, so few trial participants believed that they had been affected by it personally. At baseline, two males and six females (0.1 percent) of the 9,283 trial members were HIV-positive (Plummer, Ross, et al., 2004). In contrast, Stepping Stones was evaluated in a highly generalized or hyperendemic setting, where 21 percent of fifteen- to forty-nine-year-olds were estimated to be HIV-positive at the end of 2001, before the trial there began (UNAIDS, 2004). At baseline, 2 percent of male and 11 percent of female trial members were HIV-positive, and almost all participants had close first-hand knowledge of someone with AIDS. In addition, while both trials took place in settings where there were few if any other HIV prevention programs, it is likely that the quality and reach of national mass media interventions in South Africa (e.g., Soul City and Lovelife) were much greater before and during the trial there than the equivalent before and during the trial in Tanzania (e.g., Taylor et al., 2010).

In both the *MEMA kwa Vijana* and Stepping Stones communities, concurrent sexual relationships were common, condom use was low, transactional sex was frequent, and girls and women often had older sexual partners. However, the trial settings differed greatly in terms of crime, armed violence, intimate partner violence, and rape, which were all common in Stepping Stones communities but uncommon in *MEMA kwa Vijana* communities. Nonetheless, in *MEMA kwa Vijana* communities it was not unusual for men and boys to coerce girls to have sex through bullying, pressure, or tricks, and in most schools there was evidence that one or two male teachers had sexually abused female school pupils.

The design and implementation of the two interventions were also quite different. Stepping Stones was implemented by paid facilitators who were slightly older than trial participants, who had post-secondary school qualifications, and who were selected in part for their open-mindedness and gender sensitivity. This contrasts with the main *MEMA kwa Vijana* implementers, that is, older government health workers and teachers who carried out the intervention in addition to their regular duties, and who typically had not completed secondary school themselves. The Stepping Stones facilitators were trained for three weeks and then had monthly, day-long in-service trainings, instead of the one-week initial training, occasional supervision, and shorter annual refresher training courses experienced by *MEMA kwa Vijana* implementers. While *MEMA kwa Vijana* was carried out through existing government institutions, Stepping Stones was designed to be implemented by a non-profit organization, such as the Planned Parenthood Association. However, Stepping Stones participant selection and intervention implementation usually took place at secondary schools outside of school hours.

The *MEMA kwa Vijana* intervention involved all Year 5–7 pupils in intervention primary schools (mainly fourteen- to seventeen-year-olds). In contrast, in each Stepping Stones community forty sixteen- to twenty-three-year-old students in Years 9–11 of secondary school were selected from a group of about sixty volunteers to participate, because they lived relatively close to the school and they were considered more likely to attend than other volunteers. The Stepping Stones curriculum consisted of same-sex sessions and approximately twice as many session hours as *MEMA kwa Vijana*, but was carried out in a shorter period of time, that is, fifty hours over six to eight weeks, compared to twenty-one hours over three years in the final trial versions. There were more participatory and interactive sessions in Stepping Stones, and more sessions focused on critical reflection, assertiveness, and communication skills building. Given intimate partner violence was common in the Stepping Stones context, and this is widely recognized as a risk factor for HIV infection, that intervention also focused heavily on reducing male aggression and promoting more caring and gender equitable relationships.

It is not possible to know exactly which of the different aspects of intervention context, content, or design described above contributed to the different impacts observed in the *MEMA kwa Vijana* and Stepping Stones trials. However, the HALIRA findings suggest that Stepping Stones had several strengths relative to *MEMA kwa Vijana*. These include that participants were substantially older, more educated, and more likely to have close experience of AIDS, all of which may have contributed to deeper understanding of risk and greater personal concern about it. In addition, Stepping Stones participants were self-selected volunteers and thus presumably were more motivated to reduce their sexual risk from the onset. The HALIRA study also found that internal motivation was critical for young people who actively tried to change their behaviors; this will be discussed more in the next three chapters. Stepping Stones facilitators probably also were more capable and motivated to implement a complex and skills-based intervention than *MEMA kwa Vijana* teachers, because they were more educated, had more training and supervision, and were paid for those responsibilities.

In addition, in the Stepping Stones trial, educational authorities did not restrict the discussion of young people's sexual behavior, and particularly condom use, so intervention implementers could acknowledge and address young people's sexual relationships and risk practices much more openly than in the *MEMA kwa Vijana* trial. The Stepping Stones curriculum had several other strengths, including being developed and tested over many years prior to trial evaluation; having twice as many session hours; and devoting more time to gender relations, critical reflection, and skills building. The HALIRA findings suggest that each of those characteristics also would have made the *MEMA kwa Vijana* intervention more effective.

Comparison with the Stepping Stones Intervention Impact

The Stepping Stones trial found there was intervention impact on male intervention participants' partner number and partner selectivity. Specifically, twelve months after intervention participation, male participants reported significantly fewer partners and less experience of any casual partners than their control counterparts. There was no evidence of intervention impact on any of the other ABC behaviors. There were no significant differences between intervention arms in partner number or experience of casual partnerships for females, and also none for reported condom use for either males or females. The trial did not measure abstinence.

However, the Stepping Stones trial found there was intervention impact on other types of risk behaviors. Significantly lower proportions of male intervention participants than control participants reported transactional sex, violence against an intimate partner, attempted rape, problem drinking, or misuse of drugs. Amongst women, in contrast, a significantly higher proportion of intervention participants than control participants reported transactional sex post-intervention. It is difficult to know how to interpret the latter finding, as it may have reflected underreporting at baseline and more forthright reporting after Stepping Stones participation.

Many of the outcomes above support the HALIRA findings which have already been described, or which will be detailed in the coming chapters, including that partner number reduction and partner selectivity may be the most likely ways for young Africans to try to reduce their sexual risk, and that interventions which promote alternative forms of masculinity and heightened male risk perception are likely to be most effective in protecting both young men and young women. In their qualitative evaluation of the Stepping Stones intervention, Jewkes, Wood, and Duvvury (2010, 9) highlight that the intervention's in-depth communication and skills-building exercises seemed to contribute to men improving their relationships with women:

> . . . there was evidence that the combination of communication/assertiveness skills sessions and the experience of group discussion over several weeks built the participants' confidence and gave them skills that they used in a range of different settings and with different people. Stepping Stones also provided an opportunity for participants to reflect on their identity and essentially who they wanted to be. . . . there was evidence that after the workshops men became more caring and less violent, and a couple of the women became much more assertive in their relationships.

Jewkes, Wood, and Duvvury (2010, 9) further argue that the intervention had a critical impact on male risk perception and concern:

> In men . . . Stepping Stones instilled a clear and new perception of risk and desire to avoid it. This was manifold and apparently stemmed from the critical reflection exercises. There was no parallel discourse in the women's interviews, although some evidence of HIV risk reduction was evident. It seems likely that this reflects constraints women perceive on their agency. In other words, it was more difficult for them to be concerned about things over which they perceived

they lacked control. . . . The position of men was somewhat different as they were empowered to change their behavior and aspects of their worldview, [and] had considerable confidence that they could either persuade their girlfriends to agree to this or at least find a new girlfriend if she did not.

The authors thus propose that the Stepping Stones intervention would be more effective if it were implemented on a wider scale within each community, including adults and influencing gender attitudes more broadly. They also postulated that the intervention would be more effective for women if it were combined with other structural interventions, such as the Intervention with Microfinance for AIDS and Gender Equity (IMAGE) program, which focuses on microcredit, community action, and gender empowerment (Pronyk et al., 2006).

The impact of the Stepping Stones intervention on herpes incidence in young adults argues for its replication, adaptation, and further evaluation in other settings. However, the limited nature of the intervention's success suggests it is necessary to continue pursuing other, complementary approaches with the same target group of young adults, as well as with other groups, such as younger, less educated adolescents; young adults who do not seek out intervention participation; and older adults. It is generally recommended, for example, that interventions target young people before they become sexually active and before they have established sexual risk behaviors, which in many African contexts means prepubescent and early adolescent children (Gallant and Maticka-Tyndale, 2004; Van den Bergh, 2008; Michielsen et al., 2010). Government school systems are still likely to provide the most affordable, feasible, and sustainable way to reach such young people on a large scale. Importantly, the lessons learned from Stepping Stones outlined above can help inform and improve such school-based programs. Improvement of the broader school environment may also be essential to make such programs more effective, so this will be discussed more in the final chapter.

The next three chapters will draw on data from both intervention and control communities to describe young people who provided some of the most consistent, detailed, and plausible accounts of practicing low-risk sexual behaviors within the *MEMA kwa Vijana* trial. Each chapter will focus on a particular behavior and will be preceded by a case study series that gives an in-depth description of individual young people who practiced that behavior. Chapter 11 will then return to the findings presented in this chapter to consider how the *MEMA kwa Vijana* program and other HIV prevention interventions for adolescents in sub-Saharan Africa might be improved.

Part III

YOUNG PEOPLE WHO PRACTICED
LOW-RISK SEXUAL BEHAVIORS

Case Study Series 1

"So It Is Like This! Not For Me"
Young People Who Abstained

This case study series describes the lives of four young people in rural Mwanza who provided detailed, plausible, and consistent reports of primary or secondary abstinence. These stories illustrate some of the factors which promoted abstinence in the study population. Ng'walu's case study (1.1) describes a girl who abstained until she completed primary school in her mid-teens, because she did not desire sex and she was exceptionally assertive and confident in refusing it, despite experiencing frequent sexual pressure from men. Deo's case study (1.2) details a young man's decision not to begin sexual activity because of his educational aspirations and the influence of the *MEMA kwa Vijana* intervention. Vumilia's case study (1.3) describes how a girl decided to abstain after sexual debut because of school ambitions, positive parental and teacher relationships, and experience of one sister who had dropped out of school due to pregnancy, another who had an abusive marriage and subsequent abortion, and a third who died of AIDS. Finally, Jerad's case study (1.4) illustrates different reasons why adolescent males may be motivated to abstain either before or after initiating sex, including the external constraint of having little cash for material exchange, and the fear caused by a sexual partner becoming pregnant.

1.1. NG'WALU: A GIRL WHO NEVER HAD SEX WHILE SCHOOLING

Ng'walu was sixteen years old and at the end of Year 7 at a *MEMA kwa Vijana* intervention school when a male participant observation researcher began to live in her household. Given their differences in age and gender, Ng'walu did not discuss much in depth with the male researcher. However, over two participant observation visits she often spoke with the female researcher who was staying in the same village.

257

Ng'walu's father had died when she was a small child, after which her mother remarried and moved away to a different village with her new husband. Ng'walu and her two younger sisters instead lived with their fifty-four-year-old, widowed, maternal grandmother, and three of the grandmother's children who were in their teens and early twenties. Ng'walu's aunt (Sekelwa) was four years older than her, but she had been in the same class as Ng'walu in Year 6 and they both were participants in the *MEMA kwa Vijana* trial. However, Sekelwa became pregnant in Year 6 and then dropped out of school. At the time of the first participant observation visit, she had a four-month-old baby.

Ng'walu's family was Sukuma and Protestant. They were very poor and lived in two small mud-brick, thatch-roofed houses on land that her grandmother had been given by her grandmother's brother. The household did not have a latrine, so family members relieved themselves in bushes, in holes dug in a maize field, or in a neighbor's latrine. They farmed cassava and other produce to support the family, and the grandmother bought clothing for all of the children in her household. When Ng'walu was not in school, she was responsible for many of the chores typical of young women in rural Mwanza, such as farming, cooking, cleaning, and fetching water.

Ng'walu shared a sleeping room with her sisters and Sekelwa. During the first participant observation visit Sekelwa told the female researcher how Ng'walu assisted her when she crept out at night to meet her boyfriend for sex:

> Sekelwa said that her boyfriend picks her up at night and she pays Ng'walu Tshs 200 ($0.24) to close the door behind her and then open it again when she comes back early in the morning. Sekelwa said that Ng'walu and her younger sister are good at keeping her secret, because no one ever knew about it until she became pregnant. (PO-01-I-1-2f)

During the first participant observation visit, Ng'walu reported that she had never had sex, although male villagers often approached and tried to seduce her. She was strategic and assertive in avoiding such pressure. For example, when running errands she avoided areas which were frequented by sexually aggressive men, such as a local blacksmith's workshop. When Ng'walu nonetheless happened to be isolated by a man, she immediately tried to get out of the situation rather than engage with him. For example:

> Ng'walu mentioned how her teacher tried to seduce her near the end of her final year, when she went to the office and found him alone. She said the teacher said, "Now that you have finished schooling, why don't you give me a child?" She said that she did not tell the teacher anything, but just ran away from the office and left him alone. She said he later sometimes followed her when she was en route to the shallow pond [to fetch water], or when she returned from the market. . . . Once [another man] met her along a path and told her to have sex with him in the bushes. When she refused, he took the radio she was carrying and scared her by going with it into the bushes, so that she would go after it. She said she refused to go for the radio, even though it had belonged to her [deceased] grandfather. When

he saw that she was not moved by his act, he followed her and gave her the radio back. (PO-01-I-1-2f)

Ng'walu could not explain why she chose to abstain, other than that she did not see a need to have sex. She said her grandmother provided for most of her basic needs, and when necessary she borrowed soap or body oil from her younger sister, or sold the cassava powder she produced herself to buy underwear and pay for school expenses. Ng'walu's report that she had never had sex was independently supported by several other informants. In the course of her first participant observation visit, for example, the female researcher asked Sekelwa and individual Year 7 girls if there were any girls in that school year who were still virgins, and Ng'walu was the only girl they all mentioned. For example:

[A nineteen-year-old girl in Year 7] said that all the girls in her year have a boyfriend except for Ng'walu. She said that she believes this because the other girls talk about their boyfriends during break time, when they also show each other the money they have been given for sex. (PO-01-I-1-2f)

Ng'walu was quiet but extraordinarily assertive and determined in standing up for herself and her loved ones. For example, after she rejected the teacher mentioned above, he coerced her fifteen-year-old sister to have sex and made her sister pregnant. The researcher recorded: "Ng'walu said that she has advised her sister not to fear the teacher, for now that he made her pregnant she should ask him to meet her material needs, like body oil and soap. Ng'walu said that her sister fears him since he is so much older than her" (PO-02-I-1-2f). Feeling there were no other family member to advocate on her sister's behalf, Ng'walu herself confronted the teacher to demand that he take responsibility for the pregnancy. She demonstrated exceptional courage in speaking to an older male authority figure in this way. In that conversation the teacher refused to admit that he had caused the pregnancy, so Ng'walu spontaneously tried a different approach and told him that the female researcher wanted to speak with him about it. This strategy had some effect, as the teacher then approached the researcher and acknowledged that he had made Ng'walu's sister pregnant:

The teacher came to talk to me about impregnating Ng'walu's sister. He told me that Ng'walu told him I wanted to talk to him about it. I realized that she must have feared talking further to him about it, and she thought I could do it for them instead. I talked with him about the girl and her pregnancy, which he said was five months along. He told me he plans to take her to the district hospital so she can start attending a prenatal clinic. He also said he plans to buy her a dress and several *vitenge* (high quality, colored, patterned cotton cloth). (PO-02-I-1-2f)

Ultimately, however, Ng'walu's efforts were unsuccessful as the teacher later denied paternity and married a different girl.

Ng'walu did not pass her Primary School Leaving Examination. At the time of the second participant observation visit, she was eighteen years old and had been out of school for almost a year, and she was still living and farming within her grandmother's household. During that visit she discussed her experience of the *MEMA kwa Vijana* intervention with the male researcher:

> Ng'walu said she only remembers a few things from those lessons, like the peer educator dramas at the beginning of some classes. . . . Regarding the low-risk behaviors they were taught about, she said that she is working on them. However, she doesn't know if other girls and boys who participated in those classes are working on them, because it is hard to know what other people are doing if you do not live with them. (PO-02-I-1-3m)

Ng'walu did not specifically discuss sex with either researcher during the second participant observation visit. However, her *MEMA kwa Vijana* survey sample collected shortly before the visit suggested that she had become sexually active. During earlier surveys Ng'walu tested negative for all sexually transmitted infections and pregnancy, but in the later one she tested positive for herpes, like 21 percent of the other young women surveyed (Ross et al., 2007).

1.2. DEO: A YOUNG MAN WHO NEVER HAD SEX WHILE SCHOOLING

Deo was twenty-one years old and in Form 3 (Year 10) of secondary school when he was randomly selected for an in-depth interview at the end of the *MEMA kwa Vijana* trial. Three years earlier, when he was in Year 7, he had participated in one year of the intervention.

Deo's parents separated when he was very young, after his father married a junior wife. Deo was raised by his mother with virtually no contact with his father. Deo's mother was a Catholic, Sukuma farmer. She eventually remarried, but Deo's stepfather was often away for a year at a time. At the time of the interview, Deo lived with his mother and four siblings and half-siblings in two small houses of one or two rooms each. He commuted to secondary school every day. Deo said he was allowed to go to video shows, discos, or traditional dances, but unlike most rural young men he did not like them, so he did not go to them. Music, however, was very important to him, and he had a radio that he often used. He explained:

> *D*: It helps me so much. I love music very much. You know, entertainment is . . . essential to human life. Now, I walk with my radio and I listen to good things, even songs which may have a good message. . . . Fortunately, Tanzania has many artists who try to convey messages that are good for society. (II-02-I-315-m)

When asked what kinds of messages were good for society, Deo described a range to do with social service, human rights, prosperity, and freedom.

Deo had a chronic stomach problem that he treated at home with traditional medicines, and for which he sometimes sought medical treatment at a health facility. He said the traditional medicine his mother prepared could soothe his stomach, but he did not trust treatments provided by traditional healers, saying, "Their treatment is just a game of chance. It is not like you can go there and get reliable treatment" (II-02-I-315-m). Deo's mother provided for most of his school and household expenses. He explained: "It is only my mother who assists me. We struggle to get by together" (II-02-I-315-m). On weekends and vacations he farmed cotton and maize on his own plot, and in a good year he made enough money to pay for one-quarter of his school fees. Deo was ambitious to go far in school. He explained:

> *D*: I just love my classes, and I want to continue studying, only studying. . . . As you know, we are going through a very hard time. And if you have no education, or just a little, your life will be very hard. So if you get a chance to go to school somewhere then you must make good use of it. (II-02-I-315-m)

Deo had great respect for his teachers and called them his "directional compass." He also had one good male friend in school with whom he studied intensively.

Deo told the interviewer that he had never had sex. He was convinced that sexual activity while schooling would be detrimental:

> *D*: If I participated in wrong doing, in doing bad things, then they would definitely destroy my future. If you become sexually active then there is a very good chance you will not succeed in school. In most cases, you cannot serve two masters at the same time. So you must do one thing at a time. . . . It is not that I wouldn't enjoy it, but it is just that everything has its own time. A time will come later when I will be able to do it. (II-02-I-315-m)

Deo explained that sex while he was still schooling would be problematic because it would be both distracting and dangerous:

> *D*: The first reason is this: if you involve yourself in sexual issues, when will you get time to study? The second reason is that if you like/love someone you may have sex and get a certain disease, in this time when it is most dangerous, when there is a war against AIDS! It only takes having sex one time without protection. You cannot trust that a person does not have a disease, because he/she may have no symptoms until suddenly reaching a stage that leads to death. . . . And there are also other sexually transmitted infections which can cause childlessness, even death. (II-02-I-315-m)

Deo took initiative in avoiding sexual temptation, whether in the form of acquaintances who encouraged him to have sex or women who made it clear they would like to have a sexual relationship with him. For example:

> *D*: A certain person may happen to like/love you very much and want you to have sex with her. Maybe she starts telling you, "I have a certain problem, so I'd like

to come to your residence today. Will you have time? Please, I want to give you something." Now you can't know from that alone that it relates to sex, but there are other signs which I cannot explain [Laughter]. They are just there. Now what I do is very simple. I immediately tell her, "I don't think I'll be present when you come to my residence." Hmm, you just escape that way, cleverly, leaving a person in a good frame of mind without resenting you [for rejecting her]. (II-02-I-315-m)

Deo acknowledged that he sometimes became sexually aroused and he described having sexual dreams. He said he distracted himself when this happened and reduced his desire by tiring himself in heavy physical activities, or bathing in very cold water:

> *D*: [Sexual desire] is necessary and happens to everybody, because you can't get to adulthood without experiencing it. Desire itself is never absent. If you have grown up and are physically fit, meaning that your sexual organs are functioning, at that stage those feelings should exist. . . . But if you are in control of your life, you can discipline yourself. I don't think you will be compelled to have sex. (II-02-I-315-m)

Deo attributed his decision to abstain to his educational aspirations and the *MEMA kwa Vijana* intervention. He believed that he had participated in the intervention at a critical stage in his life when he might otherwise have begun to have sex. He explained what happened when he first experienced sexual dreams:

> *D*: I was fortunate, because *MEMA kwa Vijana* had very good lessons during that period, which convince you not to [have sex] if you are an intelligent person. Had that project not been there, AIDS would have had a much bigger chance, because pupils involve themselves in sex while still in primary school. So that is how it is. My life was saved during that time. (II-02-I-315-m)

Deo repeatedly referred to AIDS as an enemy that could make a person die prematurely:

> *D*: Really, fighting AIDS is a war, which is . . . is even greater than the world wars. This one seems to be the worst war ever. . . . Why should you die earlier than God's plan?! Why die when you knew, "If I do this then I will die?" In fact, that made me have very great fear. (II-02-I-315-m)

Deo praised the *MEMA kwa Vijana* program highly, and he was able to describe most program messages well. He understood that condoms were a means of protecting against pregnancy and sexually transmitted infections, but he had missed school on the day when his class visited a health facility, so he had never seen a condom and did not have a clear understanding of how they were used. He reported that his sexually active peers strongly believed condom use was unacceptable and a waste of time, because they believed that condoms reduce pleasure.

Deo's only disappointment in his own *MEMA kwa Vijana* experience related to the peer educator component. First, he was disappointed that he was not selected to be a peer educator, and he envied those who received training. Second, he did not consider some of the peer educators to be good role models:

> *D*: Now some of them were having sex. It is as if you say, "Don't steal," but then you participate in stealing! [In that case] I don't think you will be teaching good ethics/morals. In reality, you will just be a cheater, leading society in the wrong direction. That is the thing [about the program] that did not impress me at all. (II-02-I-315-m)

Deo believed most *MEMA kwa Vijana* peer educators and other intervention participants had continued engaging in sexual risk behaviors after intervention participation. When the interviewer asked Deo why they did not reduce their risk, Deo replied with the Sukuma expression, "A monitor lizard will not hear until blood bleeds out of its ears." Literally, this expression means that a monitor lizard—a large lizard common to Lake Victoria that can reach several feet in length—will not obey a command unless it is hit with great force, even fatally. Figuratively, it means that a person will not pay attention to warnings until they begin to suffer negative consequences, and then it might be too late.

Of the three *MEMA kwa Vijana* behavior change goals, Deo thought the most feasible and realistic for his peers was to reduce partners, after which a smaller proportion might use condoms, and only the smallest proportion could abstain completely like himself. It was not unusual for young people who plausibly reported never having had sex to believe that their sexually active peers could not abstain like themselves. Deo explained:

> *D*: [They will not abstain] because they have already established a behavior that seems important to them. For example, if a child steals sugar and tastes a little bit of it, and then you just leave sugar there and tell him not to do it again without even hitting [punishing] him, then the next day you will find more sugar is gone. . . . He will have already experienced a certain sweet taste, and he knows what advantage or enjoyment it provides. Now the same thing applies to sex. If people have already started having sex, I don't think they will be able to stop completely if you just say that they should do so. You should at least allow them to do it in a special way, in a recommended manner [Laughter]. For example, they could reduce their partner number. But that will only happen if they become fully aware of AIDS. (II-02-I-315-m)

Deo believed that he would abstain until he completed his studies, and even then he would only have sex after taking precautions:

> *D*: [The first time I have sex], it will not just happen suddenly, I will need to go through certain stages first. I think at that time I will want to get married, so I will do all that is required to marry, which as you know involves many things. The first thing is to investigate, to make sure we are both safe, because one of you might not be and might harm the other one. So medical testing should take place. (II-02-I-315-m)

Deo believed that marriage was most likely to succeed if entered into in one's mid-twenties, or later:

> *D*: When one is an adult, it is essential to have a lover, a lover with whom you may live throughout your life. . . . Some decide to marry too early, at the age of 16 or 18, but those marriages never last long because of youthful ideas. For example, [a man might think,] "Now I will just take a woman, but ah, if she goes away, I will just get another one to replace her, there is no problem." Maybe at the age of twenty-five he would be mature enough to marry for the long-term, and he will have obtained enough knowledge to know how to control his family. (II-02-I-315-m)

Deo participated in two *MEMA kwa Vijana* surveys and tested negative for all sexually transmitted infections measured for males during those surveys.

1.3. VUMILIA: A GIRL WHO ABSTAINED AFTER SEXUAL DEBUT

Vumilia was fifteen years old and in Year 6 of a *MEMA kwa Vijana* control school when she was randomly selected for a pilot in-depth interview. She lived with her mother and five of her seven siblings and half-siblings. Her father, a cattle seller, had died many years earlier. Her mother later remarried a man with two other wives, but Vumilia's stepfather only visited her household rarely. Vumilia's family was Catholic. Her mother supported the family by selling beer.

Vumilia seemed to have a close relationship with her mother, expressing respect and protectiveness toward her. Her mother in turn was concerned about Vumilia's future, encouraging her to stay in school and not allowing her to participate in activities which she thought would be harmful, such as discos or video shows. Vumilia was supported financially by her mother and one of her older brothers, but she earned extra money for exercise books, pens, and clothing by cooking and selling *uji* (maize- or millet-based porridge) in the market center with a close girlfriend. Vumilia liked to stroll with that friend in the market center some evenings, but she was not allowed to stay out past 7 p.m. Vumilia also strongly liked her teachers and school. She explained, "School pleases me. Really, when the secondary school students pass by, my heart cries out that I should also continue . . . that I should also go there" (II-99-C-33-f). She ideally hoped to become a nurse or a teacher, so that she would have a salaried position and be better able to support her mother.

Vumilia said that she had only had sex one time, when she was about ten years old, before she moved to that village and started school. She said the boy was in Year 1 but she did not know his age. Given the wide age range in rural primary schools, he might have been about her age or several years older. In any case, this boy had had unusual access to cash for a pupil, because his father had a shop. They met at his house for sex when his family was away, and afterward she used Tshs 100 ($0.12) of the Tshs 500 ($0.60) he gave to her to buy bananas. She said she buried the rest of the money at home, but when she went to retrieve it later, it was gone. As discussed in chapter 3, prepubescent sexual encounters were not unusual in rural Mwanza, including some involving vaginal intercourse, but they usually occurred outside and did not involve material exchange. Vumilia's age estimate seems likely to have been accurate because the experience happened before she moved to the village and started school. It is not clear whether the encounter involved vaginal intercourse, although it's planned nature and the monetary exchange suggests this was the case.

Vumilia's best friend had also had sex once at an early age, and both of them did not want to have sex again while still in school. Many boys and men had approached them for sex, but Vumilia reported that they consistently refused it. She said that it could be difficult to convince her suitors that she truly did not want to have sex. For example, primary and secondary school boys:

V: I don't like a boy who . . . starts provoking/teasing you. He tells you, "Sister, I like/ love you," but I don't like/love him at all. He takes your exercise book and will not give it back. Sometimes they write, "I like/love you," I don't know what, just a lot of words. . . . I met one on the way to the well, and he asked me, "Hey sister, how about my letter?" I told him, "What do you really expect me to do? I have openly told you that I don't want it." He followed me and said, "What are you afraid of? We can just have sex. Who do you think will know?" I told him, "I don't want it. I really don't like that. Maybe you should go to other girls." (II-99-C-33-f)

Vumilia also described routinely rejecting adult men who approached her for sex while she worked in the market center, or ran errands. For example:

V: Sometimes a man calls you while you are working, to try to make you go to him. You tell him, "I can't leave my customers." You tell him that you have responsibilities. He might answer, "Now you are being rude." But I have to be rude. . . . As soon as my friend and I sell all of the porridge, we just leave the center. The following day they come again, they call you again, and again you refuse to go. Yes, because you are always aware that they will try to seduce you. (II-99-C-33-f)

Some men had tried to exploit their positions of power or authority to manipulate Vumilia into having sex. For example, a shopkeeper:

V: One day I was sent by my mother to the shop where I found that man, and I asked him, "Is there cocoa powder?" He said, "Yes, there is." I asked him how much, and he told me Tshs 1,200 ($1.44). I asked him to reduce the price, because when I went there with my mother I bought it for Tshs 800 ($0.96). He said, "Give me that Tshs 1,000 ($1.20) bill," so I did. Then he said, "But sister, I like/love you." I told him, "You just leave me alone." He did not give me that powder, so I told him, "Just give me back my money so that I can go." He said, "I have all this wealth/property. Do you think I am married? I am just alone [unmarried]." I told him, "I don't have a desire to get married, no, what I want is just to continue [with school]. Maybe you should look for others, those who roam about here in the center." Mh, so he disagreed, he disagreed, he wanted to pull me into the shop, but I refused, I refused. He said, "I will give you Tshs 5,000 ($6)." I refused and went away. (II-99-C-33-f)

Vumilia reported that the closest she had come to having a post-pubescent sexual relationship was with a secondary school student who had briefly attended classes at her primary school. He and another secondary school boy tried to seduce her and her best friend, but an observant teacher intervened:

V: The teacher told us, "You girls, I used to like you, you really longed to study, but now you want to wreck your schooling completely by liking/loving boys." And we told her/him, "No, teacher, it is not like that." Mh, he/she told us, "Aren't they really your lovers?" We denied it. . . . Then the boys were questioned and told to leave the school. (II-99-C-33-f)

When asked why she had adamantly refused sex since her initial encounter, Vumilia explained that she wanted to complete school and she feared pregnancy and AIDS. She had personal knowledge of these possibilities from her sisters' experiences. One of her sisters had won a coveted place in secondary school, but she was unable to go because she became pregnant. Vumilia further explained:

V: Another of my sisters has already had an abortion, she was taught by our grandmother. She actually was married and had had her first child, and then her second, and then her third. She became pregnant a fourth time, and that is when my brother-in-law started abusing her, I don't know why. Then my sister decided, "Well, let me have an abortion and leave him." . . . After the abortion, I found her when she was ill, yes. . . . She was taken to the hospital. As soon as she recovered, she left her husband. (II-99-C-33-f)

Even more than that experience, Vumilia was deeply affected by losing a third sister to AIDS:

V: [My sister] had been married to a gold buyer. In fact, that man had AIDS. Yes, he had another wife who preceded him [died before him] . . . Then my brother-in-law became ill and my mother took him in to care for him as he didn't have relatives. . . . He died there. Then one day my sister came here while sick. My sister had sores in her mouth, she had scabs too. Yes, then her hair changed completely, and she became very thin. My mother went to see a traditional healer for divination. I think she was told that my sister had been bewitched. . . . One day my sister became critically ill and died. That is why I became shocked, thinking, "So it is like this! Not for me." (II-99-C-33-f)

Although Vumilia did not attend a *MEMA kwa Vijana* intervention school, she had once seen an AIDS education presentation by a different group that had included dramas and condom demonstrations. Vumilia could explain the basic way that HIV/AIDS could be passed between people:

V: When a person with AIDS has sex with a woman, and that woman goes to have sex with another man, they all become infected, just like that.

I: Could you also get it?

V: No. If . . . if you go [have sex] with boys, then you can get it. If the boy who seduces you has AIDS, then you can get it. But if you are not seduced, then you can't get it. (II-99-C-33-f)

Despite this basic understanding and Vumilia's personal experience of AIDS, she had important misconceptions about it. This was not unusual, especially among pupils in *MEMA kwa Vijana* control schools. Vumilia believed, for example, that a person with AIDS-like symptoms who had healthy-looking sexual partners could simply be bewitched. When describing a woman who was rumored to have AIDS in her village, for instance, she commented, "Maybe she was bewitched. We just don't know if it is actually AIDS, because her husband is still fine. Yes, and even my brother-in-law's sexual partners are still there, they are alive [and appear healthy]."

Vumilia knew condoms were worn by a man during sex to prevent pregnancy and transmission of infections, and she specifically named AIDS and gonorrhea. She had seen a condom packet at her brother's house and asked a sister about it, but she did not know if she would ever use condoms. During the interview, she repeatedly stated that the only way she knew she could stay in school and not get AIDS was to abstain completely from sex. She said that she had never felt a desire for sex, and she had difficulty envisioning marrying, although ultimately she also wanted to have children:

I: Would you like to get married later in your life, perhaps when you become an adult?

V: Not at all.

I: Why wouldn't you like to be married?

V: No, I wouldn't like to because, I mean, the world would come to an end.

I: Why do you say, "the world would come to an end?" . . .

V: You know how married life is these days, no, definitely not.

I: Would you like to have children later?

V: . . . Maybe if I ever am married by a man, then I will have children with him. But definitely I will not be made pregnant while at home [unmarried]. I am telling you, I want to continue with school instead. (II-99-C-33-f)

Vumilia was not pregnant and tested negative for all of the sexually transmitted infections measured in the two *MEMA kwa Vijana* surveys she attended before and after this interview.

1.4. JERAD: A BOY WHO ABSTAINED AFTER SEXUAL DEBUT

Jerad was a sixteen-year-old and in Year 7 of a *MEMA kwa Vijana* control school when a researcher first met him during participant observation. On a typical day, Jerad went to school, harvested cotton afterward, and strolled in the village center with his friends in the evening. He lived in his maternal grandmother's household with his mother and six siblings and half-siblings. His father was a fisherman who Jerad had not seen since early childhood. His family was Christian and Sukuma. Jerad said he hoped to marry around the age of twenty-three years, when he would be mature enough to support a wife. He hoped to ultimately have six children, which he felt was a moderate number that he could support financially without difficulty.

Jerad said that his first sexual partner was two years older than him. He explained that they had negotiated and had sex while they were herding cattle together in an isolated area. At the time, he was eight or nine years old and had not yet started school, while she was already in Year 1 of primary school. Jerad said he initiated the sexual activity and they had sex several times over a two-week period. He explained that the first two experiences were painful, because the foreskin on his penis tore, but the third time he felt pleasure. He said that these sexual encounters involved vaginal intercourse that lasted five to ten minutes until he tired and withdrew, because he did not yet ejaculate at that age. That first relationship ended when other children discovered the couple and teased them, embarrassing the girl.

When Jerad was about eleven years old and in Year 2 of primary school, he had a sexual encounter with a different girl, which was again negotiated and consummated while cattle herding. His second sexual partner was younger than him and not in school. He enjoyed intercourse with her, and wanted to continue the sexual relationship, but she ended it for unspecified reasons.

After those initial sexual encounters Jerad did not have sex again for six to seven years. As noted in chapter 3, such a gap between boys' prepubescent and post-pubescent sexual experiences was not unusual in rural Mwanza. Sexual abstinence at that stage of life often was not the boy's choice. On a number of occasions, Jerad attempted to negotiate sex with girls but did not succeed. For instance, when he was fourteen years old and in Year 5 he tried to have sex with a Year 4 girl on "LY" (Last Year) day, a celebration that marked pupils' final school day with games, food, videos, and a disco. Across rural Mwanza that day was widely known amongst youth as a day of increased sexual license. Jerad told the researcher that he and his peers had highly anticipated having sex on that day, and he had negotiated with a girl about it in advance. The researcher recorded:

> The girl asked Jerad for some money, and Jerad gave her Tshs 80 ($0.10), which was all that he had. When they started leaving for the place where they were to have sex,

they were suddenly confronted by older boys who said she had also promised to have sex with them. Jerad said that those boys started hitting the girl and demanding their money back. Jerad decided to leave without demanding his money back. He said that, after that, he believed that the girl was an *mhuni,* and he would not seduce her again even if he desired sex. (PO-00-C-3-3m)

During the first participant observation visit, Jerad said that he had heard of sexually transmitted infections and AIDS, but he believed the latter was transmitted by flies carrying germs from feces to food. He said that he did not know what a condom was.

During a second participant observation visit a year later, Jerad was seventeen years old and still in primary school. He had failed his Primary School Leaving Examination at the end of Year 7, so his mother had enrolled him under a different name in Year 6 at a school in a neighboring village. At that time Jerad told the researcher that he still had not had sex since his prepubescent experiences. However, he was trying to start a sexual relationship with a girl in Year 6 in his new school. The researcher recorded:

He has used a friend to negotiate with the girl. After the friend told the girl that Jerad wanted to have sex with her, she challenged the friend, saying, "Does Jerad not have a mouth to speak with, so that he needs to send his friend?" She told Jerad's friend that she wanted to see Jerad in person. Before they met, she wrote him a letter, including the words, "I like/love you very much, and I want to make love with you." Jerad said that, when they met, the girl agreed to have sex and asked to be given Tshs 200 ($0.24) in exchange. At that time he didn't have money, but he then got some and gave it to her. They agreed to have sex on their way back from school. (PO-01-C-3-3m)

Those plans did not come to fruition, however, because other girls accompanied the girl on her way home from school on the agreed upon day. It was not clear whether the girl genuinely had intended to have sex with Jerad or had taken his money without planning to follow through.

During the third participant observation visit, Jerad was eighteen years old and said that he had had sex during the prior year and had become more confident about it: "Jerad said that he no longer is afraid to seduce girls and he can now seduce them by talking to them personally" (PO-02-C-3-3m). Most recently, Jerad had had a sexual relationship with a school girl who became pregnant. When the teachers questioned the girl about her pregnancy, she told them that Jerad was responsible. The teachers refused to accept that Jerad could be the father, telling her that an eighteen-year-old was too young to make a girl pregnant. They pressed her to name a different partner. Eventually she named an out-of-school youth who then assumed responsibility for the pregnancy and agreed to pay the necessary compensation and marry her. The researcher noted:

Jerad said the teachers later called him into their office and advised him to stop having sex, because if they had not helped him, he would have had to pay compensation for the pregnancy and he might have been expelled from school. He thanked the teachers for their help and promised that he wouldn't do it again. Jerad said that since then he has become afraid to seduce girls, and he has decided to abstain completely. . . . Until now, he has not told people at his home what happened, because they would have strongly scolded him had they known about it. (PO-02-C-3-3m)

Jerad tested negative for all sexually transmitted infections measured for males at the three *MEMA kwa Vijana* biological surveys he attended.

CONCLUSION

These case studies have illustrated some reasons why some young people in rural Mwanza abstained from sex even when their peers did not. Motives to abstain were diverse and complex. Some of these young people practiced abstinence due to external constraints, such as lack of money or fear of punishment. Some instead took initiative and intentionally abstained for multiple reasons, including a desire to go far in school and to avoid negative health consequences. The next chapter will build upon these case studies and describe and discuss broader findings related both to primary and secondary abstinence.

Chapter Eight

Abstinence

Historically, in some settings in sub-Saharan Africa, premarital sexual activity was considered natural and acceptable, although adolescents who engaged in it may have been expected to be discreet (e.g., Tanner, 1955b; Varkevisser, 1973; Caldwell, Caldwell, and Quiggin, 1989). For example, in the mid-twentieth century in rural Mwanza, several anthropologists described permissive sexual mores for unmarried young people (e.g., Cory, 1953; Tanner, 1955a; Tanner, 1955b; Varkevisser, 1973). Based on his research there, Tanner (1955a, 124) commented: "no attempt is made to chaperon young girls who are as yet unmarried, with the result that they have comparative freedom to sleep where they like and with whom they like."

Over the course of the twentieth century many changes in rural Mwanza and elsewhere in sub-Saharan Africa influenced such practices, including the conversion of a large part of the population to Christianity, the introduction of formal education on a large scale, and the increase of average age at first marriage to late teens for girls and early twenties for boys (Caldwell et al., 1998; Żaba et al., 2009). This process essentially created an extended period of "adolescence," that is, a longer stage of life when young people are biologically mature but not yet socially treated as adults (Caldwell et al., 1998). These broad changes also contributed to new social ideals, such as abstinence for unmarried young people, and particularly school pupils. Sometimes adult practices have conflicted with this ideal, most notably when adult men have sexual relationships with unmarried adolescent girls (e.g., Luke, 2003; LeClerc-Madlala, 2008). In formal statements, however, both men and women in sub-Saharan Africa tend to advocate premarital abstinence for adolescents. In the 2004–2005 Tanzanian Demographic and Health Survey, for example, 84 to 87 percent of fifteen- to forty-nine-year-old respondents reported that young men and women should wait until marriage to have sexual intercourse (National Bureau of Statistics and ORC Macro, 2005).

As discussed in chapters 1 and 4, abstinence has also been widely promoted for unmarried youth within HIV prevention programs in sub-Saharan Africa, but such efforts have had only limited success (Gallant and Maticka-Tyndale, 2004; O'Reilly et al., 2004; Kirby, Laris, and Rolleri, 2007). Most research suggests that sexual activity is fairly common for unmarried youth, although it may be discreet or hidden to avoid stigma and punishment, especially for girls (Caldwell, Caldwell, and Quiggin, 1989; Setel, 1999b; Nzioka, 2001; Arnfred, 2004; Helle-Valle, 2004). Abstinence has rarely been promoted within HIV prevention efforts targeting adults, even, for example, in communities where spouses are often separated for extended periods of time.

Better understanding the motivations and experiences of individuals who abstain may be critical in developing more appropriate and effective abstinence promotion interventions. Most studies focused on abstinence in sub-Saharan Africa have relied on young people's self-reported abstinence in surveys, analyzing sociodemographic and other variables associated with it (e.g., Agha, Hutchinson, and Kusanthan, 2006; Kabiru and Ezeh, 2007; Molla, Berhane, and Lindtjørn, 2008; Sauvin-Dugerdil et al., 2008; Tenkorang and Maticka-Tyndale, 2008; Chiao and Mishra, 2009; Dlamini et al., 2009; Onya, Aarø, and Madu, 2009; Tenkorang, Rajulton, and Maticka-Tyndale, 2009; Sambisa, Curtis, and Stokes, 2010; Oladepo and Fayemi, 2011). Such research has found self-reported abstinence to be associated with sexual and reproductive health knowledge, younger age, female sex, religion, ethnicity, a positive attitude toward abstinence, confidence to withstand pressure, having friends with similar practices, the family environment (e.g., shared values, little conflict, parental monitoring, and positive communication), and education-related factors (e.g., parental education level, and long-term school expectations). A recent study with Tanzanian primary school pupils found 34 percent of boys and 29 percent of girls planned to remain virgins until marriage (Njau et al., 2010). Amongst males this intention was associated with the belief that girls have the right to refuse to have sex, while for females it was associated with living with both parents and the belief that they can confidently refuse sex with someone who has authority or power over them.

Given widespread adult ideals that unmarried youth should be abstinent, survey research such as that described above is likely to involve some social desirability bias, especially for girls and for school pupils, as discussed in chapters 1 and 7. For example, in a study with 2,324 twelve- to nineteen-year-old Kenyans, Beguy and colleagues (2009) categorized 20 percent of those who reported sex as "reborn virgins," because they reported having had sex in their first interview, but denied it in a second interview one year later. Another 29 percent of that study population reported that they had never had sex in the first interview, but then a year later reported an age at first sex that preceded their first interview.

Survey research on abstinence also does not offer much insight into young people's perceptions of the advantages and disadvantages of abstinence, or the motivations and experiences of "positive deviants" who abstain when their peers typically do not. Only a limited number of qualitative studies have examined such questions in sub-Saharan Africa (e.g., Hulton, Cullen, and Khalokho, 2000; Marindo, Pearson, and Casterline, 2003; Amuyunzu-Nyamongo et al., 2005; Babalola, Ouedraogo, and Vondrasek, 2006; Kahn, 2006; Izugbara, 2007; Izugbara, 2008; Winskell et al., 2011). For example, in in-depth interviews and focus group discussions in eight rural Nigerian communities, Izugbara (2007) found that eleven- to twenty-one-year-old males perceived abstinence both positively (e.g., moral, healthy, and/or decent) and negatively (e.g., dangerous, unhealthy, disempowering, and an imposition), highlighting the complex challenges potentially involved in abstinence promotion.

This chapter examines the motivations and experiences of young people in rural Mwanza who abstained, first considering those who delayed sexual initiation and then those who became abstinent after having already experienced sexual intercourse. Often abstinence is defined as voluntary forbearance, but in this chapter abstinence resulting from external constraints will also be considered, as both can result in lower sexual health risk. The discussion at the end of this chapter will consider the implication of these findings for abstinence promotion with young rural Africans; that topic will then be further examined in chapter 11.

FINDINGS

In the HALIRA study, it was not unusual for adolescents in their early to mid-teens to initially tell researchers that they had never had sex, especially girls, although over the course of an in-depth interview or a participant observation visit many changed their reports and stated that they had indeed already begun sexual activity. Some young people continued to give consistent and plausible reports of never having had sex, as seen in case studies 1.1 and 1.2. However, it was very unusual for young people to give plausible and consistent reports of secondary abstinence, that is, of having already had sex and then choosing to abstain long-term. Case studies 1.3 and 1.4 are rare examples of young people who tried to do so.

Factors Contributing to Abstinence

Young people who provided detailed, consistent, and plausible reports of abstinence often shared many of the following characteristics: a desire to continue in school (for pupils); confidence and assertiveness; active avoidance of high-risk settings; experience of negative consequences of high-risk sexual behavior for oneself or a loved one; a close friend with similar values and practices; a teacher's concern and non-punitive intervention; and/or participation in the *MEMA kwa Vijana* sexual health intervention. For girls, parental financial support, respectful communication, and close monitoring, as well as broader social ideal of girls' abstinence, sometimes also promoted abstinence. Case studies 1.1–1.4 illustrate these findings.

Importantly, none of these factors ensured that a young person was abstinent. Many adolescents had more than one of these influences in their lives, but nonetheless were sexually active. However, most abstinent youth seemed to have been strongly influenced by several of these factors in combination.

Primary Abstinence: Delaying Sexual Debut

Some adolescents in this study said that they had never had sex because they did not feel a need or desire for it. For boys, this was most commonly reported by early adolescents, but it was also occasionally reported by middle to late adolescents. Physically, abstinence thus seemed to be relatively easy for some adolescents and more challenging for their same-aged peers, who seemed to require more self discipline and restraint in maintaining it. Female adolescents of all ages rarely mentioned physical desire for sex, whether they were sexually active or not. Only a small minority of young women reported physical pleasure as a strong motivation to have sex.

A number of boys and girls who reported abstaining said that they experienced sexual desire, but they ignored it, engaged in physical exertion, masturbated, and/or went to sleep until it passed. This was true both for young people who abstained voluntarily and for some who did so for other reasons, such as a young man who said he masturbated on evenings when he was unable to find a sexual partner. Similarly, one young married woman who had tested negative for all sexually transmitted infections measured in *MEMA kwa Vijana* surveys acknowledged that she experienced sexual desire sometimes before marriage, but explained: "I used to just leave it alone and just sit. I just went to sleep, that's all" (II-02-I-314-f).

Girls and Young Women Who Had Never Had Sex

As discussed in chapter 3, abstinence was a social ideal for school pupils in rural Mwanza, so young people—especially adolescent girls—received positive reinforcement for it from most adults, which could contribute to their pride and determination in abstaining. However, most adolescents who had never had sex also experienced strong pressure and ridicule from same sex peers, and girls additionally experienced frequent and intense sexual pressure from boys and men. To persevere in being abstinent in such circumstances often required an extraordinary resolve, confidence, and ability to disregard negative comments. Critically, girls who were determined to stay abstinent did not simply need to resist pressure on one or two occasions, but typically needed to strategize and assert themselves to resist it on a frequent basis, something that many girls found too difficult to do long-term. Several girls who reported abstinence said that they sometimes were rude or insulting to convince men to leave them alone, something that was challenging for them as it went against Sukuma values of female subservience to males, and young people's respect for older people. Most boys and girls who abstained reported that they were not allowed to attend—or they intentionally avoided—video shows, discos, or nighttime *ngoma* events.

One example of consistently and plausibly reported abstinence involved a fifteen- to sixteen-year-old girl (Pili), who a researcher came to know over two participant observation visits. Pili lived with her mother, her polygynous father, and several siblings. She was frequently approached by boys and men who sought to have sex with her, but the researcher observed that she firmly and consistently rejected them. Pili was unusually opinionated and confident about these issues with her peers and her parents alike. This was something that could bother her twenty-year-old unmarried sister, who also lived in their parents' household and who had a secret lover. The researcher noted:

> Pili's sister told me that, if you go out with Pili, when she returns home she will reveal everything. She said that even if a boy approached you [for sex], Pili will just say it, even in front of their father and mother. Pili's sister said it is not good for parents to know about that. (PO-01-I-4-5f)

Pili said that she had never felt a desire for sex, and she also had not felt pressured by her peers to have sex. Instead, in a recorded in-depth interview she explained:

> *R*: What makes me refuse sex is that some girls are made pregnant and then are deserted [by their partners]. So I refuse.
>
> *I*: You are afraid of getting pregnant?
>
> *R*: Yes. . . . I just don't want it. . . .
>
> *I*: Are you going to get married later in life?
>
> *R*: No, I will just stay like this [single].
>
> *I*: What has made you prefer not to get married?
>
> *R*: It is because of this disease . . . the one that has spread all over, AIDS. (PO-02-I-4-5f)

Later, Pili qualified her statements to say that she probably would get married, but it was too far in the future for her to imagine clearly, and she intended to be abstinent until that time. Pili had learned about AIDS in her *MEMA kwa Vijana* classes and possibly also from her brother, who was a *MEMA kwa Vijana* peer educator.

A small minority of girls were very enthusiastic about schooling and aspired to go as far as possible in formal education, which motivated them to abstain. For example, during participant observation in a *MEMA kwa Vijana* control community, a fifteen-year-old Year 5 pupil (Rebeka) told a researcher that she greatly enjoyed studying, and she was one of the top pupils in her school year. Rebeka said she had never had sex and she intended to remain abstinent because she wanted to stay in school. She feared that if she had sex she would become pregnant and have to drop out. However, she often was pestered by school boys who sought to seduce her. The researcher recorded the following quote from Rebeka in her fieldnotes:

> Boys here never stop trying to seduce girls. Many have already tried to seduce me, but I always evade them. They like to provoke me and my friend when we are studying. If you are not careful they will make a fool out of you. They say evil things, they even hit you. I don't like those matters, not when I am still in school. If you begin [sex] early, you may even become pregnant [and have to drop out]. (PO-00-C-9-5f)

Rebeka later explained that education and sexual relationships are difficult to maintain simultaneously, because, "If you hold two things at one time, one of them will slip away" (PO-01-C-9-6f). Several other boys and girls who reported abstaining also said that schooling and sexual activity conflicted in a fundamental and detrimental way, as seen in case study 1.2. In another example, an eighteen-year-old boy in Year 7 said, "I don't [have sex] because when you are studying you shouldn't involve yourself in two things. . . . I have a goal [to succeed] in school, so all I can do is study" (II-99-I-21-m).

In addition to Rebeka's personal educational ambitions, she was strongly motivated to abstain because her father was very strict and—unusually for parents of girls in rural Mwanza—he had high expectations that she would excel in school. It was not unusual for girls who had very strict parents to strongly declare their abstinence, particularly if their fathers were likely to beat them in punishment if this were discovered. However, if such girls did not also have a strong personal motivation to abstain—as in the example of Rebeka's educational aspirations—they usually were sexually active but exceptionally secretive about it. Even in the strictest households, girls rarely were so well monitored that they could not have sex if they wanted to do so.

Finally, some abstinent girls reported that they were motivated in part by a great fear of sexually transmitted infection based on their family members' experiences, as seen in case study 1.3. In another example, a sixteen-year-old Year 6 pupil (Shikalile) reported a memorable experience when her sister had a painful sexually transmitted infection, for which her sister had sought treatment from both a traditional healer and a hospital. Shikalile explained: "The *MEMA kwa Vijana* teacher also told us that, even if a girl has sex one time, she can get pregnant. Men say to me, 'Hey you, girl, I like/love you. I want to have sex with you', and I just refuse" (II-00-I-105-f). When Shikalile completed primary school eighteen months after that interview, she married a farmer in a *bukwilima* (traditional Sukuma wedding) event. She tested negative for all sexually transmitted infections measured in each of the three *MEMA kwa Vijana* surveys.

Case studies 1.1 and 2.1 describe other girls who actively delayed their sexual debut after most of their peers had become sexually active.

Boys and Young Men Who Had Never Had Sex

Adolescent boys who had never had sex usually attributed this to external constraints, most importantly the difficulty they had convincing girls to have sex with them, particularly if they had little to offer in exchange. Two examples:

> [A sixteen-year-old in Year 7] said that he has never had intercourse, because he tries to seduce girls, but every one that promises to meet him [for sex] fails to appear. He said that he sometimes follows any available school girl . . . but they refuse and some insult him. (PO-00-C-9-3m)

> [A twenty-one-year-old] said he never had sex until he failed his Primary School Leaving Examination in one school and went to repeat a grade at a different school when he was seventeen. He said that when he was in his first school, he desired sex, but he couldn't do it because he was shy and did not know how to seduce girls. . . . He said that his peers seduced girls by writing them love letters, but he did not know how to read and write, so he couldn't do it and was compelled to remain [abstinent]. (PO-00-C-3-3m)

A minority of adolescent boys reported that they had delayed their sexual debut by choice. One sixteen-year-old who had dropped out of school reported that he had never had sex because he did not desire it and he believed he was too young for it, so he rejected a girl who once wrote him a love letter in school. In addition, however, this boy's decision to abstain seemed to have been influenced by his older brother's disturbing experience of a sexually transmitted infection. He explained: "My brother noticed some sores appeared on his private parts . . . eventually the whole area was full of sores. They became big and started excreting pus. Finally they had to take him to the district hospital for treatment" (II-99-I-27-m).

In another example, a sixteen-year-old boy in Year 6 explained that he felt sexual desire but he always resisted temptation because his Pentecostal faith considered premarital sex to be a sin. In a third example, a sixteen-year-old boy in Year 3 (Ernest) explained that he abstained due to educational aspirations:

R: I have never even tried [to have sex].

I: But you had the desire, and you resisted it?

R: Yes, yes. . . .

I: Now, when you sit with your peers, do they laugh [because you abstain]?

R: My peers? Yes, they must laugh at you. Whether they do or don't laugh at me, I just see it as normal. I have never made a plan to do something just because they laughed at me.

I: And why do you abstain?

R: It is because of school. When I complete school, then I shall start having sex. . . . There is one [girl] in the village. She is beautiful, and her heart is good. What attracts me is her good behavior. . . . I intend to marry her one day. (II-99-I-22-m)

Ernest tested negative for all sexually transmitted infections tested for males in each of the three *MEMA kwa Vijana* surveys.

Finally, in a fourth example, a twenty-one-year-old farmer (Ndebile) reported that—apart from some prepubescent sexual play—he also had abstained from sex, despite intense peer pressure:

R: Youth who have sex see youth who do not have sex as impotent . . . and [the abstinent youth] asks himself, "Is it true that I am not a real youth if I do not have sex?" Even me, when I was the class prefect, many girls came to me [for sex], but I was disciplined. Some youths started to say, "You are not a real man, your penis doesn't work, you are completely a woman." I answered, "Ah, if I am a woman then leave me to be female, leave me the way I am." Other things they say are that [abstinent boys] are crazy, or that they don't have money to bribe a girl. I have managed to tolerate what they say until now. . . . There are church friends with whom you talk about God, and how to build your lives, and there are other village friends, those who talk about sexual issues. Me, I like my church friends. (II-02-I-298-m)

Ndebile attributed his decision to abstain to his religion, his *MEMA kwa Vijana* classes, and his fear of AIDS. Importantly, he did not see abstinence as the only way he might avoid HIV infection before marriage. He explained:

R: I'm afraid of AIDS. When I was in Year 7, we learned a lot about protection against AIDS, and they said, "If you want to have sex, you should use a condom and be with a trusted lover. If there is no protection, then leave, don't even try to have sex." If I decide to have sex, I intend to use a condom. For instance, in this village condoms are sold in shops, but in [a neighboring village] you'll get condoms for free at the hospital. Likewise, in this village there are some youths who were given condoms for distribution to other youths. So it will be very easy to get condoms. (II-02-I-298-m)

Ndebile participated in two of the *MEMA kwa Vijana* surveys, and tested negative for all sexually transmitted infections measured at those times.

Case studies 1.2 and 2.2 describe other male youth who actively delayed their sexual debut after most of their peers had become sexually active.

Secondary Abstinence: Abstaining after Sexual Debut

The vast majority of young people in this study said that it was too challenging to abstain after sexual debut. For most young men, abstaining after having already experienced sex was considered very difficult physically, and also detrimental to masculinity and well-being. Only a small minority of young men thus reported voluntary secondary abstinence. There was even less evidence of female secondary abstinence, as in the entire study there were only a handful of young women who consistently and plausibly reported that they had abstained from sex for a long period after their first post-pubescent sexual experiences. Once a girl had had sex, she no longer had an incentive to abstain to preserve her virginity or related respectability, but she typically had substantial reasons to continue sexual activity. First, girls were constantly approached by boys and men seeking to have sex, and sometimes they were strongly pressured to do so, as already discussed. Second, material exchange for sex was a fundamental way for girls to meet their basic needs and desires in adolescence, so much so that the vast majority did not consider not having transactional sex once they had engaged in it.

Despite these general findings, a few young people reported abstaining after sexual debut, usually attributing this to possible negative consequences of sexual activity, school ambitions, and/or participation in the *MEMA kwa Vijana* sexual health intervention. For example, a twenty-year-old woman (Maimuna) reported that she had only had one sexual relationship, over a one year period, with a farmer who had left school several years before her. That relationship ended when she completed school. She explained that she then became abstinent for one year because she greatly feared becoming pregnant out-of-wedlock. She said that she was motivated to abstain after she witnessed her father beat and throw out an unmarried cousin who became pregnant, and she knew other single mothers who were enduring similar hardships:

> R: After completing school, I thought, "Eh, let me stop it." I thought I was going to become pregnant and suffer with the baby after delivery. I used to see many people becoming pregnant and delivering their babies, and now they're facing problems with those babies alone. After all, if [a baby] gets a fever, you don't have money [as a single mother]. (II-02-I-252-f)

Eventually Maimuna eloped with a man from a different village. It is unclear how much contact they had had prior to eloping, but this was probably minimal given how far away he lived and the strict nature of her parents' household. Maimuna tested negative for sexually transmitted infections in the first *MEMA kwa Vijana* survey. She did not participate in any subsequent surveys, so no other biological data were collected for her.

A few young people reported having had sex one time due to curiosity, desire, or pressure, and then choosing to abstain for years afterward because they did not enjoy their initial experience. For example, a sixteen-year-old girl who had tested negative for sexually transmitted infections in a recent survey reported that she had had sex once only, when she was fourteen years old and in Year 5. Her partner gave her Tshs 400 ($0.48) for the encounter, which she used to buy an orange, two buns, an exercise book, and a pen. However, the experience was so painful that she had not had sex again. She explained: "I didn't enjoy it . . . no, I didn't enjoy it. I felt pain there, in my vagina. . . . We only had sex that day, and then stopped for good, because he was older . . . his penis was too big" (II-00-C-112-f). Similarly, when female group discussion participants were asked if they had ever known a young woman who abstained after sexual debut, the only scenario they could envision hypothetically involved a girl who first had sex when her vagina was too small, and then abstained until she matured more.

A twenty-one-year-old man in his first year of secondary school (Stephano) also reported that he had abstained after sexual debut because he disliked his first experience of vaginal intercourse at age nineteen. Stephano said that he had enjoyed the girl's company over many weeks before they had sex, and that they ultimately only had sex because she and his friends put a lot of pressure on him to do so. He experienced both pleasure and pain during the encounter, the latter reportedly because the foreskin of his penis tore. The researcher's fieldnotes:

> [Afterward] Stephano said he began asking himself why he did such an act, because he thought it was neither necessary nor advantageous. He decided not

to continue having sex, because he was afraid of his teachers finding out and losing their respect and confidence in him, because he had good relationship with them. Also, he said he remembered the instruction of his religion, the [Protestant] Africa Inland Church, that having premarital sex is a sin. Stephano said that at present he is still a student, thus he doesn't want to mix things. Some of his friends laugh at him and say that he is impotent. However, he says he has a friend in Form Four [Year 11] at school who encourages him to do away with sex until he completes his education, a situation that enables him to stick to his principle of abstaining. (PO-00-C-3-3m)

A few young men reported trying to abstain after causing an unplanned pregnancy or contracting a sexually transmitted infection, as seen in case studies 1.4 and 3.3, but it is unclear how long they maintained their abstinence. Occasionally, a young man reported abstaining after sexual debut because he did not want to spend his limited money on sexual partners. For instance, a participant in a group discussion:

P: I started [being sexually active] slowly, but later I heated up to the point that other youths were talking a lot about me, saying, "Ah! Somebody has become very promiscuous, he has sex with the girls who reject us, I don't know why, perhaps he gives them a lot." I got messages at home like, "Nowadays you are overdoing it to the point that you will get ill." . . . I calculated the amount of money that I had already spent on sexual partners. If I had stopped for three or four months, where would I be? I would have bought something, like new clothes, I would have been wearing them at this moment. I just decided to stop and rest. When I started [abstaining], I became very troubled. You may dream perhaps that you are talking or having sex with your lover and when the dream is over you find . . . you have ejaculated, ah, you take a handkerchief and rub, it ends like that. When I completed a month, my sexual desire reduced. When I finished two months, it really disappeared, and the third month I started seeing women just like my fellow men . . . until I completed a year. (GD-02-I-1-m)

Like the young man above, several youths who reported secondary abstinence said it was most physically difficult in the first weeks after abstaining, but it became more manageable over time, until they reached a point when sexual desire no longer bothered them.

Finally, a small number of unmarried young men reported that they voluntarily practiced secondary abstinence after they converted to an evangelical Christian denomination. Importantly, these individuals professed a strong personal faith, unlike some young people who formally converted to a new religion with their parents but did not seem to feel a strong personal commitment to it. In one example from a *MEMA kwa Vijana* control village, a twenty-five-year-old man described how he had had many partners by his mid-teens, but he decided to stop once he converted to the Apostolic Church.

When discussing this he used a metaphor of trapping and eating doves to represent seducing and having sex with women:

> He said, "Before I was saved, I used to trap doves. I used to trap them in a net and eat them right there, and then return home empty-handed." . . . I asked him if he will abstain until he dies, and he said he doesn't know yet. . . . He said, "Jesus separates you from earthly matters," which he listed as drunkenness, theft, witchcraft, and adultery. He said if you are adulterous you can get sexually transmitted infections, such as gonorrhea, syphilis, chlamydia, and AIDS. He explained that he had been taught about AIDS in his church. (PO-00-C-9-5f)

This young man believed that traditional medicine could be used to successfully treat AIDS and other sexually transmitted infections, especially if a person did not truly have AIDS, but instead had been bewitched with an AIDS-like illness. He gave the example of a deceased woman who initially was believed to have died of AIDS, but who later was believed to have been bewitched with an AIDS-like illness, because her husband continued to appear healthy and had remarried a woman who also appeared healthy.

Case studies 1.3, 1.4, and 2.2 describe other young people who tried to abstain for an extended period after initiating sex.

DISCUSSION

In this study, adolescents who intentionally delayed sexual debut were usually relatively young, in early to mid adolescence. Boys and girls sometimes had similar motivations to abstain, such as religious beliefs or commitment to schooling, as has been found elsewhere in sub-Saharan Africa (e.g., Chiao and Mishra, 2009; Onya, Aarø, and Madu, 2009). However, in the HALIRA study boys and girls often experienced quite different external influences that promoted abstinence, such as boys having very little money to exchange for sex, and girls anticipating relatively great punishment and stigma if they have sex.

Among young people there was a strong belief that, once someone became sexually active, it was extremely difficult to abstain again, although the reasons attributed to this for young men and women were again quite different. For young men, secondary abstinence was considered too physically challenging, while for young women sex was considered too important to give up as a primary way to meet their material desires and needs. These findings suggest it would be most effective to promote abstinence and other low-risk behaviors prior to sexual debut, rather than attempting to change risk behaviors once they are established, as has also been found elsewhere in sub-Saharan Africa (Gallant and Maticka-Tyndale, 2004). Nonetheless, the HALIRA study did find a very small number of young people intentionally abstained after sexual debut, particularly boys. Those individuals sometimes reported that their earlier sexual experiences had been unpleasant or insufficiently satisfying, particularly when compared to potential cost to their finances, health, or school careers. Others reported actively managing or ignoring their sexual desires, similar to studies elsewhere in sub-Saharan Africa which found young people abstained due to schooling or marital goals and strategically managed their abstinence, for example, by engaging in sports (e.g., Marindo, Pearson, and Casterline, 2003; Amuyunzu-Nyamongo et al., 2005).

Some young people who gave plausible reports of primary or secondary abstinence said they became convinced to abstain after coming to understand their risk of HIV and sexually transmitted infections through intervention participation and/or personal experience of infection (i.e., their own or a family member's). This suggests that a school-based curriculum such as the *MEMA kwa Vijana* program can be effective in reducing sexual risk behaviors for at least a small minority of young people. Importantly, however, some youth who abstained because of possible sexual health consequences still had important misconceptions about them, for example, believing that someone who appeared healthy could not have been infected by a sexual partner with AIDS. While such misinformation was most evident amongst control participants, intervention participants sometimes also were confused about such issues, highlighting that basic information should be provided and reinforced in multiple ways when intervention participants have little or no prior understanding of mathematics or biology.

Boys and girls in this study experienced quite different incentives and pressures to initiate and continue sexual activity, so abstinence promotion is likely to be most effective if tailored to their particular needs. Examples will be discussed separately below.

Reduced Pressures and Incentives for Girls to Have Sex

Adolescent girls often were pressured for sex by men and boys in rural Mwanza, including early adolescent girls, and the ubiquitous and intense nature of this pressure made it difficult to resist long-term. At an individual level, abstinence promotion with girls should reinforce positive social influences, such as parental attitudes, while also building girls' skills to resist pressure from female peers, boys, and men. However, promotion of girls' abstinence is unlikely to be effective if it only focuses on developing girls' confidence and negotiation skills. It must also challenge the broader community about its tolerance of boys and men who routinely and intensively pressure girls for sex, and then develop strategies to reduce this. Abstinence promotion efforts also need to directly engage with parents about the common expectation that daughters increasingly provide for their own material and monetary needs in adolescence, specifying how this may often lead to unwanted sexual consequences.

Positive Attitudes and Practical Strategies for Male Abstinence

Abstinence promotion with adolescent boys may be most effective if it focuses on developing positive attitudes toward abstinence, strategies to manage sexual desire, skills to resist pressure from same-sex peers, and other ways to demonstrate masculinity, such as financial independence or physical self-control. For example, many boys and young men in this study were interested in becoming financially independent in order to be able to eventually support a wife and family. Abstinence promotion could emphasize how much money a boy might save over time if he does not give his money to girls for sex, but instead invests it in schooling or a small business, and then discuss practical strategies to do so. Similarly, given boys' and young men's concerns about masculinity, mastering their sexual urges through abstinence might be promoted as a positive demonstration of masculine strength, self-control, and autonomy. In a qualitative study with eleven- to twenty-one-year-old males in Nigeria, for example, Izugbara (2008) found that some young men perceived abstinence as a marker of strong will and manliness because of the self-discipline it involved.

In addition to fostering more positive attitudes toward abstinence for boys, abstinence promotion may be more successful if it addresses how boys might safely relieve their sexual desire. As noted in chapters 3 and 7, masturbation was almost never acknowledged as a safe alternative to unprotected intercourse in rural Mwanza, and boys and young men instead sometimes considered it to be a sign of inability to seduce partners as well as being unmasculine, unnatural, and even harmful. Similar findings have been documented elsewhere in sub-Saharan Africa. For example, when 716 Zambian secondary school students were asked to write down questions they had about sexual or reproductive health, many expressed concern that masturbation is sinful, immoral, or shameful, and that it might spread disease, shorten life, or reduce fertility (Warenius et al., 2007). Similarly, in a large scale qualitative study with 216 Kenyan adolescents, participants who met in small groups over a six month period reported experience of masturbation, and some of the older youth claimed to be "experts," but even they associated masturbation with embarrassment and shame (Balmer et al., 1997).

Recent studies in Tanzania also suggest that many adolescents have experience of masturbation and have questions and concerns about it. One study found that, among 885 ten- to nineteen-year-olds who reported having had sex, 36 percent of boys and 17 percent of girls also reported experience of masturbation (Kazaura and Masatu, 2009). In a different study of 715 primary and secondary school students in Mwanza and Dar es Salaam, when respondents were asked to write two questions about sex and relationships that they would like to have answered, 7 percent chose to ask a question about masturbation (Mkumbo, 2010).

The *MEMA kwa Vijana* intervention, like most adolescent sexual health programs in sub-Saharan Africa, did not acknowledge masturbation because it was considered to be a private, sensitive, and potentially controversial issue. However, masturbation is an obvious, safe way to relieve sexual desire, and if it is not frankly acknowledged within sexual health programs, young people may feel confusion or shame to the extent that they have unprotected intercourse rather than masturbate. If instead it is acknowledged, for example, by having highly respected young men with unquestioned masculine credentials refute young men's beliefs that masturbation undermines masculinity, it may be helpful in promoting both primary and secondary abstinence. Ideally, discussion of masturbation would take place within a broader discussion of puberty and related issues, such as privacy and hygiene.

Notably, in a recent questionnaire survey with 187 parents of ten- to thirteen-year-olds in Mwanza and Dar es Salaam, 75 percent of parents supported the provision of sexual and relationships education in schools and overall rated the topic of masturbation as "somewhat important" (urban parents) or "important" (rural parents) for programs to address (Mkumbo and Ingham, 2010). In many African settings, however, government officials, religious leaders, health workers, parents, and others may have preexisting notions that masturbation is immoral, shameful, or dangerous, which could make frank and positive discussion of this topic within adolescent risk reduction programs more challenging (Warenius et al., 2006). This highlights the need for any interventions with young people to be contextualized within broader awareness-raising interventions with adults, which will be discussed more in the final chapter.

Importantly, the recommendations outlined here for the promotion of premarital abstinence could be relevant in other circumstances. For example, interventions could frankly address short-term abstinence strategies when targeting young men who need to abstain for six weeks post-circumcision, or married couples that wish to abstain during the postpartum period or due to geographical separation. Chapter 11 will outline broader intervention recommendations which also have implications for abstinence promotion, such as programs which provide alternative sources of income for girls, organized sports for boys, and increased access to schooling for both.

Having described the HALIRA study's findings on young people who abstained in this chapter, the next series of case studies and the chapter following it will focus on young people who tried to limit their partner number and/or practice fidelity.

Case Study Series 2

"This One is Enough"
Young People Who Limited Their Partner Number and/or Were Monogamous

This case study series describes the lives of three young people who provided plausible and consistent reports of reducing their number of sexual partners and/or being faithful. Shija's case study (2.1) illustrates how fear of negative consequences of premarital sexual activity led some girls to abstain in school, and then to marry their first sexual partners soon after leaving school. For Shija, those consequences included parental punishment, reduced ability to marry, and sexually transmitted infection, which she had learned about in her *MEMA kwa Vijana* classes. Rajabu's case study (2.2) describes a young man who also had a relatively late sexual debut but then alternated between brief, monogamous relationships and long periods of abstinence. At that stage of his life, Rajabu was primarily focused on building a small business, and he seemed to adopt this practice as a way to occasionally satisfy his sexual desire with a woman while reducing his risk of exposure to HIV and other sexually transmitted infections. Finally, Elizabeth's case study (2.3) describes a young woman who enjoyed having sex and multiple partners while she was in primary school, until she was forced to drop out due to pregnancy. After delivering her child she married a new partner, and two years later she seemed content in her long-term monogamous relationship with him.

2.1. SHIJA: A YOUNG WOMAN WITH
LATE SEXUAL DEBUT WHO BECAME MONOGAMOUS

Shija was a sixteen-year-old girl in Year 7 of an intervention school during the first year of the *MEMA kwa Vijana* program. Several months after she completed school she was randomly selected for an in-depth interview. The same researcher then interviewed her again two years later.

Shija's parents were Catholic, Sukuma farmers, and she was the fifth of their eleven children. During her first interview, she said that her parents paid for all of her school expenses, except that she bought shoes and clothing with money she earned from her own small plot of land. There she grew maize or cotton, for which she had earned Tshs 1,000 ($1.20) and Tshs 5,000 ($6) respectively in the seasons before the first interview. While still a pupil, Shija had also participated in an all-female *rika* that shared agricultural tasks and hired itself out for a fee. Shija said she had never gone to a video show or disco.

When Shija was in Year 7 her mother delivered twins and died soon afterward. Shija's father remarried a few months later. Near the end of Year 7, Shija met a young man from a neighboring village at a market and eloped with him one month later. Shija reported that her husband had been one year ahead of her in school, but she did not know his age.

As noted in chapter 2, women who participated in in-depth interviews both before and after marriage often reported premarital sexual activity before they married but denied it afterward. Shija was married at the time of both of her interviews, so it is not possible to examine the consistency of her reports before and after marriage. During both interviews she consistently reported that she had never had sex before meeting her husband. Shija said that, during the month after she first met him, she saw him in agricultural fields and at the water hole, when he sometimes gave her Tshs 500–1,000 ($0.60–$1.20). Three weeks after they first met they had sex for the first time, when he snuck into the room she shared with her younger siblings and stayed from 10 p.m. to 5 a.m. He gave her Tshs 1,000 ($1.20) the next day. When first asked what made a girl like/love a boy, she said gifts, but when later asked why she decided to have sex that first time, Shija said, "Because we liked/love each other, due to our conduct" (II-00-I-106-f). Before eloping one week later, Shija only told one sister about her sexual relationship. When Shija eloped, her husband picked her up near her home at 10 p.m. and they went to one of his relative's home for a week. Her husband then visited her father and negotiated the elopement fine of two cows and some money. The dates Shija reported for the elopement and the subsequent delivery of her baby nine to ten months later suggest that she became pregnant soon after eloping, rather than that she eloped due to pregnancy.

Shija's husband was a farmer, and they lived in a two-room house in his mother's compound. At the time of the second interview Shija had established a small business buying bananas for a low price when they were green, and then re-selling them at the evening market once they had ripened. Her husband similarly had a small business buying, husking, and re-selling rice.

Shija said she had learned in her *MEMA kwa Vijana* classes that condoms could be used to prevent pregnancy and the transmission of AIDS and other sexually transmitted infections during intercourse. She said she had never seen a condom, but she knew they could be bought at kiosks and she had a basic understanding of how they worked: "It is made of rubber. We were taught at school. The teacher took some socks. He/she demonstrated on his/her hand, and said that is what a condom looks like" (II-00-I-106-f). Shija clearly explained sexually transmitted infections as "discharged pus and abnormal fluids coming from the private parts, including scabs [transmitted] through sexual intercourse" (II-02-I-306-f). She reported that a health worker had visited her school: "He/she told us, 'If you feel any symptoms of sexually transmitted infection, come to the facility for treatment'" (II-02-I-306-f). However, Shija had not participated in a class visit to a health facility.

Shija missed some *MEMA kwa Vijana* classes after her mother delivered twins, because she stayed home to help her mother and then to care for the babies after her mother died. This seemed to have left her with more gaps in her sexual health knowledge than most intervention participants. For example, unlike most intervention participants, she believed that AIDS could be transmitted through casual contact:

> S: AIDS is transmitted through sexual intercourse. Even by what—even by mouth, when talking like we are doing now, or when yawning. Or if you rub yourself with a sponge when bathing, and then someone else comes to bathe and uses the same sponge. (II-02-I-306-f)

When asked if the *MEMA kwa Vijana* program had helped her in any way, Shija said that it had, because it taught her, "even if you have a lover and you want to refuse to have sex with him, you can just refuse" (II-02-I-306-f). Although Shija said she herself had abstained from sex until shortly before she married, she believed most of her classmates had already experienced sex, and she did not believe that abstinence was a feasible option for young couples once they had become sexually active, except when a young woman was in late pregnancy. She explained: "He/she can't [abstain], because they have already become acquainted [had sex]. And it becomes difficult to stop the boy" (II-02-I-306-f).

However, Shija believed it was feasible for a young woman with multiple partners to reduce her partner number, especially once she married. She explained that a young woman with more than one sexual partner might "just choose one that she likes/loves the most and leave the rest" (II-02-I-306-f). In contrast, she did not think men with multiple partners were likely to reduce them: "Because even if he wants to reduce [his number of partners], he may leave one but just continue with others. And if he quarrels with one of them, again he will just leave her but continue with another" (II-02-I-306-f).

When asked why she had only had one lifetime sexual partner, Shija explained: "They were very strict at home. If they knew you had sex, they would punish you severely. Both of them, father and mother" (II-02-I-306-f). She also explained that she eloped soon after beginning her sexual relationship, because she believed a woman's chance of marrying a man diminished if they had an extended premarital sexual relationship: "If you have sex very often and become very acquainted like that, he may refuse to marry you. It is not good" (II-02-I-306-f).

During her first interview Shija reported that she had never been to a hospital or to a traditional healer. For minor ailments she purchased manufactured medication recommended by a kiosk owner or used free traditional medicines prepared by a neighbor. In the second interview, Shija reported that she had had a baby at a local hospital, and afterward attended it for both her own and her child's health care. She said she had used oral contraceptives since her child was five-months old, and described this in plausible detail, including monthly trips to renew her free supply over the last year.

Shija generally believed it was feasible for men who engaged in unprotected sex to adopt condom use. For example: "He can just go buy it, then if he doesn't know how to use it, he can ask how it is used there at the shop" (II-02-I-306-f). In her own situation, however, Shija found it difficult to imagine ever using a condom with her husband. If he proposed it, she said, he would need to explain why it was necessary before she consented: "You will first ask him why. . . . Because a person comes to tell you to use condoms when you have never used condoms together . . . definitely, you have to ask him" (II-02-I-306-f).

In both interviews, Shija seemed confident that she was not at risk of HIV infection, because she was monogamous. In her first interview, she explained: "If you don't have sex with other men, you can't get it" (II-00-I-106-f). Similarly, in her second interview:

I: Do you think you can get [AIDS]?

S: Me? No.

I: What kind of people do you think can get AIDS?

S: There are those women who have sex with every lover they can get. From one lover, she goes somewhere else and has another lover. She may even have sex with a lover who is suffering from AIDS, in that case, he can infect her. (II-02-I-306-f)

In both interviews Shija said she had never experienced symptoms of sexually transmitted infection. However, in the survey conducted four months prior to her second interview, Shija provided samples which later tested positive for herpes and trichomonas, similar to 21 percent and 27 percent of all young women who participated in that survey, respectively (Ross et al., 2007). Neither of these infections was tested in earlier surveys, so it is not clear when Shija became infected. In any case, her positive results do not necessarily mean that her reports of one lifetime partner were false. Even if her husband was also monogamous during their relationship, he may have contracted the infections in prior relationships. Alternatively, the marriage may not have been mutually monogamous, in which case she could have become infected through his extramarital relationship.

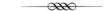

2.2. RAJABU: A YOUNG MAN WHO ALTERNATED BETWEEN ABSTINENCE AND MONOGAMY

Rajabu was twenty-two years old when he was randomly selected for an indepth interview in a *MEMA kwa Vijana* control community at the end of the trial. At the time of the interview, he had been out of school for over two years and he was farming and maintaining a small business.

Rajabu was the last of his parents' four children. His father had died the same year he was born, so Rajabu had no memory of him. His widowed mother had remarried and divorced twice. Rajabu lived with her and his three younger half-siblings. Originally they had all shared a two-room house, but when he and his younger brother reached late adolescence they had each built their own two-room houses within the same compound.

Rajabu grew his own peanuts and rice, for each of which he had earned about Tshs 60,000 ($72) the previous seasons. He also had a small maize buying and re-sale business. He contributed to the household income, including purchasing clothes for himself and his mother. Rajabu was focused on building his small business and was not interested in marrying soon. He explained: "I think my age doesn't permit me to get married. I mean, there is no special age to get married, but it is a matter of deciding, 'Now I should get married,' and I just have not decided that yet [Laughter]" (II-02-C-318-m).

Rajabu's family was Sukuma and Muslim, and he followed some Muslim practices, such as not farming on Fridays. He described having one good male friend, the twenty-eight-year-old Village Executive Officer, who also had grown up in that village. Rajabu said they enjoyed telling one another stories and discussing issues related to their small businesses. He explained that he did not go to *ngoma* or discos:

R: Video shows are the one I like the most, but even those I attend rarely. I am just not interested in *ngoma*. Even the discos. There is too much dust at them, and then people sometimes fight each other, they chase one another around. Personally I just don't enjoy them. (II-02-C-318-m)

Rajabu told the interviewer he had had two sexual relationships. During the first relationship he was nineteen years old and in Year 6 and the girl was fourteen years old and in Year 4. Rajabu said she took some initiative in starting the relationship:

R: She told me to go to her house, to just walk straight in. Now if she hadn't told me to do that, I wouldn't have done it. She used to tell me, "If you don't want to come in alone, I will come collect you." So I waited for her at a place near her home, and she came to collect me. I don't know why she did that. (II-02-C-318-m)

Rajabu said he had sex with that girl four times over a two-month period, until she moved away with her family.

Rajabu said his second relationship occurred ten months before the interview, when he was twenty-one years old and out of school. He said his second partner was a fifteen-year-old Year 6 pupil who also took some initiative in starting their sexual relationship, even though she was formally engaged to another man. The two of them had sex in her room at night three times in the course of a week. They ended the relationship when she got married.

Rajabu said he had not used any contraception with his partners. After most of the sexual encounters he gave them money. He explained:

R: You have to give some women Tshs 2,000–3,000 ($2.40–$3.60), it is necessary. But I only gave them Tshs 500–1,000 ($0.60–$1.20).

I: Mm, why did you decide to give them money?

R: I just gave it to them. Are you suggesting that you can convince a person to have sex and have sex with her without giving her anything, just like that?

I: Yes.

R: Can you? [Laughter]

I: What do you think would happen if you didn't?

R: You would definitely be bewitched [Laughter]. . . . Yes, girls can learn witchcraft from their mothers, don't underestimate them. Of course you would get trouble. (II-02-C-318-m)

Rajabu said that he liked both of his sexual partners, but he did not feel a strong emotional attachment to either of them. He said the main reason he had sex with them was physical desire:

R: It is only desire that makes us have sex. It makes all such things happen. We think, 'Let me try to have sex with this one too.' . . . The pleasure, the pleasure is always there. Mister, I had pleasure throughout my whole body the last time I had sex [Laughter]. (II-02-C-318-m)

When asked whether he had ever had concurrent partners, or whether he could see himself doing so in the future, Rajabu said he could not. He explained:

R: Some youths will seduce any girl, whoever they may see. It becomes impossible. Some have just one. The youth who only has one feels, "Ah, this one is enough," and not that he should have one now and another when he wants one again later. . . . Personally I feel that, if I seduce this one, then she will be the only one. (II-02-C-318-m)

For an unmarried, out-of-school twenty-two-year-old, Rajabu reported abstaining for unusually long periods between sexual partners, despite his desire and pleasure having sex. He attributed this to HIV/AIDS education he received in school. While most *MEMA kwa Vijana* control schools did not have HIV prevention lessons, Rajabu's school was an exception. He explained the education's influence on him:

R: I stopped [having sex] because of my conscience. Nowadays there are so many diseases, like AIDS or syphilis, so I had to stop. . . . There was a lesson about AIDS at school, a teacher from our school taught it every week. We were told to protect ourselves against what? Against AIDS. I mean, to avoid careless sexual intercourse and to use *Salama*. (II-02-C-318-m)

Rajabu believed it is feasible to abstain from sex after sexual debut, not only for himself but for others also, if they have the conviction to do so.

R: These days I don't even desire to have sex. Maybe I desire it once a week, or twice. In that case the desire will be there, but if you continue like that for one to four months, then you will just experience it as normal. . . .

I: Do you think that other youth who have already started having sex can also stop?

R: Yes, they can stop. . . . There are some who think, "Well, not today. No women right now." And really, they can manage. (II-02-C-318-m)

Rajabu could name some sexually transmitted infections and describe general symptoms of them. He also had a basic understanding of how HIV/AIDS could be transmitted through unprotected sexual intercourse. Nonetheless, he also reported some incorrect beliefs, for example, that AIDS could be transmitted by a shared toothbrush. In addition, although Rajabu knew condoms could protect against AIDS and other sexually transmitted infections, he could not describe a condom: "I can't explain them very clearly. I have heard people say there are three in each packet. But I have never opened a packet. I don't know what one looks like. I don't even know its shape" (II-02-C-318-m).

Rajabu reported that he had never had signs or symptoms of sexually transmitted infection. He also tested negative for all infections measured in the *MEMA kwa Vijana* surveys he attended.

2.3. ELIZABETH: A YOUNG WOMAN WHO REDUCED HER NUMBER OF PARTNERS AND BECAME MONOGAMOUS

Elizabeth was randomly selected for an in-depth interview from all of the girls who were pregnant during the first *MEMA kwa Vijana* survey in 1998, when she was in Year 4. Her school records listed her birth year as 1979, suggesting that she was nineteen years old during that first survey. However, school records were often inaccurate and that seems possible in this case, because Elizabeth would have been extraordinarily old for a girl in Year 4. In her first in-depth interview eighteen months after that survey, Elizabeth herself did not know how old she was or the year when she was born, but she guessed she might be eighteen or nineteen years old. At the time of that first in-depth interview Elizabeth was no longer in school and she had recently married a man who was not her baby's father. When she was surveyed again eighteen months later, she was still married to the same man and again had a positive pregnancy test. Several months after that and one week after delivering her second child she participated in a second in-depth interview. At that time Elizabeth guessed that she was twenty years old, although according to the school records she would have been twenty-three.

Elizabeth was the second of her parents' ten children. Her parents had divorced sometime in her childhood. After that, her father formed a polygynous marriage with two other women, although the marriage to his second wife did not last long. At the time of her first interview, Elizabeth lived with her father, his third wife, and eight other family members in five mud-brick and thatch-roofed houses. Her father owned cattle and farmed maize, peanuts, beans, and cassava. He had given Elizabeth a small plot where she grew the same crops, but during the first interview she said she had only earned Tshs 500 ($0.60) from this the prior season, which she used to buy body oil and kerosene. She emphasized that she earned very little: "How much do I grow per season? Maybe enough to fill four or five small bowls [Laughter]. I don't sell it, it is more like I give it away. I take very little for it" (II-00-I-113-f). Elizabeth said that she had never been in a *rika* or gone to a disco, and she had only attended a video show once.

Elizabeth reported that she first had sex the year before she started primary school, approximately six years before her first in-depth interview, when she had first moved to her father's village and was in her early teens. She said she had had a total of five sexual partners, including her husband. Elizabeth's description suggested she had been with each partner for a fairly extended period, having sex with him many times before the relationship ended and she began a new one. She described her first partner as a shopkeeper and her subsequent partners as young farmers and cattle traders of about the same age or a bit older than her. Elizabeth said they usually had had sex in her room at home, which she did not share with anyone else. Elizabeth said that, after each sexual encounter, her partners had given her Tshs 500–1,000 ($0.60–$1.20), soap, lotion, or body oil. She explained she never told anyone about her premarital sexual relationships: "Nobody knew about them. I never told anyone, I just hid them. If others had known I would have been the subject of much gossip, because people say: 'So-and-so is with so-and-so'" (II-00-I-113-f).

Elizabeth said that she liked/loved each of her partners, and—unusually for female pupils in this study—she also sexually desired them and experienced physical pleasure with them during sex. Elizabeth told the researcher that she was embarrassed to discuss sexual issues, but when asked why a girl decides to have sex she laughingly explained: "The boy's thing makes a girl have sex. Girls enjoy sex. Yes, they do enjoy it. They enjoy the man's thing . . . his penis" (II-00-I-113-f). Similarly, later in the interview when Elizabeth was asked whether it is possible for unmarried, sexually active young people to abstain, she replied: "They can't stop completely. They can't because of **luhya** (sexual desire). There is no stopping it. We are just created like that" (II-02-I-313-f).

Elizabeth said her first four relationships ended when she had disagreements with her partners. She reported that she had never had concurrent partners, but she also seemed uncertain about which partner had fathered her first child, so if her relationships did not overlap then at least two were close together. She said a certain man had been forced to take responsibility for her first pregnancy: "He was apprehended and taken to my school. He had to pay the school, I have forgotten how much. And he also paid my father in shillings and two cows" (II-00-I-113-f). This payment was perceived as a fine and not bridewealth, because Elizabeth's father did not like the man and refused to let him marry her. Instead, after Elizabeth delivered her baby, she became involved with her fifth sexual partner and married him soon afterward.

At the time of her first in-depth interview Elizabeth repeatedly referred to herself as married, although she was still living in her parents' household. She did not explain this situation, but it seems likely that she was transitioning to marriage over a matter of weeks or months. In some marriages, for example, the husband paid a portion of the bridewealth and was then entitled to conjugal visits with his wife in her parents' household, but she did not move into his household until he had completed further payments.

At the time of the second in-depth interview Elizabeth was living in her husband's uncle's household with her husband, her second child, and five of her in-laws. All of the adults in the household worked in the family's agricultural plots. Elizabeth regularly went to markets and also said she had gone to *ngoma* events many times since moving to her husband's home, but she had never attended discos or video shows. Like most married men and women, she did not attend *ngoma* events with her spouse, but instead went with another young woman who had married into Elizabeth's husband's family. Elizabeth said she did not have a close girlfriend in her new neighborhood, unlike when she had lived in her parents' home. She had delivered her second child at home with the assistance of a female relative one week before the interview. Since then she had experienced some pain and discomfort, which her husband was treating with traditional medicine he obtained for her locally.

During her second interview Elizabeth reported that she had a history of chronic stomach pain, which in this context could have meant either abdominal or genital pain, as women often used the term "stomach" when referring to genital problems. Elizabeth explained that she first sought treatment at a hospital, where she was treated for worms. However, her symptoms worsened and she became concerned that they affected her fertility:

> *E:* My stomach pains have bothered me for a long time. They just itch, they itch a lot. Whenever they erupt, they bother me every day.
>
> *I:* Do you know what causes them?
>
> *E:* What causes them? . . . When you are bathing with someone and she tells you, "Take a piece of stone and scrub my back to clean it." If she has got it, you may also catch it and become ill. It could take a year, then you become ill. . . . I went to the hospital for treatment. I was told to have five injections, but I stopped at four because I was not getting healed. . . . Then I was unable to get pregnant, so last year I went to a traditional healer.
>
> *I:* When you went to the traditional healer, didn't you already have a child?
>
> *E:* I had had the first child, but I had to struggle to get this one. . . . I told the healer I was ill, that every day when I woke up, I had [symptoms]. My stomach was not

getting healed. . . . He/she told me, "**Nzoka ja buhale** is troubling you" and gave me traditional medicines. He/she did a good job, because I became pregnant and gave birth. (II-02-I-313-f)

In rural Mwanza the female condition referred to as **nzoka ja buhale** was typically characterized by severe menstrual pain and perceived infertility, and traditional medicine was believed necessary to cure it. It is possible that some of these women had endometriosis or pelvic inflammatory disease (Allen, 2002), the latter of which can be caused by sexually transmitted infections. Indeed Elizabeth's description of a condition that "erupted" and itched could have been symptoms of a sexually transmitted infection. However, she tested negative for all of the infections which were measured in the *MEMA kwa Vijana* surveys, so if she did have such an infection it was likely to have been one that was not tested, such as Human Papilloma Virus, which can cause genital warts.

Elizabeth had been a pupil in a *MEMA kwa Vijana* intervention school but she dropped out before she participated in the program. When asked if she had heard of AIDS, she replied:

E: I have heard that if you have sex with a man with AIDS, he will infect you with it.

I: Do you think that you might ever get AIDS?

E: Yes. Of course I could get it. Just through having sex with a man, if he has got AIDS.

I: Do you know if there is any way to protect someone from getting AIDS?

E: Mm. There is none. . . .

I: Have you ever heard anything about condoms?

E: Condoms. . . . I have only heard people mention them on the radio, but I don't know what they are. I have never seen one. I have just heard, 'Use condoms to prevent diseases.'" (II-02-I-313-f)

Elizabeth did not want to prevent pregnancy and she had never used contraception, but she knew some women in her village who used injectable or oral contraceptives. She reported that she had not had another partner since she married. She said her household lived on the food that all of the household members produced on their farm, and when she occasionally needed money for something her husband gave it to her. She seemed satisfied in her intimate relationship with him as well, and reported that she had no interest in taking another lover.

CONCLUSION

The young people in these case studies varied in the extent to which they adopted monogamy passively as a social ideal or actively as an intentional way to reduce their sexual health risk. Importantly, they also differed in their interpretation and practice of monogamy, and their sexual health risk related to it. Shija, for example, said she had never had sex until she practiced long-term fidelity with her husband. Nonetheless she had two sexually transmitted infections by the end of the study, illustrating how someone with one lifetime sexual partner can still be at risk. In contrast, Rajabu was mainly abstinent but he had had two short-term monogamous relationships, one of which was with a woman who most likely had a concurrent sexual relationship with her fiancé. Finally, Elizabeth's experience of a series of monogamous relationships before marriage, and longer-term fidelity with her husband afterward, highlights how fidelity is the only ABC behavior that allows for reproduction, something that was valued very highly in the study population. The next chapter will describe and discuss these and other broad findings related to partner reduction and/or fidelity within the study.

Chapter Nine

"Being Faithful"

Limiting Partner Number and/or Practicing Fidelity

In sub-Saharan Africa most adolescent sexual health interventions have focused on abstinence and/or condom use. Far less attention has been given to reducing partner number and/or increasing fidelity (Shelton et al., 2004; Grills, 2006; UNAIDS, 2007; Wilson and Halperin, 2008; Leclerc-Madlala, 2009; Lurie and Rosenthal, 2010; Green, 2011). For example, a 2004 review of school-based HIV/AIDS prevention in Africa identified four programs which targeted abstinence only, and six which targeted both abstinence and condom use, but none which specifically focused on limiting partner number or fidelity (Gallant and Maticka-Tyndale, 2004).

Research on these behaviors in general populations in sub-Saharan Africa has also been relatively limited. For example, when one of the main search engines for public health and medical journal articles (PubMed) was used to identify papers on each behavior in 2010, 71 percent of retrieved articles related to condoms, compared to 18 percent for abstinence, and 11 percent for being faithful and/or limiting partner number.[1] Some sub-Saharan African studies have examined all of these risk reduction goals together, and they might not be listed in such an individualized search (e.g., Ferguson et al., 2004; Amuyunzu-Nyamongo et al., 2005; Okware et al., 2005; Pool, Kamali, and Whitworth, 2006; Steele et al., 2006; Landman et al., 2008; Selikow et al., 2009; Sambisa, Curtis, and Stokes, 2010). However, such studies have also typically given less attention to limiting partner number and practicing fidelity than to abstinence or condom use. In addition, the vast majority of these studies have consisted of surveys with adults. Very few have involved in-depth, qualitative research focused on young Africans' perceptions and experiences.

DIVERSE INTERPRETATIONS OF "BEING FAITHFUL"

Studies of people's motivations and experiences of "being faithful" in sub-Saharan Africa may be sparse partly because of how challenging it is to define and measure this behavior. "Fidelity" is often used interchangeably with "monogamy," but this can be problematic. Monogamy is a condition or a practice of having only one sexual partner for a given period of time, whereas sexual fidelity implies a loyalty or obligation to a partner not to have other, non-agreed upon partners, and someone can have a monogamous relationship due to circumstance rather than a sense of loyalty or obligation. For example, adolescent boys may want to have multiple partners but only be able to convince or provide material exchange to one girl. Similarly, in much of sub-Saharan Africa polygynous men may practice fidelity with multiple wives by not having extramarital relationships. However, even this interpretation of fidelity is ambiguous, as studies have found that people sometimes interpret "faithfulness" to partners as respect, discretion, and/or trust, but not necessarily sexual exclusivity (Leclerc-Madlala, 2009; Lillie, Pulerwitz, and Curbow, 2009; Baumgartner et al., 2010; Kenyon et al., 2010).

Even if "fidelity" is taken to mean "monogamy," it can be interpreted and practiced in diverse ways which have very different implications for HIV risk. Monogamy is likely to be most safe if both partners test negative for HIV before having unprotected sex, and then have a long-term, mutually monogamous relationship. In practice, however, many monogamous relationships do not involve HIV testing, are not long-term, and/or are not mutually monogamous, all of which can contribute to greater HIV risk. For example, an individual may practice monogamy by having a series of brief relationships, with small gaps between them. Practicing serial monogamy in this way can substantially increase risk of exposure to infection if condoms are not used, increasing the chance that a person has contact with someone with HIV or another sexually transmitted disease. In addition, if there is only a short period of time between sexual relationships, there is a greater chance of transmitting infections received from one partner to a subsequent partner, including bacterial infections which have a limited period of infectivity, and viral infections which have an initially brief but intense period of infectivity, such as HIV (Kraut-Becher and Aral, 2003; Pilcher et al., 2004; Wawer et al., 2005). Alternatively, a monogamous person might have a long-term relationship with a partner who entered the relationship HIV-positive, or who contracted it from another partner during the relationship. Indeed, in such circumstances sexual fidelity may be a high-risk practice (Painter et al., 2007; Landman et al., 2008; Hageman et al., 2010). However, expectations of trust within mutually monogamous relationships can make it difficult to raise such concerns, or to insist upon condom use (e.g., Parikh, 2007; Jana, Nkambule, and Tumbo, 2008; Hirsch et al., 2009; Shai et al., 2010).

Research and intervention work focused on "being faithful" is further complicated because it typically is assumed to include the behavioral goal of limiting partner number. However, a person may lower his sexual health risk by reducing his concurrent partners from four to two, even if he is not practicing monogamy or fidelity. Alternatively, an individual who maintains the same number of partners and frequency of sex for a given time period—for example, having three partners over a one year period—but who shifts from concurrency to serial monogamy, is also practicing a lower risk behavior, at least for the earlier partners who cannot be indirectly infected by later partners. The goal of limiting partner number may also involve quite different approaches depending on the target population. In a high-risk population, for example, it may involve reducing existing partner number (e.g., from multiple concurrent partnerships to one), while in an early adolescent population the goal might be to have few lifetime sexual partners once participants become sexually active.

Finally, the protective potential of limiting partner number is clearly greatest if condoms are used consistently within sexual relationships. However, the majority of sexually active young people in sub-Saharan Africa do not use condoms (Bankole et al., 2009), so most of the following discussion considers these practices in the absence of condom use. Condom use will be examined in depth in the next chapter, while the potential for individuals to employ different low-risk practices together, or to use different strategies at different times of their lives, will be returned to again in chapter 11.

The discussion above highlights how the goal of "being faithful" can be complex and ambiguous, and thus warrants careful examination. In this book the term will be assumed to encompass both partner number limitation and partner exclusivity, with the latter including monogamy, polygyny, and/or fidelity.

RESEARCH WITH MEN IN SUB-SAHARAN AFRICA

Until very recently, research on limiting partner number and/or partner exclusivity in sub-Saharan Africa has mainly involved asking survey respondents how many sexual partners they had over a given time period. Such data can be problematic, as some respondents may under- or overreport their partner number if they believe this to be socially desirable (e.g., Catania et al., 1990; Agnew and Loving, 1998; Devine and Aral, 2004; Beguy et al., 2009; Turner et al., 2009). Even if respondents strive to provide honest answers, they may have difficulty with accurate recall, especially those who have had many partners (e.g., Brewer, Garrett, and Kulasingam, 1999). In addition, such survey questions rarely clarify the duration and overlap of partnerships, or the frequency of sexual encounters within them, all of which can have important implications for sexual health risk.

Recognizing these limitations, survey data nonetheless provide some insight into factors which may be associated with low partner number and/or monogamy. For sexually experienced boys and men in sub-Saharan Africa, these behaviors have been associated with parental disapproval of early and premarital pregnancy; later sexual debut; later marriage; low lifetime partner number; marriage and/or cohabitation with a sexual partner; satisfaction with one's main sexual relationship; belief that a partner is faithful; the partner knowing one's best friends; belief that a best friend practices marital fidelity; older age; religion; rural residency; ethnic homogeneity of community; limited travel away from home; never having used condoms, alcohol, or tobacco; and never having had sex with a female sex worker (e.g., Ferguson et al., 2004; Babalola, Tambashe, and Vondrasek, 2005; Mpofu et al., 2006; Steele et al., 2006; Carter et al., 2007; Benefo, 2008; Jana, Nkambule, and Tumbo, 2008; Bingenheimer, 2010; Clark, 2010; Sandøy, Dzekedzeke, and Fylkesnes, 2010; Kenyon et al., 2010). A recent multi-study comparison also found that, in some countries, men residing in poorer households, with lower levels of education, and without wage-earning jobs were less likely than others to have multiple partners (Bingenheimer, 2010).

Many of the associations listed above have been found consistently in different sites, but some variables have had inconsistent findings. Early in the AIDS epidemic, for example, numerous African studies found that men with higher education reported more partners than those with less education, but this pattern has largely reversed in recent years (Mmbaga et al., 2007; Sandøy, Dzekedzeke, and Fylkesnes, 2010). It may be that existing HIV prevention programs have been more successful in promoting partner reduction amongst men with higher education level, or that they have come to see it as more socially desirable to underreport this in surveys. In another example, surveys in Zimbabwe and Zambia found that urban men were less likely to have multiple or concurrent partners than their rural counterparts (Sambisa, Curtis, and Stokes, 2010; Sandøy, Dzekedzeke, and Fylkesnes, 2010). The Zambian survey further found that single men were less likely to have concurrent partners than married men, even when polygynous relationships were excluded (Sandøy, Dzekedzeke, and Fylkesnes, 2010).

Chapter 3 described how polygynous marriages were fairly common in rural Mwanza, and polygyny was practiced in diverse ways by people of different faiths, both formally and informally. Similarly, in recent Tanzanian surveys 11 to 12 percent of married men and 23 to 24 percent of married women reported that they were currently in a polygynous marriage (National Bureau of Statistics and ORC Macro, 2005; TACAIDS et al., 2008). The vast majority of those marriages involved two wives only. Older, rural, and/or less educated men and women were more likely to be in polygynous unions than others, as were relatively poor women (National Bureau of Statistics and ORC Macro, 2005). Polygyny is also common in many other parts of sub-Saharan Africa (Caldwell, Caldwell, and Quiggin, 1989).

By definition, polygynous marriages involve concurrency, which broadly suggests a higher potential sexual health risk than monogamous marriages. However, like monogamy, polygyny can be practiced in diverse ways which have very different implications for sexual health. In African settings where both monogamous and polygynous marriages tend to follow strict religious and social ideals, for example, polygyny may be a formal and uniform practice. In other settings, polygynous marriages can be informal and highly variable. For instance, a union may form when a married man makes an extramarital partner pregnant and she gradually comes to be perceived as his junior wife, whether or not she formally marries him, and whether or not she lives in the same household as his senior wife.

Although polygyny involves concurrency and it is widespread in sub-Saharan Africa, it has rarely been closely examined within HIV prevention research and interventions. Researchers and intervention developers may be particularly wary of raising questions about polygyny where it is a legal practice that is supported by strong religious and traditional beliefs (Caldwell, Caldwell, and Quiggin, 1989). The relative risks of different forms of polygyny compared to monogamous marriages or out-of-wedlock sexual relationships are thus not clear (Reniers and Tfaily, 2008; Vissers et al., 2008; Bove and Valeggia, 2009; Clark, 2010; Reniers and Watkins, 2010). However, there is little doubt that the general principles of limiting partner number and being faithful to reduce sexual health risk are relevant to polygyny. A polygynous marriage can be low risk, for example, if no spouses have sexually transmitted infections and if their sexual network is closed, that is, if none of them have extramarital relationships.

Only very recently have in-depth, qualitative studies specifically examined men's perceptions and experiences of multiple partnerships, polygyny, other forms of concurrency, limiting partner number, and/or practicing fidelity in sub-Saharan Africa (e.g., Amuyunzu-Nyamongo et al., 2005; Samuelsen, 2006; Pool, Kamali, and Whitworth, 2006; Lewinson, 2006; Izugbara and Modo, 2007; Leclerc-Madlala, 2009; Harrison and O'Sullivan, 2010). In research in Uganda, for example, 53 percent of 168 respondents reported that they had reduced their number of sexual partners since becoming aware of AIDS, and almost one-third of them attributed this to fear of AIDS (Pool,

Kamali, and Whitworth, 2006). In that study, 35 percent of the men who reported partner reduction said they reduced their number of partners because they could no longer afford multiple partners, while some said that they had lost interest or had become too old and "weak" to engage in extramarital relationships. Some women who had had multiple partners as teenagers instead reported that they became monogamous when they married.

RESEARCH WITH WOMEN IN SUB-SAHARAN AFRICA

Little information has been published about women's multiple or concurrent partnerships in sub-Saharan Africa, in part because few women report multiple partners in surveys, possibly due to social desirability bias (Gersovitz et al., 1998; Nnko et al., 2004; Sandøy, Dzekedzeke, and Fylkesnes, 2010). The limited research has found women's self-reported monogamy or low partner number is associated with older age at first sex; financial, emotional, and sexual satisfaction within a main relationship; little or no alcohol or tobacco use; and monogamous marriage (e.g., Mpofu et al., 2006; Hattori and Dodoo, 2007; Jana, Nkambule, and Tumbo, 2008). For example, a study in Kenyan slums found that women in polygynous marriages, single women who lived with a man, and especially widowed, divorced, or separated women were more likely to report multiple partners in the last year than women in monogamous marriages (Hattori and Dodoo, 2007).

These survey findings offer some insight into risk, partner number, and partner exclusivity, but it is difficult to know the extent to which they are biased, given marital fidelity is a widespread ideal for women in sub-Saharan Africa. As noted in chapter 3, for example, many never married women who reported sexual partners in a first in-depth interview in the HALIRA study, who then married a different man before a second interview, initially denied having ever had any partners other than their husbands in the second interview. It was only after they were reminded of their earlier reports that some of these women acknowledged they had indeed had other, premarital partners.

This book has already described how transactional sex was an important way for unmarried young women to meet their basic material needs and desires in rural Mwanza, as has also been found in many other parts of sub-Saharan Africa (e.g., Kaufman and Stavrou, 2004; Luke, 2003; Dunkle et al., 2004; Maganja et al., 2007; Tawfik and Watkins, 2007; Swidler and Watkins, 2007; Béné and Merten, 2008; Hunter, 2009; Wamoyi et al., 2011a). Research similarly suggests that extramarital relationships are one of the main ways for both polygynous and monogamously married women to obtain supplemental income when needed (Caldwell, Caldwell, and Quiggin, 1989). Women in polygynous marriages, and especially those who live in separate households than their co-wives, may be particularly likely to have extramarital relationships, because their husband's support is shared between households and they have more freedom of movement than women who live with their husbands full-time (e.g., Nnko et al., 2004; Hattori and Dodoo, 2007; Vissers et al., 2008).

HISTORICAL RESEARCH WITH THE SUKUMA

Historical anthropological research on Sukuma sexual behavior and monogamous and polygynous marriages has some relevance to this discussion. As noted in the last chapter, for example, anthropological research in the mid-twentieth century found that unmarried teenage boys and girls were allowed some sexual freedom as long as they were discreet (e.g., Tanner, 1955a; Tanner, 1955b; Cory, 1953; Abrahams, 1967; Varkevisser, 1973). Indeed, those researchers found that it was not unusual for young men and women to have had multiple sexual relationships prior to marriage. Cory (1953, 39–40) described expectations of unmarried adolescent girls:

> The behavior of the girls is not criticized by the community as long as they ob-serve the conventions of their position which demand not chastity but discretion. As far as their relations with men are concerned, the girls have only one duty, which is to inform the "lady of the house" if they change a lover. If changes happen too often, a girl is warned that she is likely to get a bad name for fickle-ness; but it is also not proper for a girl to consort with the same lover for any considerable time, because the parents fear that the girl and her lover may finally decide to live in concubinage, a step which would spoil the marriage prospects of the girl and deprive her family of an immediate payment of bridewealth. The ideal behavior of a girl . . . is to have a few lovers, so as to gain sufficient experience for a good wife.

Importantly, the "lady of the house" mentioned above was not one of the girls' mothers, but usually a grandmother who shared sleeping quarters with teenage girls from different families, and who sometimes had an informal role of advising the girls on sexual matters, such as traditional contraception (Varkevisser, 1973). As was found in the HALIRA study, teenage children typically did not discuss sexual matters with their parents, because parents and their children had what anthropologists refer to as an "avoidance relation-ship," that is, a relationship characterized by authority on one side and respect and obedience on the other, including a taboo against children speaking of sex

in front of their parents (Radcliffe-Brown, 1950; Varkevisser, 1973). Historically, once Sukuma young people married, wives were expected to be faithful
to their husbands, and if a woman was unfaithful then this was considered
grounds for her husband to divorce her. In contrast, a husband was entitled to
have extramarital partners as well as multiple wives (Cory, 1953).

As noted in the previous chapter, there were many social changes in
rural Mwanza during the twentieth century, including the conversion of a
majority of the population to Christianity, the introduction of formal education on a large scale, and the increase of average age at first marriage
to late teens for girls and early twenties for boys (Caldwell et al., 1998;
Żaba et al., 2009). These changes contributed to new social ideals, such
as abstinence for school pupils and marital monogamy for Christian men.
It is unclear, however, whether these shifting ideals had much impact on
actual practices. Rather than reducing sexual activity, for example, unmarried Sukuma adolescents may have become more intent on hiding it
from adults than their counterparts had been in the past. This practice also
inadvertently may have made a young person's current and prior sexual
partners less aware of one another than they might have been in the past,
effectively hiding multiple partnerships.

The next section of this chapter will examine the motivations and experiences of young people in the HALIRA study who tried to limit their sexual
partner number and/or to have exclusive relationships. It will be followed by
a discussion of how interventions might better promote low partner number,
monogamy, and/or fidelity with young rural Africans; this topic will then be
further examined in chapter 11.

FINDINGS

In the HALIRA study, it was unusual for young people to report intentionally limiting their sexual partner number after previously having had several
partners, unless they got married. Many unmarried youth instead reported
that they were at low risk of sexually transmitted infection because they had
never had many sexual partners, or they had always been monogamous. It is
possible that a large proportion of the population actively tried to be monogamous. However, individual interpretation and practice of monogamy varied
greatly, as described in chapter 3, and this could result in quite different
sexual health risks. Only a small minority of sexually active unmarried youth
seemed to have one monogamous sexual relationship over an extended period
(e.g., one year). Even they, however, could not be certain that their partners
were also monogamous.

Factors Contributing to Low Partner Number and/or Fidelity

Economic factors sometimes played a role in whether unmarried young men and women were monogamous and/or had few partners over an extended period of time. Young women who were relatively secure financially could be more selective and have fewer partners because they were less likely than other young women to seek partners simply for material exchange. Relatively poor young men, in contrast, sometimes had fewer partners than men with more money—and/or stayed in monogamous relationships for longer—because less was expected in material exchange after the first one or two sexual encounters with a partner.

Other factors which seemed to promote a low number of partners and/ or partner exclusivity included: personal belief; religious teachings; social ideals of fidelity (especially for females); participation in the *MEMA kwa Vijana* intervention; experience of sexually transmitted infection; emotional commitment to a partner; fear of losing a partner because of one's infidelity; and/or satisfaction with the sexual activity or materials provided within one relationship. Case studies 2.1–2.3 and 3.3 illustrate some of these findings.

As was the case for factors contributing to abstinence, none of the factors above were prescriptive and ensured that a young person had a low partner number and/or practiced fidelity. Many adolescents had more than one of these influences in their lives but had multiple and/or concurrent partners. Nonetheless, most young people who actively tried to reduce their partner number and/or to be monogamous had been strongly influenced by several of these factors in combination.

Practicing Monogamy before Marriage

As noted above, many sexually active unmarried youth considered mutual monogamy desirable, but few seemed to achieve it long-term. A number of factors contributed to this. First, as discussed in chapter 3, it was not unusual for individuals to have concurrent relationships but not to recognize them as such. Even when a couple had a steady, semipublic sexual relationship for a year or more, for example, one or both partners might occasionally have casual sexual encounters with someone else. These could be onetime encounters or opportunistic encounters with a prior partner. In addition, unmarried couples sometimes stopped having sex because of external reasons, such as geographic separation due to school or work. In such scenarios the two individuals did not necessarily expect to continue their sexual relationship. In the meantime, they took new partners but then resumed having sex with one another again when the opportunity arose later. Such relationships technically constitute concurrency, but the individuals involved might have perceived themselves as having had a series of monogamous relationships, albeit some with the same person at different stages of their lives.

A second reason why few unmarried couples achieved mutual, long-term monogamy is that, even when couples were truly faithful to one another, it was not unusual for relationships to end after a couple of weeks or months. As noted in chapter 3, couples often knew very little about one another before having sex, and as they got to know one another better they sometimes came into conflict about material support, infidelity, or other issues, and then quickly broke up. Alternatively, unmarried individuals sometimes sought new partners for sexual satisfaction or prestige (males) or material gain (females). After an unmarried couple separated, it was not unusual for the individuals to begin new sexual relationships within a week or a month.

In contrast to these general findings, HALIRA researchers occasionally documented strong evidence that at least one member of a couple was monogamous in a long-term premarital relationship. For example, a nineteen-year-old pregnant woman (Diana), who had recently returned to her village after dropping out of secondary school, reported that she had only had one sexual partner, a kiosk owner who worked near her school:

> Diana said she met her boyfriend when she was in secondary school. She said she used to go to his shop and pose like any other customer, and while there she would talk with him. She said she decided to have sex with him because she trusted him. She said it was not necessary for him to give her gifts, because as long as she liked/loved him she would have accepted him [as her lover], even without a gift. But she said he did give her body oil and anything else she told him she needed. . . . She wrote to him recently, so she assumes he now knows that she is pregnant, but he has not replied to her letter. (PO-99-C-5-2f)

No data were collected from Diana's partner directly because he lived in another village. However, extensive participant observation research found that male kiosk owners typically had many concurrent sexual relationships, because they had frequent contact with many girls and women, and they could easily offer goods and cash in exchange for sex. There is thus a strong possibility that Diana's partner was not faithful to her during their relationship.

In this study it was challenging to clearly identify unmarried couples in long-term sexual relationships who were mutually monogamous, partly because it was difficult to collect in-depth information on both members of a couple, as seen in the example above. When in-depth data were collected from both members of a long-term premarital relationship, the relationship usually did not seem to be mutually monogamous. In one example, a twenty-one-year-old man (Msafiri) explained to a male researcher that he was devoted to his girlfriend of three years (Sabina), who lived with their two-year-old daughter in the village center. The researcher recorded the following:

> Msafiri said that Sabina has rented a room and he sometimes pays her monthly rent of Tshs 1,000 ($1.20). He wants to marry her, but . . . his father says Sabina is too sickly and that she is an *mhuni*. Msafiri said that as far as he knows Sabina is not an *mhuni*, because she does not have other men in the village apart from him. I asked him how he knows this, and he said he stays overnight with her all but one or two nights per week. He said that he likes/loves her a lot, and that is why he does not have another girlfriend. (PO-01-C-2-1m)

Sabina had lost substantial weight in the months preceding that participant observation visit, and some villagers speculated that she had AIDS. Villagers also discussed Msafiri's extraordinary devotion to her. Some considered him to be married to her. For example, on one occasion the female researcher in that village noted:

> Today we passed Msafiri and Sabina where they were uprooting cotton seedlings. As we did my companion said, "That is Msafiri's wife." She said she did not know where Sabina comes from, because she migrated to the village and then Msafiri made her pregnant. She said Msafiri's father didn't want him to marry her, and that his father accepted the child but not the woman. . . . My companion said Msafiri publically refuted what his father had said and declared that Sabina was his wife. She said Msafiri must have great love for Sabina, because any other youth would not have defied his father like that. (PO-01-C-2-5f)

When the researchers returned to the village one year later, Msafiri's father had sent Msafiri to Tanzania's commercial capital to join the army. During the preceding year both Sabina and her child had become severely ill with diarrhea, vomiting, and weight loss, until Sabina lost consciousness and was brought to a traditional healer. Sabina later recovered her strength and told the female researcher that the healer had cured her of her ailment. During that same year a different man had claimed to be the father of Sabina's child. His claim was considered valid enough that the child was living with him at the time of the new participant observation visit, suggesting that Sabina had not been monogamous during her relationship with Msafiri.

Limiting Number and/or Type of Premarital Sexual Partner

In the HALIRA study, a small number of unmarried youth said they tried to reduce their sexual health risk specifically by limiting their number of sexual partners, and some of them attributed it to what they had learned in the *MEMA kwa Vijana* program. A fifteen-year-old *MEMA kwa Vijana* peer educator in Year 7 provided an example:

> He told me that he used to have three lovers, all of whom are now in Year 7. He said each of those relationships lasted one to two months. Last year he began his current relationship, with a girl who is now in Year 6. He said he is pleased with his lover and that they have never quarreled. He said that he decided to remain with one lover after being taught by *MEMA kwa Vijana* that he should only have one reliable partner. He said that those lessons taught him that having one faithful partner helps to protect against sexually transmitted infections. (PO-01-I-7-3m)

Some young men said they reduced their partner number and/or only had unprotected sex with low-risk partners after a frightening personal experience of sexually transmitted infection, as seen in case study 3.3. Others said they stopped having sex with certain kinds of partners after discovering a partner had other partners. Generally such young men said they stopped having sex with women who were rumored to have multiple partners, and/or those who worked in a position where this was believed to be common, such as barmaids or guesthouse workers. Instead, some men sought partners who they thought had had few or no other lovers, such as pupils or other young adolescent girls. For example, the young man in case study 3.3 said he resisted the temptation to have sex with women who he perceived to be high risk—or he used condoms with them—but he had unprotected sex with women who he perceived to be low risk.

It was very unusual for an unmarried young woman to shift from having many partners to only having one long-term partner while remaining single. If young women wanted to do this, they almost always married the man in question.

Limiting Partner Number and/or Being Faithful in Marriage

The HALIRA study primarily focused on young people's unmarried sexual relationships, but those relationships often led to marriage at a young age. Indeed, as already noted, the most common way that young people actively tried to reduce their sexual partner number and/or to be faithful was by marrying, as seen in case studies 2.1 and 2.3. Approximately half of women married by their late teens and half of young men by their mid-twenties, but few young people who married soon after completing school were in polygynous marriages. Young men generally had neither the resources nor the interest to take a junior wife at that stage, while young women typically did not join polygynous marriages as junior wives unless they were very poor or their marriageability had been reduced due to divorce or an out-of-wedlock pregnancy.

Importantly, about half of the married young people in the HALIRA study had married someone who they had met only about one month earlier, as described in chapter 3. Even when two individuals had known one another for a longer premarital period, they typically had had very limited opportunities to spend time alone, and thus entered into marriage without great familiarity or emotional intimacy. In this way, marriage for many young people in rural Mwanza seemed to be a "leap of faith" that involved leaving old sexual relationships and childhood homes behind in the hopes of creating a more satisfactory life with a promising new partner.

HIV testing was very difficult to access in rural Mwanza at the time of the HALIRA study, but in rare instances engaged couples tried to lower their sexual health risk by having HIV tests before marriage. This procedure seemed to be limited to formal marriage within some branches of the Protestant African Inland Church. Virtually all young men entered into marriage expecting their wives to be sexually faithful, and some were motivated to marry specifically to reduce their own sexual health risk. For example, during participant observation a researcher heard the following report from a twenty-six-year-old man:

> He said his lover lives in another sub-village, but he meets her whenever he feels like having sex, usually twice per week. He said he likes/loves that girl very much because he took her virginity and they have been together a long time. When he has sex with other girls he is afraid of getting diseases, so he plans to marry that girl instead. (PO-00-I-4-4f)

Most young women also entered marriage hoping that their husbands would be faithful to them and any co-wives they might have, although they were generally less confident that this would be the case. For example, a young woman who adamantly reported she had never had an extramarital sexual relationship said she did not assume the same for her husband. She took a fatalistic approach to this: "If God has planned that I will die of AIDS, perhaps my husband will bring it. It may happen. These days you can't deny it" (II-02-I-252-f).

As noted in chapter 3, extramarital sexual relationships were not unusual, especially for men, but during the first years of marriage young men and women generally seemed to have fewer partners than they had had before marriage, especially if the couple was not separated for long periods. Newly married young women were less likely to have extramarital sexual relationships because their husbands met their ongoing material needs, and their movements were closely monitored within their husbands' households. For example, in a first in-depth interview an unmarried seventeen-year-old woman (Mpelwa) described having had two prior sexual relationships, each of which lasted a couple of months and did not overlap. The first relationship was with a shopkeeper in her home village who she met for sex on market days between 3 p.m. and 4 p.m. in a grassy area near the market. She met her second partner, a farmer, when she was staying with relatives in another village. They also met for sex on market days, but they met between 6 p.m. and 7 p.m. on the grounds of a secondary school.

In a second interview two years later, Mpelwa reported that she had married a different farmer in a third village not long after her first interview, mainly because she did not have a place to live and wanted to find a secure home. At the time of the second interview Mpelwa was six months pregnant with her first child and living with her husband in his parents' household. She described how her movements were restricted:

> R: I never go to video shows, because I'm married, aren't I? Even if I were not married, it is bad to attend video shows. . . . Some women say they are going to watch videos but in fact they are going for other things . . . like [meeting] men. . . .
>
> I: And have you traveled to other villages?
>
> R: No, only long ago, before I got married. Like I used to travel far to stay with my uncle. . . . If we women are married, we can't just leave home and go for a visit. Perhaps you are forbidden by your husband. If I ask mine, he will say he doesn't need me to go and visit anyone right now. (II-02-I-103-f)

Mpelwa said she had not had any extramarital partners. She reported that sex with her husband had been painful for her and she did not see any reason for sex during pregnancy, so when she became pregnant she asked her husband to abstain from sex with her, and he had agreed. Shortly before her second interview, Mpelwa had tested positive for gonorrhea and herpes during the 2001–2002 *MEMA kwa Vijana* survey.

Newly married young men generally had more opportunity for extramarital sex than young wives. However, they typically enjoyed the novel experience of having sex with a wife every night if they wanted, without needing to hide the relationship or immediately provide her with money or gifts, and this could contribute to them having fewer partners than they had had before marriage. In addition, when some young men married they said they had tired of the effort involved in having multiple sexual relationships, as described by one male group discussion participant:

> P: I don't know if there are two stages of puberty, if the first time you have just begun to be with girls and you reach a time when people say, "He is going out

a lot" [has a lot of sex/partners]. And then you may become tired of it, and even decide to marry and settle down. (GD-02-I-1-36m)

A twenty-one-year-old farmer and small businessman (Charles) who had married a week before his interview explained that he expected his sexual behavior to be different in marriage. He reported that he started having sex at the age of fourteen, and that in total he had had sex with seven girls in five villages, in most cases one time only. Charles described his history with his wife: "I seduced her a long time ago, when she had come to visit this village. . . . Three months ago she went back home and began cultivating there. Then she came back to this village again a few weeks ago, and I took her [eloped]" (II-02-I-248-m). The timing Charles described suggests that he had sex with at least one of his other partners after he first had sex with the woman who became his wife. However, when asked whether he had ever had concurrent relationships he repeatedly said that he had not and he did not intend ever to do so. He explained his intention to be monogamous in marriage: "I have not had a girlfriend since I got married. Those matters are not important. They are just indulgent, they are not beneficial" (II-02-I-248-m). Charles tested negative for all sexually transmitted infections measured for men in each of the three *MEMA kwa Vijana* surveys.

In rural Mwanza, men's sexual fidelity often seemed greatest soon after marriage. Within several years, however, the data suggest that most young husbands had experienced at least one extramarital relationship, and sometimes multiple ones. The husbands who seemed least likely to engage in extramarital sex were those who did not travel for work, and those who did not have lucrative businesses that brought them into frequent contact with women seeking goods or services, as was the case for shopkeepers or bicycle taxi drivers. Nonetheless it was not unusual even for relatively poor and stable men to occasionally have extramarital sex.

Separation and divorce were fairly common among married young people in rural Mwanza, as discussed in chapter 3. Several factors were reported to cause divorce, such as infidelity, or disappointment with a spouse or new living circumstances after having married someone largely unfamiliar.

DISCUSSION

For young rural Africans, "being faithful" may be the most culturally appropriate, feasible, and desirable of the ABC behavioral goals. First, it is strongly supported by existing social ideals. Second, it allows for sexual pleasure, and particularly the experience of "flesh-to-flesh" intercourse that was highly prized amongst young people in this study. Third, it does not prevent pregnancy, something many young people actively sought and others wanted to leave to chance. Some research elsewhere in sub-Saharan Africa has also found that intensively promoting low partner numbers and/or fidelity may be effective with at least some sexually active youth and adults (e.g., Thornton, 2008; Todd et al., 2009; Sandøy, Dzekedzeke, and Fylkesnes, 2010). For example, while there has been some debate about which factors caused the dramatic decrease in incidence of HIV infection in Uganda during the 1990s, many researchers believe that reduced partner number and increased partner selectivity played important roles (e.g., Singh, Darroch, and Bankole, 2003; Stoneburner and Low-Beer, 2004; Okware et al., 2005; UNAIDS, 2005; Pool, Kamali, and Whitworth, 2006; Thornton, 2008). Some have argued that early and intensive promotion of the Ugandan concept of "zero grazing" was critical. As Thornton (2008, 19) explains:

> . . . The slogan referred to the practice of tethering a cow to a peg in the middle of a patch of good grazing. As the animal ate the grass that its tether permitted it to reach, it would clear a circular area around the peg. . . . It simply meant "Eat (have sex) as much as you like, but don't roam too widely." As it turned out, this simple rule may have turned the tide in Uganda because it altered the configuration of the sexual networks on which the spread of HIV depends.

Thornton (2008) further argues that the decrease in incidence of HIV infection in Uganda reflected an overall decrease in sexual network connectivity, especially for links between the general population and highly infected persons or groups, such as soldiers or transportation workers. Recent research in migrant mining zones in Guinea also suggests that faithfulness to partners contributed to the remarkably low and stable HIV rate found in that country (Kiš, 2010). Similarly, it has been stipulated that a reduction in concurrent partnerships in Zambia has contributed to the decline in HIV prevalences there (Sandøy, Dzekedzeke, and Fylkesnes, 2010). Such findings have led to new initiatives to intensively promote partner reduction, such as the Tanzanian initiative *Sikia Kengele: Tulia na Wako* (Listen to the Bell: Stick to Your Partner[s]), which targets high-risk individuals along transport corridors in Tanzania (Mahler and Ndegwa, 2008). This intervention uses mass media, community mobilization, and interpersonal communication strategies to promote partner reduction and fidelity from a secular perspective.

The findings in this chapter and the broader HALIRA study have implications for interventions seeking to promote lower sexual partner numbers, increased partner selectivity, and fidelity with rural African youth. These include: improving intervention participants' understanding of risks related to multiple partnerships; intensively promoting HIV testing; developing alternative forms of masculinity; increasing awareness and acknowledgment of youth sexual activity; and building stronger premarital and marital relationships. Each of these will be discussed more below.

Understanding Risks Related to Multiple Partners

Young people in this study who actively tried to limit their partner number and/or to select a faithful partner often had a better sense of their sexual health risk than most rural youth and adults, either because of intervention participation (including intensive training as a peer educator), or because of personal experience of a sexually transmitted infection. This stresses the importance of young people developing an in-depth understanding of local prevalences of HIV and other sexually transmitted infections, the nature of disease transmission within networks, and the different risks involved in multiple partnerships, concurrency, serial monogamy, and having short gaps between partners.

Interventions should also engage with participants about the different ways that "fidelity" can be interpreted and practiced, so that, for example, participants understand that the protective potential of fidelity is undermined if occasional, opportunistic sexual partnerships overlap with a main long-term relationship. Given many young people may highly value a partner's fidelity but do not consider it equally important to be faithful themselves, interventions must also stress how individuals expose themselves to risk when they engage in unprotected concurrent partnerships. Programs could thus potentially promote personal commitment to fidelity in two ways, first as it is commonly understood as an issue of loyalty or obligation to a partner, and second also as an issue of self-preservation, protection, and fidelity to one's self. Most importantly, interventions must clearly convey that fidelity is only protective if it is mutual between two partners who have tested HIV-negative.

A recent study with fourteen- to twenty-year-olds in urban Dar es Salaam and rural Iringa, Tanzania also found that young people interpreted fidelity in diverse ways, so that simple "be faithful" program messages were ambiguous. The authors proposed several alternative messages, such as "test together before starting a new relationship," "be faithful to one tested partner," and "avoid overlapping partners" (Baumgartner et al., 2010). They additionally recommended the promotion of partnership spacing, that is, taking more time between ending old relationships and starting new ones (Pilcher et al., 2004).

Intensive Promotion of HIV Testing

At the time of the *MEMA kwa Vijana* trial in 1997–2002, HIV testing services in Mwanza Region and elsewhere in Tanzania were largely limited to specialized services in district and regional hospitals. In the last decade, however, HIV testing has become far more accessible in Tanzania and elsewhere in Africa (Padian et al., 2011; Doyle et al., 2012). In Tanzania, for example, the proportion of fifteen- to twenty-four-year-old females who had had sex in the last year and who were tested and knew their results increased from 6 percent in 2004–2005, to 24 percent in 2007–2008, to 39 percent in 2010.

The increased availability of HIV testing has important implications for fidelity promotion within HIV prevention programs. Critically, it is no longer necessary for individuals to begin a sexual relationship without knowing their own or their partner's HIV status, and they can also test themselves at intervals in the course of a relationship. An HIV-negative couple can thus make an informed and relatively safe decision to have unprotected sex within a mutually monogamous relationship, while HIV-positive individuals can knowingly protect their partners through condom use. This is particularly important as the number of discordant couples increases, that is, the number in which only one person is infected with HIV (Eyawo et al., 2010; UNAIDS, 2010).

While HIV testing has become more common and accessible in sub-Saharan Africa in recent years, there is great potential for improvement in those areas and for increased use of mass media and community mobilization to raise general awareness and reduce stigma related to HIV testing and status. Historically, HIV testing programs have mainly targeted individuals and occasionally married or cohabitating couples (e.g., Kamenga et al., 1991; Allen et al., 2007; Njau et al., 2011). Few such programs have specifically targeted unmarried couples. There is a need to develop and test strategies to do this within interventions promoting monogamy with unmarried youth.

Alternative Forms of Masculinity

In a study with fourteen- to twenty-five-year-old South Africans, Kenyon and colleagues (2010) found that the extent to which a sexual relationship was "structurally embedded"—that is, the extent to which sexual partners knew and were close to each other's friends and family—influenced whether either partner has concurrent relationships. Specifically, the authors found a considerable reduction of African women's reported concurrency rates if a partner knew the friends or family of the respondent, but they did not find a similar association for African men. Noting that male sexual concurrency is often tolerated or encouraged in southern Africa, Kenyon and colleagues (2010, 41–42) comment:

> . . . embeddedness mediates its impact on concurrency via peer pressure, loss of reputation and the like. Thus in a society where the norm is acceptance and even

expectation that one gender has multiple concurrent partners, then we would expect that embeddedness would either have little protective effect or even encourage concurrency in that gender. . . . Thus encouraging individuals and their friends to get to know their partners' friends is only likely to have any chance of reducing concurrency in communities where concurrency is not regarded as acceptable behavior.

Similarly, a small study with fifteen- to nineteen-year-old Ugandan youth found that young men aspired to have multiple partnerships because they provided them with the pleasure, sexual experience, and relationship control that were central to their notions of masculinity (Joshi, 2010). To promote partner exclusivity for both men and women, it may thus be necessary to develop and promote other forms of masculinity than sexual conquest of new partners, such as physical self-control, educational achievement, or financial independence. Young men in this study who seemed successful in reducing their partner number and/or being monogamous tended to be confident, ambitious, and capable of rejecting peer pressure.

At a community level and through the mass media, youth leaders and role models might promote male sexual exclusivity as smart, cool, and/or modern by encouraging young men to perceive peers who have many unprotected partners as ignorant and backwards, because they foolishly risk exposure to disease. Ideally such efforts would target different groups of young men with tailored messages and role models. A program addressing masculinity for adolescent school boys with relatively little sexual experience, for example, would be different from a program for young men in their twenties, particularly those who are likely to have many partners because of high access to women and discretionary incomes, such as kiosk owners, mill workers, bicycle taxi drivers, and traveling traders. Limiting one's sexual partner number need not be presented entirely as a matter of restraint and self-discipline, as the potential to enhance pleasure within a relationship with fewer partners could be emphasized (e.g., Undie, Crichton, and Zulu, 2007). Ideally, this kind of intervention would help shift young male norms to foster a sense of responsibility and accountability.

Greater Acknowledgment of Youth Sexual Activity

The secrecy of non-marital sexual relationships in rural Mwanza was a fundamental barrier to sexual risk reduction, because it facilitated multiple and concurrent relationships. Some other African studies have had similar findings (e.g., Jana, Nkambule, and Tumbo, 2008; Kenyon et al., 2010). Greater acknowledgement of young people's sexual relationships may thus be important in promoting fidelity and/or lower partner numbers for both men and women. With greater openness, sexual partners would be better able to monitor their partners' behavior, and individuals might be less likely to have concurrent partnerships for fear of discovery and damage to their reputations and/or their main relationships. This would mean directly addressing the culture of discretion in which presenting oneself differently in different social contexts (e.g., appearing to be monogamous while having concurrent relationships) is more important than following particular practices (e.g., truly being monogamous). Critically, the intention of greater openness would not be to promote more youth sexual activity, but rather to acknowledge and address what is already taking place in secrecy.

However, it would be challenging to achieve such acknowledgment in an African setting (e.g., Pattman and Chege, 2003; Francis, 2010). Probably one of the most important reasons why partner reduction and fidelity have hardly been promoted with unmarried adolescents to date is that this requires acknowledging adolescent sexual relationships, which some may feel undermines abstinence promotion. Promotion of monogamy for sexually active adolescents could conflict with adult ideals of school pupil abstinence, female sexual respectability (particularly as relates to maximizing future bridewealth), parental authority, and the need to maintain discretion about sexual relationships. There is also a possibility that, if one "official" relationship is acknowledged as legitimate, other relationships may simply become more secretive. The complexity of this issue was illustrated in Uganda, where HIV prevention campaigns increased the moral stigma of extramarital relationships, but in some instances this had the unintended consequence of increasing sexual secrecy (Parikh, 2007). Finally, the transient and exploratory nature of adolescence may seem incompatible with long-term monogamy, unless the young people are married.

Despite these formidable challenges, it is worth developing and testing interventions that encourage parents to acknowledge if their children are sexually active, and to openly recognize a sexually active young person's boyfriend or girlfriend. They might be persuaded to do this by the compelling evidence that sexually transmitted infections are common among young people, and the research findings that secrecy promotes greater risk behavior. Where there is historical and cultural precedence for greater openness about premarital sexual activity, as was the case amongst the Sukuma in the early twentieth century (e.g., Cory, 1953; Abrahams, 1967), this might be drawn upon to legitimize a potentially controversial issue with parents. By parental endorsement or at least tolerance of an adolescent's sexual partner, it would help the adolescent's relationship strengthen through more social contact and simultaneously would discourage other relationships. It would also open up possibilities for parents to encourage safer sex, however indirectly. If parents are too uncomfortable directly addressing safer sex with their children, there might be potential for grandmothers or other appropriate adults to take on such a role, as may have sometimes happened informally in Sukuma girls' dormitories in the early twentieth century (Cory, 1953; Varkevisser, 1973). Such interventions will be discussed more in the final chapter.

Stronger Premarital and Marital Relationships

Young people in this study who were in long-term monogamous partnerships typically said they experienced emotional, sexual, and material satisfaction within those relationships. Interventions could thus focus on promoting partner selectivity before relationships begin and encouraging potential partners to get to know one another better before having unprotected sex and/or marrying, to reduce the chance of dissatisfaction, conflict, and quick partner change later. Strategies to promote stronger sexual relationships both before and after marriage will be discussed more in chapter 11.

Since monogamy is most protective when it is mutual between two uninfected partners, monogamy promotion is also likely to be more effective if it targets couples as well as individuals. As noted earlier, couple-oriented interventions could promote HIV testing before having unprotected sex, as well as communication and problem-solving skills to build stronger and more enduring relationships. For example, a qualitative study of how South African couples discussed HIV testing found that concerns about existing children, or the desire to later have and raise children, provided a legitimate basis for partners to discuss HIV risk (Mindry et al., 2011).

In the HALIRA study, the main way young people attempted to reduce partners and/or to practice mutual fidelity was by marrying. There is evidence that a similarly strategic approach has been adopted in response to the AIDS epidemic in southern Africa (e.g., Reniers, 2008). In rural Mwanza, some young people—particularly young men—had extramarital sexual relationships, but overall newly married couples probably did reduce the number and frequency of their concurrent partnerships in the years immediately after marrying. This seemed to relate to both external and internal factors, including increased sexual access for new husbands, and reduced freedom of movement and dependence on transactional sex for new wives. Other studies in sub-Saharan Africa similarly have found that married young people report fewer extramarital partners than their single counterparts (Ferguson et al., 2004; Hattori and Dodoo, 2007).

The HALIRA study did not closely examine fidelity within long-term marriages, but the findings broadly suggest that extramarital sex may increase after the first few years of marriage, particularly for husbands. A survey in Mbeya, Tanzania also found that married men under thirty years of age were less likely to engage in extramarital relationships than thirty- to thirty-nine-year-old married men, who in turn were less likely to do so than married men over thirty-nine years of age (Mbago and Sichona, 2004). Thus the protective nature of marriage cannot be assumed. Interventions should explore any possible protective effects that marriage may have for young people, and ways that they can be further enhanced (e.g., mutual HIV-testing and fidelity promotion before and during marriage), but such interventions also need to be carefully evaluated to ensure that they do not have unintended consequences. The prevalent double standard for men and women's sexual activity and the relative tolerance of husbands' infidelity are of particular concern, as they may mean that unfaithful husbands dispro- portionately expose faithful wives to HIV through unprotected sex (Painter et al., 2007; Landman et al., 2008; Hageman et al., 2010).

This chapter described the HALIRA study's findings on young people who tried to limit their partner number and/or to be faithful. The next case study series and chapter will now focus on young people who tried to re- duce their sexual risk by using condoms. The final chapter will then outline broader intervention recommendations which are relevant to the promotion of all of the ABC behaviors.

NOTE

1. Specifically, on May 11, 2010, key word searches for "Africa and condom" resulted in 2,179 journal articles, compared to 544 for "Africa and ('abstain' or 'ab- stinence'; 'sexual debut,' 'sexual initiation,' or 'sexual onset')," and 330 for "Africa and ('fidelity' or 'faithful'; 'monogamy' or 'monogamous'; 'partner reduction' or 'reduce partner'; 'partner limitation' or 'limit partner'; or 'partner exclusivity' or 'sexual exclusivity')." The latter figures are actually smaller than implied, as listings for abstinence sometimes referred to alcohol use, and those for fidelity / monogamy sometimes related to religion or the natural sciences. Similar searches on search engines for other disciplines (e.g., Sociological Abstracts and Anthropology Plus) resulted in similar proportions of articles by behavior.

This case study series describes three young people who provided plausible reports of having used condoms on multiple occasions. Their stories illustrate some of the factors which promoted ongoing condom use, at least with some partners. In Lubango's case study (3.1), several factors seemed to contribute to his condom use, including a guardian's concern for his future and his own strong future aspirations; a belief that pregnancy would inhibit him from achieving those goals; and intensive training as a *MEMA kwa Vijana* peer educator. Christina's case study (3.2) also suggests that multiple factors contributed to her condom use, including a strong desire to avoid pregnancy; a confident expectation that she could control her life and her future; a strong ambition to become a successful, independent businesswoman; and her training as a *MEMA kwa Vijana* peer educator. Finally, Makoye's case study (3.3) describes an adolescent boy who had unprotected sex with multiple partners until he became infected with syphilis. Over the ensuing decade, Makoye actively tried to reduce his risk of new infection using several approaches: first by being abstinent, then by having unprotected sex with only one partner, and finally by using condoms with high-risk partners while having unprotected sex with low-risk partners.

3.1. LUBANGO: A YOUNG MAN WHO CONSISTENTLY USED CONDOMS

Lubango was twenty-two years old and a Year 7 *MEMA kwa Vijana* peer educator when a researcher met him during participant observation. Lubango explained that his father had been a soldier in the Tanzania-Uganda war in the late 1970s and had died soon after Lubango was born. His mother eventually remarried a teacher, but he also died. As a child, Lubango had moved between an uncle's household and his mother's households in different villages. He repeatedly started

Year 1 in those different settings, the final time at the age of fifteen, when he had moved to his current village with his mother and four siblings and half-siblings. Lubango's family was Sukuma and Christian.

Lubango had strong ambitions to complete primary school and to become financially secure before marrying and starting a family. He explained that some of his peers had married soon after completing school, and they had not been able to support their wives and families, which led some of the wives to become unfaithful and the marriages to break down. The researcher noted: "Lubango's uncle also advises him not to get married right after completing school, but that instead he should prepare himself well first. Lubango said that he plans to establish a tomato farm and then to use the profits as capital for a small business" (PO-01-I-1-3m).

Lubango was one of eighteen pupils in his school and 1,124 pupils across the region who had been trained to be *MEMA kwa Vijana* peer educators. In that role, Lubango said that he performed dramas and answered pupils' questions in class afterward, but he did not engage in any other peer education. He believed that the *MEMA kwa Vijana* intervention addressed common problems:

> Lubango said that most of the matters taught in the *MEMA kwa Vijana* lessons happen in the village, such as the drama about a girl who becomes pregnant and then is rejected by the young man who impregnated her. Lubango said it is true that some of the men and boys who make girls pregnant refuse responsibility, and then the girls really experience problems. (PO-01-I-1-3m)

Lubango did not believe, however, that many youths adopted the low-risk behaviors promoted by *MEMA kwa Vijana*:

> Lubango said that very few young people take their *MEMA kwa Vijana* lessons seriously. He believes most consider them to be humorous, saying that the dramas teach them how to seduce girls. Lubango said that those few who take the *MEMA kwa Vijana* class seriously find it teaches good things. . . . He said those who understand the importance of condoms do use them, but they are very few in number compared to those who don't. (PO-01-I-1-3m)

Lubango explained that he was sexually active, but that unlike most of his peers he used condoms and he avoided committed relationships. The researcher noted: "Lubango doesn't like to bring his lovers home and instead he sleeps alone. He said no one else will sleep in his bed until his wife does, after he gets married. Usually he has sex with his lovers before supper while on his evening walks, in bushes, or any place where people don't pass by" (PO-01-I-1-3m). Lubango said he always used condoms to prevent pregnancy and infection. He said that he began using them sometime after participating in the *MEMA kwa Vijana* intervention, specifying that a *MEMA kwa Vijana* trainer had taught him and other peer educators how to use them after the training course had ended. Lubango said it was easy for him to obtain condoms, because he received them for free from a friend who was a *MEMA kwa Vijana* condom distributor.

In the two *MEMA kwa Vijana* surveys that Lubango attended, he tested negative for all sexually transmitted infections measured.

3.2. CHRISTINA: A YOUNG WOMAN WHO
USED CONDOMS WITH WILLING PARTNERS

Christina was sixteen years old and a *MEMA kwa Vijana* peer educator at the beginning of Year 7 when she was randomly selected for an in-depth interview in 2000. She was reinterviewed by the same interviewer in 2002, when she was farming and managing petty businesses in her home village and regularly commuting to another village for a tailoring course. Christina then participated in a phone interview with the same interviewer in 2009, when she was living and working as a shop attendant in Dar es Salaam, Tanzania's commercial capital.

Christina's reported sexual history was not always consistent across her three interviews. This was not unusual for respondents who participated in multiple interviews, particularly when the interviews took place over many years, possibly because of limited recall and changing perceptions of what is socially appropriate. In addition, there were technical difficulties during Christina's third interview, as the telephone connection was frequently lost, disrupting the flow of the conversation, and some of the discussion was not recorded. In this analysis, when Christina's statements were unclear or inconsistent, both reports are presented below or her detailed early interview reports are taken to be more valid than her relatively vague long-term memories.

Christina's parents had divorced when she was very young, and at the time of the first interview she lived with her mother and several younger siblings and cousins in three two-roomed houses made of mud and thatch. Christina's mother, a retired nurse, was a member of local committees for a woman's association, a health and sanitation organization, and a children's rights non-governmental organization. In those positions, she sometimes earned allowances. Christina's family was Sukuma and active in the Protestant African Inland Church. However, like many villagers Christina had relatives of other faiths, including a brother who was training to be a Catholic priest, and a cousin who was Muslim.

Christina said her mother paid for her clothing and school costs, although she also drew on her own earnings to pay for them. Christina farmed her family's rice paddy and had a small plot of her own where she grew spinach, tomatoes, and onions. She occasionally sold a basin of spinach for Tshs 500 ($0.60), and she also had a small business crocheting sofa, stool, and table covers for about Tshs 1,000 ($1.20) each. In her free time, Christina liked to play checkers or other games with neighbors of varying age and sex. She reported that she was not allowed to attend discos or video shows, in the first

interview attributing this to a teacher's intervention, and in the second to judgment from her religious community:

> C: My mother refused after a teacher saw us coming from the video show one time.
> . . . Later he/she came to tell our mother, "These children of yours shouldn't be go-
> ing to video shows, they doze so much in class the next day. If they imitate what
> they see in the streets, they won't profit from it." (II-00-I-85-f)

> C: We are Christians [Laughter]. We are really Christians. Mm, we are strongly
> forbidden to go to video shows. It is also difficult to dance at the discos held at the
> end of some weddings. First of all, the shame: a child of a Christian entering a disco!
> They would talk in the church [Laughter]. You will know they are talking about you,
> so it is difficult. (II-02-I-285-f)

Christina could describe many *MEMA kwa Vijana* intervention topics. For
example: "Only by using condoms will sperm not go in the vagina. [If semen
enters it] and a man has sexually transmitted infections, the woman can also
get it" (II-00-I-85-f). However, at the time of her first interview Christina had
never seen a condom, because educational authorities did not permit it in
the peer educator training or the school program. Later in Year 7, Christina's
class visited a health facility where intervention health workers gave them a
condom demonstration. Christina explained in her second interview: "There
was a stick [Laughter], they had carved it. Now everyone was sent to put the
condom on it. They were saying, 'If you don't want to stop having sex, use a
condom, and this is how you put it on'. So, we were taught about it" (II-02-
I-285-f). Christina said she also appreciated her teacher's unusual approach
when teaching *MEMA kwa Vijana* classes, explaining: "We are beaten in other
lessons, but not during the AIDS lesson. There you are not beaten, even if you
make a mistake" (II-00-I-85-f).

During her first interview, Christina described having many friends, but particularly one close fifteen-year-old girlfriend. She said that recently that girl had
become pregnant and had dropped out of school. Christina explained:

> C: She did not tell me that she was pregnant. Now it is obvious. . . . I think she
> regrets it. She hasn't told me.

> I: What does she say when you talk with her?

> C: Mm, now to see her! It has become very difficult. She just stays at home. She
> doesn't go out. (II-00-I-85-f)

Christina believed that most girls who became pregnant out-of-wedlock had
had sex due to financial need:

> C: Most often pupils get pregnant because of money. That is what troubles them.
> A girl can be seduced by a boy who has money. You also find some have been
> given the go-ahead by their parents. Even if you are my age, some parents tell you
> to look out for yourself. When my friend [who got pregnant] was still in school, she

was paying the fees herself. One time she even paid for me when my mother was away. (II-00-I-85-f)

During her first interview, Christina reported that boys and men had tried to seduce her since she was twelve years old and in Year 3. In that interview she did not mention that she had also been sexually assaulted when she was fourteen years old, but she described such an experience in her phone interview nine years later. At the time of the assault, she had been working as a maid for people her mother knew in a nearby town, in exchange for room and board during school holidays. Christina said that one Sunday morning when no one else was at home the head of household had assaulted her:

> *C*: He tried to pull me into his room. . . . He assaulted me but he did not succeed in raping me. I mean, he only touched me. When I tried to make noise, he covered my mouth and told me to be quiet. But I was still making noise . . . so the neighbor ran inside, thinking I had been bitten by a snake. When she came in, that's when he let go of me. . . . I told that neighbor [what happened], but she refused to hear it, saying, "Don't tell his wife," and that man also told me not to tell his wife. Then he started cursing me and saying he could not have done such a thing. . . . Later his wife told me I had falsely accused her husband. . . . Even today when I think about that experience it really hurts my spirit. (II-09-I-485-f)

At the time of her first interview, Christina said that she had only had sexual intercourse once, two months earlier, with a former schoolmate who was about the same age. The young man had repeatedly given Christina Tshs 500 ($0.60) during the school year, and then he gave her Tshs 7,000 ($8.40) during the Christmas break. Christina said this boy was good-looking and seemed well-behaved, and she had a girlfriend who had strongly encouraged her to have sex with him. However, she only had sex with him after he found her alone one day and threatened her with public shaming. She described this experience as follows:

> *C*: One day I was going to his house to have my skirt tailored, because they make school uniforms at his house. My mother had sent money to his father and told me, "Now go pick up your skirt." Once I was inside the house he shut the door. He just said many things. . . . I refused to have sex, but he told me, "If you refuse, I will lock the door and go away, leaving you here. You will have to sleep right here, and then you will be beaten at home [for not coming home at night]." . . . I just decided to do it, because he was disturbing me so much. (II-00-I-85-f)

At that time of her second interview, Christina was eighteen years old and taking a tailoring course in another village. She said her mother continued to be the main household earner but Christina also had her small crocheting business and a rice paddy from which she had culled Tshs 50,000 ($60) worth of rice the last season. Christina said that she liked to stroll and talk with unmarried girlfriends in her free time. She explained, "We talk to broaden our thoughts about life issues [Laughter]. We just think to ourselves: 'Now I want to start this business, and then do something else.' We just talk about many things" (II-02-I-285-f).

During the second interview, Christina mentioned that a married teacher had asked her to have sex when she was sixteen or seventeen years old, as soon as she had completed school. Christina explained: "He wrote me a letter. . . . He wanted to seduce me, and I refused. He didn't write me again" (II-02-I-285-f). Instead, at the time of the second interview Christina said she had two ongoing sexual relationships with men with whom she used condoms. One partner was a bus driver who passed through her village on a regular basis. He lived in Mwanza City, and Christina did not know his age. That man made it possible for Christina to travel on the bus system for free, and he also frequently left Tshs 5,000 ($6), clothes, or shoes for her when he passed through her village. Christina said that they had sex in a guesthouse about once every three weeks, when she was en route to her tailoring course. This man had formally proposed marriage when Christina was in Year 7, offering her mother three cows and some money, but Christina declined. She seemed to take the suggestion lightly, commenting, "Ah, you know the Sukuma tradition. It is all about cows. I didn't want to just stop school and get married. [Laughter]. Even mother didn't want me to get married. She wanted me to attend school" (II-02-I-285-f).

The other new sexual partner Christina described during her second interview was a former schoolmate who was training to become a priest. She had sex with him for the first time two or three months before the interview, when he snuck out of the mission where he lived to meet her at a guesthouse during Christmas festivities. That young man gave Christina Tshs 5,000 ($6) for the encounter. Since then they had sent one another letters to try to arrange another sexual encounter, but they had not yet been able to meet alone.

At the time of the second interview Christina explained her perspective on her two partners in the following way:

C: I like/love the driver [Laughter]. Now, with the priest, it is just stealing. . . .

I: And does the driver know that the priest is also your lover?

C: No, he doesn't know.

I: And does the priest also know that you have another lover?

C: Mm. He doesn't even know him.

I: And does he also tell you he wants to marry you?

C: Yes, yes. Once he told me, "I want to marry you," but he was telling lies. Since when can a priest get married? I myself know that priests are not permitted to marry. (II-02-I-285-f)

During this interview Christina provided plausible and detailed accounts of consistently using condoms with both of these partners. For example, the bus driver:

C: I told him, "You should use a condom." Because the first time [we met for sex] he didn't have one, so I refused. I went away. The second time we met he had it. I just didn't want [sex without a condom], because I was a pupil. I was scared of pregnancy. And diseases. I am still afraid of it. Why should I give birth? I haven't reached the stage of giving birth.

I: And did you say you used condoms all the time, or does he sometimes come without it?

C: I mean all the time. Even he has become used to it. I can put it on to him. I have never put it on to the priest, but I have put it on to the driver. . . . I just know it well [Laughter]. You open the condom itself . . . and then here in front you squeeze it like this [gesturing]. After squeezing it then you place it on the penis and pull it down like this. (II-02-I-285-f)

In addition to wanting to prevent pregnancy, Christina said that she used condoms because she had learned from *MEMA kwa Vijana* that even a trusted, healthy-looking sexual partner could pass on HIV:

C: You could have sex with a man you trust, but he has AIDS. Now, if you were told that he has AIDS, you might say, "He has got a good [healthy] body, no, I can't believe it," and have sex with him, flesh to flesh [unprotected]. . . . But he might have it. So if you don't want to get AIDS, use condoms. (II-02-I-285-f)

Despite Christina's extraordinary confidence about condom use, she believed that buying or selling condoms was inappropriate for girls and women. When the interviewer asked the price of condoms sold by *MEMA kwa Vijana* condom distributors, she replied: "Mm, now I didn't ask that. A girl asking, that would be strange. We girls were just taught about condoms in general, we were not selling them. It was boys who used to sell them. It is the person you are having sex with who brings them along" (II-02-I-285-f).

At the time of her second interview, Christina perceived condoms as a feasible risk reduction behavior not only for herself but also for other sexually active young people, particularly if a girl insisted on it: "I think others could use condoms also. If some young man has never used a condom, he could get a girl who takes him by surprise" (II-02-I-285-f). She was less confident about the potential for unmarried young people to practice other forms of contraception, abstinence, or partner reduction. For example, contraception: "I hear that if you have never given birth you will not be given contraceptive pills at the hospital. I have never seen a person who takes them" (II-02-I-285-f). Christina was particularly doubtful about secondary abstinence:

C: It is actually difficult [to abstain]. Maybe those who . . . who have sex and then become nuns . . . maybe they stop, mm. But even some of those who are training to become nuns are still having sex. So, actually you can't tell.

I: But normally, for someone who is not a nun, do you think it is possible for him or her to stop having sex?

C: Mm. It is difficult. Maybe if he/she has been sick with an illness, just any illness [Laughter]. Maybe if he/she has been overwhelmed, can't talk, and can't do anything. (II-02-I-285-f)

It is unclear how long Christina's relationship with the priest trainee lasted, but in her third interview she said that her relationship with the bus driver had lasted two years and ended not long after the second interview. During the third interview, Christina said different men had pursued her sexually in the intervening years. She mentioned that a second man had formally proposed marriage to her while she was still living in her village. She said her aunts and brothers had strongly encouraged her to accept the man's proposal, but Christina did not feel he was financially stable, so she turned him down. Christina described having had one other sexual partner before moving to Dar es Salaam, a man attending a teacher's training college with whom she had a five-year sexual relationship:

C: It just happened that I liked/loved him. . . . We were together for a long time . . . it was very good. Every once in a while he still phones me. He tells me to go back there.

I: So will you go back?

C: Where, there? Ah, it is not easy. I may go there to visit my family, but not to live. (II-09-I-485-f)

Two years before her third interview Christina had moved to Dar es Salaam when a woman visiting her village offered her a place to stay and a job in her *vitenge* shop there. The woman initially offered to pay Christina Tshs 80,000 ($64) per month, but she never actually paid her that much, and some months she did not pay her at all. Christina sent most of the money she earned to her mother, and then after one year she moved out of the woman's house and into a rented room of her own, taking a new position working as a shop attendant for a different woman.

Of the twelve randomly selected female respondents who participated in a third in-depth interview in 2009, Christina was only one of two who did not have a child (the other respondent said she had struggled with infertility) (Wamoyi and Mshana, 2010). Christina was also the only one to have moved away from northwestern Tanzania. When asked why she had made such an unusual choice, Christina said she had a strong ambition to become an independent businesswoman and she prioritized this over marriage or having children:

C: [Some women my age in my village] already have three children. I have just decided [to do otherwise]. People in my village think I am waiting for a wealthy husband, but that is just what people say. I know my own principles. I don't need that in a person. I mean, if he were a wealthy man, then fine, that would be his luck, he should have a decent life. But even if a person is wealthy you might not be happy. . . .

I: So what are your goals?

C: My really big goal is to have a shop, my own place of business. I mean a place that is truly mine. When you are working for someone else, people disregard you. . . . I believe my field/calling is in business. And honestly I don't know if there is any man who could agree to that, so that we could be fully compatible. (II-09-I-485-f)

At the time of the third interview, Christina was finding it very difficult to achieve her goal. She explained, "I am really struggling. Life is very difficult these days. You know a lot of girls in the city have such problems. We talk about them a lot. . . . Every day in the city is expensive" (II-09-I-485-f).

Over the years Christina had also found it more difficult to consistently use condoms than she had believed in the second interview, mainly because she found it challenging to convince her partners. At the time of the third interview, for example, she was involved with a man who refused to use condoms. Since she did not want to become pregnant, she had arranged to have Depo Provera injections at a health facility instead. However, she experienced heavy bleeding for six weeks after her first injection, so she did not return for a second injection as scheduled after three months. She eventually became pregnant, but had a miscarriage. It is not clear whether Christina was using contraception at the time of that interview.

During her first interviews Christina reported that she had never had a sexually transmitted infection, and during the second one she said she did not think she would tell anyone if she did, noting, "No one has ever told me they were ill with a sexually transmitted infection [Laughter]. It would be difficult. I myself wouldn't tell my friend that I was ill with such-and-such disease, no" (II-02-I-285-f). However, in her third interview Christina reported that she had experienced symptoms of an infection when she was involved with the man from the teacher's training college:

C: My genitals itched. I went to an old woman in my village who knew traditional medicine. She boiled some medicine, two containers of five liters each. I drank that, and when I finished it I felt better. She told me if I got the sexually transmitted infection again I should go to a hospital for an injection. . . .

I: So did you also go to a hospital?

C: Yes, I went to a dispensary to get an injection. I mean, I hadn't felt the problem for a long time [after taking the traditional medicine]. I didn't know it, but it had stayed there for a long time. . . . [At the dispensary] I was given an injection and then the problem stopped. (II-09-I-485-f)

In the 2001–2002 *MEMA kwa Vijana* survey Christina tested positive for herpes, like 21 percent of the other young women in the survey (Ross et al., 2007). In addition, by the time of Christina's third interview in 2009, HIV testing services had become more common in Tanzania and she reported that she had been tested three times. She did not say if she had specifically sought out such services, or if they had been offered to her when she attended health facilities for other issues. She also did not specifically say that her HIV test results were negative, although her casual mention of the tests suggests that they were.

Several unusual factors seemed to contribute to Christina's early use of condoms, including her confidence, her ambition to become financially independent, her strong desire to avoid pregnancy, and what she had learned about sexually transmitted infections and condom use in her intensive training as a *MEMA kwa Vijana* peer educator. Her partial use of condoms may have protected her to an extent, particularly when she had a sexual relationship with a bus driver, whose lifestyle probably placed him at high risk of infection, as noted in chapter 3. However, Christina's ability to use condoms consistently and long-term ultimately depended on the cooperation of each of her individual partners, and she found this more difficult to negotiate as she got older.

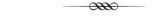

3.3. MAKOYE: A YOUNG MAN WHO USED CONDOMS WITH HIGH-RISK PARTNERS

Makoye was randomly selected for an in-depth interview in 2000, when he was eighteen years old and in Year 7 of a *MEMA kwa Vijana* intervention school. He was then reinterviewed by the same researcher in 2002 and again in 2009, when he was working in the fishing industry in a larger village.

During the first interview, Makoye lived in a compound of three mud-brick, thatch-roofed houses which he shared with his parents, seven siblings, and two others. His parents were Catholic, Zinza farmers who grew bananas, cassava, and maize. Makoye's father had a junior wife in another village who he occasionally visited; she had one child with him. After school Makoye usually carried out household tasks, such as farming the family plot or taking grain to the mill. In the evening he often sat with the men of his household around a fire after they shared a meal.

Makoye's father paid for his school fees, uniforms, and related costs. As a pupil Makoye also earned money for his clothing, soap, and entertainment in several ways. First, he could earn Tshs 500–1,000 ($0.60–$1.20) for half a day of fishing. Second, his parents gave him three chickens and one hectare of land where he grew cassava and corn for the household and cotton for his own sale. Third, he and his brother had a small candy selling business. During his free time, Makoye enjoyed playing soccer and strolling with his friends in the village center. At night he sometimes attended discos and video shows. Early in the first interview Makoye volunteered that boys tried to negotiate sex with girls at these events, using one another as intermediaries when they were young, shy, and sexually inexperienced. He explained:

> *M*: Maybe a youth is somewhat timid, thinking, "If I go there and tell her myself, she may insult me." . . . He may give you a letter to take, or he just sends you to say, "That young man likes/loves you. He wants to have a little conversation with you."
>
> *I*: Now suppose she refuses. What will you do? . . .
>
> *M*: I will tell her, "You should not refuse people. You must have a good heart." If she refuses completely then you just leave her. . . .
>
> *I*: And, if you have made the arrangements, will he pay you money?

M: No, because he is your friend, and sometime you may also send him [to negotiate on your behalf]. (II-00-I-75-m)

Makoye said that he first had sex with one of his classmates in Year 4, when he was probably fourteen or fifteen years old. He said that he did not actually want to have sex, but his older brother pressured him, selecting the girl and making the arrangements, and Makoye went along with it. Makoye met the girl at a disco, gave her Tshs 500 ($0.60), and they went to his house to have sex. He explained, "I felt shy, I had to make an effort. At the beginning, I did not feel much pleasure" (II-00-I-75-m). He said that his relationship with that girl continued over the next several years, although they had sex infrequently. When he was in Year 7 she married someone else and their relationship ended.

When Makoye was in Year 5 or 6 he also had sex with a Year 5 pupil from another village, who he met at a sports event during the December holidays. He gave her Tshs 1,000 ($1.20) and they left the event to have sex at his friend's house. Since then he had occasionally seen her at the market of a larger village, and when she asked him he had given her relatively small amounts of money, such as Tshs 200 ($0.24), but they had not had sex again.

While in Year 5 or 6 Makoye also had a onetime sexual encounter with a third primary school girl, who he met at a disco at a wedding celebration. She was visiting relatives in his village. He reported that he had gained confidence in sexual negotiation by that time, so he approached her directly. He gave her Tshs 1,000 ($1.20) and they left the disco to have sex in his room.

Sometime after the last sexual encounter described above, Makoye said he felt pain in his genitals and experienced an unusual discharge from his penis. He tolerated the symptoms for two months but then told his parents, who took him to a hospital. He was diagnosed with syphilis and treated over many hospital visits. Makoye explained that his father had been angry about the illness: "My father said, 'You must reduce your speed [frequency] of having sex.' I did decrease having sex. Since I was cured I have not had sex again" (II-00-I-75-m).

Makoye went on to say that, recently, a young woman had sent intermediaries to initiate a relationship with him, but he had declined. When the interviewer asked Makoye if he was ever tempted by sexual desire, opportunity, or the knowledge that his peers were sexually active, Makoye replied, "Right now I am not interested at all. I just remain calm, relax, and eventually [desire] disappears. I just remain alone" (II-00-I-75-m). Makoye also said he was motivated to abstain because of sexual health education he had received from *MEMA kwa Vijana*. His comments about the program will be reviewed at the end of this case study.

At the time of his second in-depth interview, Makoye was twenty years old and had spent most of the intervening two years farming rice in his home village. He had also earned money raising and selling chickens and goats. However, one month before the second interview an older cousin had recruited him to work in a job in the fishing industry, so Makoye had moved to a larger village for that. There he lived with eleven other people in the four small houses of his cousin's homestead. Makoye worked nights buying and packing Nile perch in ice, and about once per week he traveled to Mwanza City with a full boat of fish. In his first month on the job, Makoye had earned Tshs 20,000 ($24), which was as much as he had earned from his rice crop the entire year before.

During his second interview Makoye told the researcher that, despite his earlier decision to abstain, he had eventually resumed sexual activity. However, to reduce his chance of infection he tried to select a low-risk sexual partner and to be monogamous with her:

> *M*: I reduced my number of lovers. I remained with one only, because I saw those things caused me to get that disease.
>
> *I*: What led you to continue with her and not others?
>
> *M*: I decided to reject the others because they had many partners. I chose her because I trusted that she did not have many partners. I believed in her.
>
> *I*: Why do you say that you believed in her?
>
> *M*: Because after I was treated and recovered [from syphilis], I continued having sex with her and I didn't get that disease again. (II-02-I-275-m)

Although Makoye said he was trying to be monogamous, in the course of the second interview he revealed that he still occasionally had onetime, unprotected sexual encounters with girls or women he hardly knew. His most recent experience of this occurred a couple of weeks before the interview, after he had moved to his new village. That time he gave a young beer seller Tshs 2,000 ($2.40) and they had sex in his room one night.

When the researcher interviewed Makoye for a third time seven years later, Makoye's job involved buying large quantities of fish at fishing camps and islands and then transporting them by canoe and truck to factories, for which he earned about Tshs 150,000 ($120) per month. At that time Makoye had a two-year-old child by one woman and a five-month-old baby by another. He had married his second child's mother about one year earlier.

Makoye considered his fishing village and nearby fishing islands to be locations where the chance of getting a sexually transmitted infection was high, because he believed many people had unprotected sex and frequently changed partners in those places. He gave an example of how new women in the village were sought-after sexual partners:

> *M*: If a new girl or woman arrives in this village, the first thing she's told is, "Let's pass by the dock where the boys are." She'll pass there, and you, too, in order to be seen as a real man, you won't resist calling out to her. . . . Of course there will be many boys doing this, so you are just following suit. (II-09-I-475-m)

Makoye said that the men who were most successful in negotiating sex were those who offered the most money or gifts in exchange. Although Makoye earned a good living, he said he could not compete with what *dagaa* fishermen could offer women:

M: *Dagaa* fishermen have an advantage, because they can just give a woman *dagaa* for free. Of course they defeat you, the one who only offers money. . . . Because if a woman gets a sack full of *dagaa* she can sell it for Tshs 25,000 ($20), or as much as Tshs 50,000 ($40) if they are scarce. . . . Whereas I'd give her Tshs 10,000 ($8) and someone else would give her Tshs 15,000 ($12). (II-09-I-475-m)

Makoye emphasized that women also took initiative in sexual negotiation in fishing communities. For example:

M: When you go to the island, of course, women there regard you as having money. . . . They try to attract you, so that you approach them and spend your money. They may start teasing you: "You are not active [virile]." And they call, "Hey, could you please buy me some tea?" (II-09-I-475-m)

Because of his concern about sexually transmitted infections, Makoye said that he tried to be selective and only to have unprotected sex with women he considered to be low risk. He explained his strategy of recent years:

M: Once I separated from a woman, I usually did not find another one right away. I'd stay for a while, reflecting. I'd move around observing: "This one behaves in such-and-such a way. And how does that one behave?" Personally, I needed to confirm that a person did not show off [flirtatiously] like her fellows. The one who didn't is the one I'd approach. But if she started being familiar with me right away, I'd leave her too. (II-09-I-475-m)

In addition, Makoye said he used condoms with women he considered to be high risk:

M: I have used condoms with some women because I didn't trust them much. Because . . . you know, I found the ones I used to have sex with here, they had become so accustomed to this place. So I said to myself: "These people have already had a lot of experience in this place. Now I'm attracted to them, but there are others who've been attracted to them [and had sex with them] before me. I must use a condom." (II-09-I-475-m)

Makoye's description of condoms suggested he was quite familiar with them. He detailed where he bought condoms, their price, and correct condom use, including opening the package carefully so as not to tear the condom, squeezing air out of the bubble at its tip before putting it on, and using a new one for each new act of intercourse.

During that final interview Makoye described several of the sexual relationships he had had in the prior seven years. One was with the guesthouse worker:

M: We used to anchor here, so when she came over to fetch water I would see her . . . I asked a colleague to relay my message [of interest]. . . . I stayed with her for about two months and then we got into conflict. You know, when I hear my lover has other lovers, of course I won't have sex with her. . . . Maybe [I would] if she breaks up with the other lover, then we could continue together. But she did not do that, so we broke up.

I: So you heard that she had another lover?

M: I saw him with my own eyes. . . . Some days I'd go to the guesthouse but she would have an appointment with another guy in the same place. I saw her go [with another man] with my own two eyes, and I thought, "Well, everything is fine, but I just cannot pursue her any further." (II-09-I-475-m)

One partner who Makoye considered to be low risk was a Year 6 pupil with whom he had unprotected sex one time. When she became pregnant he was fearful that legal steps would be taken against him: "Her father threw her out of his house, so she went to live at my parents' home. My family told me, 'Hey, she's a pupil, so you'll be imprisoned for this'. So I left to work on an island. . . . Then [after four months] the girl went back to her parents' home" (II-09-I-475-m). Makoye was skeptical at first about whether he had made this girl pregnant, because they had only had sex one time and he thought his earlier syphilis infection had made him sterile:

M: When she told me: "You got me pregnant," at first I disagreed, thinking, "Mm . . . I suffered from that disease . . . how can I get a child?" Then I thought: "Well, let me wait for the child to be born." So when the child was born and it resembled me, I said, "Hey, nothing in me was ruined!" (II-09-I-475-m)

Makoye described another onetime sexual encounter, but because the woman was a bar maid, he used a condom:

M: Both of us started drinking beer. It was a way of seducing her. Now the good thing about taking a barmaid [for sex] is that it only lasts one day. It is not like she becomes yours [permanently]. One day and then when you go, that's it. . . .

I: How much did you pay her?

M: About Tshs 5,000 ($4) . . . and the drinks. . . .

I: And where did you have sex with her?

M: Right there, of course. It is both a bar and guesthouse. . . . First she informed me herself: "I cannot have sex without *Salama*." And I said, "That's completely fine." I mean, how I needed to hear that! I had prepared for it a long time earlier . . . the condom was just in my pocket. I wouldn't try without it—I didn't know her, I had just found her there working in a bar. (II-09-I-475-m)

Men like Makoye who wanted to use condoms generally had fewer problems negotiating them with their partners than women did, but this excerpt highlights how they also could have difficulty broaching the topic.

At the time of the third interview, Makoye was living with his twenty-year-old wife and their five-month-old baby in a rented room. He said that his wife had moved to the village to live with her sister and sell *dagaa* about a year before they became sexually involved. Makoye said he had never felt it necessary to use condoms with her because she had not been in the village for long. They had sex about once per month for five months before she became pregnant. He explained:

M: Before getting married, you know, we used to have sex secretly. Her sister didn't like me at all [Laughter]. Then I got her pregnant. Her sister threw her out using strong language, saying, "Get out, move out of my house." Then I thought, "This person might suffer a lot. Let me just be with her [marry her]". . . . Her parents agreed. How could they refuse? [Laughter] . . . We were told to pay Tshs 300,000 ($240) [in compensation to her parents]. Of course, we've only paid half of it. (II-09-I-475-m)

Makoye mentioned that he had had one other sexual partner since getting married, another woman who sold *dagaa* like his wife. He said that they had had sex on two occasions after his wife had her baby, but he ended the relationship because he did not trust that the woman would be faithful to him:

M: I used to have a girl, but then she left for the islands and I thought: "This is not worth it. I have a wife." So I abandoned it [extramarital sex] completely. . . . Now she is back and I don't care about her, so she asked me, "What has gone wrong with you?" I answered, "Now I've abandoned outside matters [extramarital sex]. I cannot trust you because you'll have sex with someone else out there, and there are so many diseases." . . . Right now I don't want to have any lovers other than my wife. (II-09-I-475-m)

During the third interview, Makoye said that *MEMA kwa Vijana* was the only sexual or reproductive health program he had experienced. He remembered the program positively, particularly the dramas and games. He further explained:

M: That was my favorite subject. . . . I learned a lot about sexually transmitted infections. And I thought: "Hey, so that is what made me ill when I had sex with that girl" . . . For instance, when they mentioned feeling pain during urination, it reminded me of the disease I'd contracted. (II-09-I-475-m)

Makoye also said that he greatly valued the *MEMA kwa Vijana* principle that, if he gave a woman a gift, he was not obliged to have sex with her. This intervention message was primarily intended to empower girls to refuse sex if they did not want it, even if they had accepted a gift, but Makoye said he reminded himself of it sometimes when he agreed to buy a drink or food for a woman who requested it, but with whom he did not want to have sex.

In each interview, Makoye demonstrated some correct information about sexual health. For example, he referred to HIV when explaining how "AIDS" was transmitted between people, something few villagers mentioned unless they had participated in the intervention. Nonetheless, Makoye also believed some false information, for instance, in his first interview he said that pregnancy could be prevented if a girl took aspirin or traditional medicines immediately after having sex, and in his second interview he said that traditional medicine could cure sexually transmitted infections if those infections had not yet spread within the body.

In all three interviews, Makoye was able to list the *MEMA kwa Vijana* behavioral goals, although his sense of which was personally most feasible and desirable changed over time. During his first interview he said he most valued and aspired to the intervention goal of abstinence, while in the second he said this for having unprotected intercourse with only one, committed, low-risk partner. In the third interview Makoye reported that the most important message he learned from *MEMA kwa Vijana* was "not to make love carelessly," which he explained meant using condoms for premarital sex and "protecting your marriage" once married. When asked what he meant by "protecting your marriage," Makoye explained it meant having unprotected sex with his wife and "not going outside of marriage for sex" (II-09-I-475-m).

Makoye attributed his active attempts to reduce his sexual health risk to his *MEMA kwa Vijana* intervention participation and his early experience of syphilis. Notably, however, he seemed most worried about sexually transmitted infections at the time of his first interview, possibly because he had only recently recovered from syphilis. Looking back on that time a decade later, Makoye reflected: "I became afraid . . . I regarded women as enemies . . . At that time, even if you had asked me to carry a message to a woman, I wouldn't do it" (II-09-I-475-m). In contrast, by Makoye's second and third interviews his concern about sexually transmitted infections seemed neither as strong nor immediate, and he was willing to knowingly take some risks. For example, when asked in the second interview if he might ever get AIDS, he replied: "I think I can get it, because I am having sex" (II-02-I-275-m).

Makoye was found negative for all sexually transmitted infections tested for males in the *MEMA kwa Vijana* surveys he attended. In the third interview he reported that he and his wife also had tested HIV-negative the year before. They had been tested separately: Makoye when he was being treated at the regional hospital for liver damage related to schistosomiasis, and his wife when she delivered her child at a private, mission hospital.

CONCLUSION

A very small number of young people in the HALIRA study were highly motivated to use condoms, but these case studies illustrate how even they had difficulty practicing consistent condom use long-term. Christina, for example, was only able to use condoms if her partners consented and actively participated in the practice. Makoye instead had more control over his condom use, but he felt he only needed to use them with women who he considered to be high risk, and his ability to assess someone else's risk was inevitably limited. The next chapter will describe and discuss these and other broad findings related to condom use within the HALIRA study.

Chapter Ten

Condom Use

Male condoms are very effective in preventing both pregnancy and sexually transmitted infection if used during sexual intercourse (Davis and Weller, 1999). While this practice sounds straightforward, using condoms correctly and consistently over time requires becoming familiar with a new technology and having ongoing access to it, as well as intention and discipline on behalf of one or both sexual partners, and the man's active participation. Thus, like "being faithful," the "condom use" goal of the widely promoted ABC behaviors is more complex than it immediately appears.

Until recently, research on condom use in sub-Saharan Africa has mainly involved asking survey respondents simple questions, like if they have ever used a condom, or if they used a condom at last intercourse. Both of these experiences are fairly easy for respondents to recall accurately. Use of a condom at some point in the past is a salient experience, and use of a condom at last sex usually involves remembering a recent experience, which can be easier to recall than specific sexual encounters in the distant past. The question about condom use ever can provide useful insights into general condom knowledge, attitudes, and access, but it does not reveal much about whether a person actively practices low-risk behaviors in an ongoing way, because someone might have only used a condom once out of hundreds of sexual encounters. The question about condom use at last sex is often taken to be more representative of a person's typical behavior, in the assumption that most people's last sexual encounters will not have been particularly unusual or special (Cleland and Ali, 2006). Nonetheless, this variable also only crudely indicates the frequency of a person's condom use.

In survey research examining these questions, reported condom use has been associated with: relatively high education level; not being married; sex with a new and/or casual partner; positive attitudes toward condoms;

337

perception of a pregnancy as problematic; perceived risk of HIV infection; belief in one's own ability to negotiate and use condoms; and communication with a partner about risk (e.g., Adetunji, 2000; Prata et al., 2006; Maharaj, 2006; Hendrikson et al., 2007; Bogale, Boer, and Seydel, 2010). Survey questions on experience of condom use ever, or at last sex, have also provided insight into intervention impact on condom use. For example, a review of sixty-two condom promotion evaluations in Asian and African countries found some positive intervention impact on reported condom use, especially among commercial sex workers and their clients (Foss et al., 2007). Of fourteen interventions which targeted young people, eight found small but statistically significant increases in reported condom use at last intercourse. Generally, however, reported condom use has not been very high in sub-Saharan Africa, even in casual relationships and even after condom promotion interventions (e.g., Lagarde et al., 2001; Cleland and Ali, 2006; Wellings et al., 2006; Foss et al., 2007; Rutherford, 2008; Papo et al., 2011). The review mentioned above found that, after an intervention, condom use was particularly low in primary partnerships, unless one partner was known to be HIV-positive (Foss et al., 2007).

Increasingly researchers have attempted to collect more complex and nuanced data about condom use, such as the factors associated with the intention to use condoms, differences between consistent and inconsistent condom users, and the circumstances in which people do or do not use condoms (e.g., Katz, 2006; Sayles et al., 2006; Tassiopoulos et al., 2006; Bankole, Ahmed et al., 2007; MacPhail et al., 2007). Studies have generally found consistent condom use to be rare in sub-Saharan Africa. For example, a study with 252 men working in the informal sector in Kenya found 39 percent had had multiple partners in the last year, but only 3 percent used condoms consistently with all of them (Ferguson et al., 2004). Similarly, a study with 194 participants in rural Uganda found that 48 percent had used condoms at least once, but only 7 percent currently used condoms regularly. In a third study involving 120 rural adolescent boys in Nigeria, Izugbara and Modo (2007) found that awareness of condoms was high, and 21 percent of respondents who reported more than one current sexual partner said they had used condoms the last time they had sex, but only 4 percent reported consistent condom use with all of their partners.

A comparative study of adolescents in Burkina Faso, Ghana, Malawi, and Uganda found that consistent condom use was associated with a small age difference between partners, not having multiple partners, urban residence, being in school, having a higher education level, and exposure to mass media (Bankole, Ahmed et al., 2007). Research with young men in Nigeria instead found that consistent condom use was associated with having two or more partners, as well as always purchasing condoms, rather than sometimes receiving them for free (Sunmola, Adebayo, and Ogungbemi, 2008). Studies in rural South Africa further found that young people's consistent condom use was associated with having just one partner, little relationship conflict, and higher gender equity in relationships (Hoffman et al., 2006; Shai et al., 2010).

As discussed in chapter 1, it is difficult to know how valid such findings are given that condom use, like abstinence and being faithful, may be overreported due to social desirability bias, particularly in areas where respondents have been exposed to public health interventions which promote condoms (Goodrich, Wellings, and McVey, 1998; Geary et al., 2003). For example, in in-depth interviews with forty-seven rural South African eighteen- to twenty-four-year-olds, Harrison and O'Sullivan (2010) found that one-quarter to one-half of men and women initially reported consistent condom use, but many of those respondents later acknowledged that condom use with their primary partner was inconsistent.

At the beginning of the *MEMA kwa Vijana* trial in 1998, when participants were fifteen years old on average, 2 percent of all participants and 5 percent of those who reported sexual experience said that they had used condoms (Todd et al., 2004). As described in chapter 7, at the end of the trial, of those participants who reported having had sex, a significantly higher proportion of male intervention participants (39 percent) than control participants (28 percent) said they had initiated condom use during the trial, as did a significantly higher proportion of female intervention participants (38 percent) than control participants (28 percent) (Ross et al., 2007).

The next section describes the motivations and experiences of young people who gave plausible and consistent reports of condom use during HALIRA qualitative research. It first describes findings on the proportion of young people who had used condoms, and then broad differences between individuals who used condoms a few times and those who had used them on many occasions. Differences between young people who used condoms primarily for pregnancy prevention and those who used them primarily for protection against infection will also be described. The chapter will end with a discussion of ways to improve condom promotion with adults and young people in rural Africa; that topic will then be further examined in chapter 11.

FINDINGS

Prevalence and Consistency of Condom Use

By the end of the *MEMA kwa Vijana* trial, intervention participants had a better understanding of condom use and its protective value than control participants, and they were also more likely to have seen a condom, as described in chapters 5, 6, and 7. Both the quantitative and qualitative interviews further found that intervention participants were more likely to report condom use (e.g., table 7.1). For example, of the thirty-three randomly selected intervention participants who participated in a second in-depth interview at the end of the trial, twenty-three reported sexual experience; of those, thirteen (seven male, six female) said they had used a condom at least once. In contrast, of the thirty randomly selected control participants in that interview series, twenty-five reported sexual experience, but only three of the males in that group said they had ever used a condom.

Participant observation findings suggest that a smaller proportion of trial participants used condoms than reported it in formal in-depth interviews or survey questionnaires during the trial. Participant observation research found that very few sexually active villagers had tried using condoms by their late teens—including intervention participants—suggesting that condom use was overreported in formal interviews. This may even have been the case in surveys in control communities, where young people may have known from radio programs, health facility posters, and other sources that condoms were promoted for public health purposes.

In addition, overall the qualitative research suggests that most youth who had tried condoms had only used them for a relatively small proportion of their sexual encounters. For example, many intervention participants in the second in-depth interview series gave plausible accounts of having used a condom once, but only four reported having used condoms many times, and none reported having used condoms every time they had had sex. In the entire HALIRA study there were very few people who plausibly and consistently reported having always used condoms, with the exception of a small number of people who had only had sex a few times. It was also very rare for someone to report consistently using condoms with all current partners, as seen in case study 3.1.

Factors Contributing to Condom Use

The HALIRA study found that several factors influenced sexually active young people to use condoms, including a desire or willingness to prevent pregnancy; experience of negative consequences of unprotected intercourse for oneself or someone close; *MEMA kwa Vijana* intervention experience (particularly for those who received intensive training as peer educators or condom distributors); ambitions other than farming and marriage; planning and obtaining condoms in advance of sexual encounters (almost always the male); and a partner's insistence. Notably, a few intervention participants reported it had been fairly straightforward for them to negotiate condom use with a particular partner, because they had both participated in the intervention. For example, a fifteen-year-old girl in Year 5 explained that she and her boyfriend of two months, a boy in Year 6, used condoms:

> She said their teacher taught them that condoms prevent sexually transmitted infections, AIDS, and pregnancy. She mentioned that Year 5, 6, and 7 pupils went to the local dispensary for a demonstration of how condoms are used. . . . She said her boyfriend gets free condoms from the dispensary and uses them with her to prevent pregnancy. . . . She explained the first time they had sex, he just came with one without asking her permission to use it. (PO-99-I-1-2f)

Young women who initiated condom use were unusually confident and assertive, and also were prepared to end a sexual encounter rather than have unprotected intercourse. Even if a young man did not initiate condom use, his consent and active participation was essential in using them. In contrast, some young women reported being uncertain of whether a partner had used condoms during intercourse, or said they passively allowed a partner to do so even if they disliked the idea.

Many adolescents and young adults had more than one of these factors influencing their lives but never used condoms. However, most young people who tried to used condoms once or twice, and especially those who used them many times over an extended period, were strongly influenced by several of these factors in combination.

Using Condoms to Prevent Pregnancy

In both participant observation and in-depth interviews, almost all of the adolescent girls who said they had initiated condom use had participated in the *MEMA kwa Vijana* intervention (particularly peer educators), did not want to contract a sexually transmitted infection, and also were determined to avoid pregnancy while still in school. Girls who were considered "hard-to-get" and who insisted upon condom use seemed to be most successful in negotiating it. For example, the former peer educator in case study 3.2 describes ending a first sexual encounter with a man prior to intercourse specifically because he did not have a condom, which ensured that he brought one the next time they met for sex.

In another example, a nineteen-year-old girl (Adija) in Form 3 (Year 10) reported that she had had three sexual partners and she had used condoms with each of them. This included a villager with whom she had a sexual relationship for one year in primary school, a secondary school student with whom she had a one to two year relationship in secondary school, and a farmer with whom she had a onetime sexual encounter during that same period. She explained:

> *R*: You just tell him that he should use a condom to prevent pregnancy. If you tell him something like that, he will do it. . . .
>
> *I*: Did you use a condom every time that you had sex with your first partner?
>
> *R*: Sometimes we used condoms, sometimes not. I mean, we did not use them when he did not bring them. He would tell me, "Today I couldn't get them at all. I have tried but I haven't got them." He used to get them from the dispensary and from small shops. . . .
>
> *I*: And with your second partner?
>
> *R*: Yes, sometimes we used them and sometimes not, if he did not get them. . . .
>
> *I*: And how about the one with whom you had sex only once?
>
> *R*: Even him, I just told him, "You must use it." Then he agreed. . . .
>
> *I*: And have you ever gone to buy a condom yourself?
>
> *R*: No.
>
> *I*: But do you think that you could go look for them?
>
> *R*: [Long pause] . . . I could go look for them, but where I would find them, I don't know. . . . I have never tried to get them before. (II-02-I-287-f)

Adija tested negative for all sexually transmitted infections measured in the three *MEMA kwa Vijana* surveys she attended. Like Adija, other girls who initiated condom use almost always relied on their partners to obtain the condoms, because they felt it was inappropriate or potentially embarrassing to get them themselves. Such girls tended to be less adamant about using condoms over time if their partners did not bring them reliably.

Several male informants also reported that they had used condoms in isolated instances because a school girl insisted that they do so to prevent pregnancy. For example, a twenty-two-year-old farmer:

> . . . said that he has used condoms only once. . . . He had had no intention of using a condom, except that his lover [a pupil] told him to use it. . . . He said that the pleasure was just the same as when he is not wearing them, except for the inconvenience of putting on the condom, which delayed him starting sex. (PO-01-I-1-3m)

As discussed in chapter 3, in their first years of marriage young couples rarely actively attempted to prevent pregnancy. When they did, this usually took place after a couple had already had one or two children, when women sometimes used oral or injectable hormonal contraceptives. Only two of the randomly selected women who were married during the second in-depth interview series reported having occasionally used condoms for contraception with their husbands, and one of those was married to a *MEMA kwa Vijana* condom distributor. Similarly, when a former peer educator was asked if he used condoms with his wife, he replied, "Now why would I use condoms with my wife? I want us to have children" (II-02-I-317-m). That young man tested negative for all infections measured for male participants in the trial surveys.

Using Condoms to Prevent Sexually Transmitted Infection

Most of the young men who reported initiating condom use to avoid infection were in their twenties and thus were too old to have participated in the *MEMA kwa Vijana* intervention at the time of the HALIRA study. However, they had learned about condoms from their peers, the radio, or information acquired when traveling to larger villages and towns where some HIV prevention programs targeted high-risk settings, such as bars and guesthouses. Often these young men had work and an income that facilitated multiple partnerships, such as shopkeepers, bicycle taxi drivers, and fishermen.

These young men usually said they used condoms with new sexual partners who they perceived to be high risk, such as bar maids, guesthouse workers, or local women with reputations for being promiscuous. They almost invariably also said they did not use condoms with their wives or steady partners. A male researcher documented one example from a conversation at a blacksmiths' workshop:

> A blacksmith who was holding a piece of iron in his hands told another youth that the iron looked like a circumcised penis. He commented that it is better to have a circumcised penis during sex than an uncircumcised one, especially when wearing a condom. I asked him if people in the village use condoms when having sex. He said there are a few villagers who use them and that he also uses them, particularly when having sex with women other than his wife. He said that there is no difference in pleasure when having sex using a condom. Some of the other smiths who were present disagreed with him while others supported him. (PO-01-I-1-3m)

Although villagers often broadly associated AIDS with people in towns and cities, they rarely were concerned that specific urban visitors might pose a higher risk of infection than local people. To the contrary, as discussed in chapters 3 and 7, young male and female visitors to villages often were much sought after as sexual partners, including those who came from urban areas.

Occasionally, however, young men reported initiating condom use to be more careful with an urban visitor. A participant observation researcher recorded the following example:

> [A twenty-seven-year-old man] told me that there are two girls who have come to the village to be cured of an unspecified disease by the traditional healer. He said that he and another villager talked to the girls and they had agreed to have sex. . . . When they later met to have sex he said he put on a condom, but after the girl saw this she said she would not have sex with him if he wore a condom. . . . After a long argument, she finally agreed . . . but while they were having sex, she attempted to take the condom off. He said . . . they had a big quarrel and he chased her away. (PO-99-C-2-1m)

Sometimes young men said that they used condoms with a particular partner specifically because they had heard or believed she might have a sexually transmitted infection. For example, a nineteen-year-old farmer (Athumani) explained that he had not used condoms with his first five sexual partners, but he had used them during the several encounters he had had with his most recent partner, a woman who sold peanuts at the market:

> *I*: Why do you use condoms with her?
>
> *R*: Because I don't trust her. . . . Perhaps she has a sexually transmitted infection. . . .
>
> *I*: But why do you use condoms with her, when you didn't with your earlier partners?
>
> *R*: I don't trust her . . . and also I did not understand how to use them earlier.
>
> *I*: Who taught you how to use them?
>
> *R*: When I went to [a certain shop], the youth there taught me. (II-02-I-241-m)

Athumani said that he had learned that condoms protect against sexually transmitted infections in his *MEMA kwa Vijana* lessons, but he had not understood how to use them until the shopkeeper taught him. He participated in all three *MEMA kwa Vijana* surveys and tested negative for sexually transmitted infections in each of them.

Importantly, men's assessments of new partners as high risk were quite subjective and open to change. For example, some men initially considered certain sexual partners to be high risk because of how they met or where the women worked. However, if a man developed a liking for such a woman over a few sexual encounters and was open to an ongoing relationship with her, he typically decided the woman was no longer high risk, so condom use was no longer necessary.

Despite taking initiative to reduce their risk of infection, young men who used condoms often still had misconceptions about them. In one example, a twenty-four-year-old man (Edward) from a control community believed a widespread myth that condoms have minute holes which allow the transmission of sexually transmitted infections. Edward reported that he had had six sexual partners, including a regular partner over a three year period, but he believed that he had been infected with syphilis on the only two occasions when he had used condoms. Edward explained:

> *R*: I used condoms with one who was not trustworthy, with that girl who was new to my village.

> *I*: And you feel that she infected you, even though you used condoms?

> *R*: Yes, because I heard that inside the condoms there are some holes, small holes. . . . A doctor examined me last year. He said, "You have syphilis." He started treating me. . . . I know she is the one [who infected me]. I had sex with other girls, but they are all still fine. They don't have any problems. (II-02-C-276-m)

Edward had tested negative for sexually transmitted infections in the first *MEMA kwa Vijana* survey and he did not participate in any later surveys, so no subsequent trial biological data were available for him. Unlike Edward, some young men who personally experienced a sexually transmitted infection were motivated to use condoms afterward, as seen in case study 3.3.

In this study, few data were collected directly from female bar workers and guesthouse workers. However, several men reported that such women had initiated condom use with them in the past, suggesting that HIV prevention interventions which targeted bars and guesthouses had had some impact.

Pleasure, Trust, and the Discontinuation of Condom Use

As noted earlier, the HALIRA study found that most young people who had used condoms had only used them once or a few times out of multiple sexual encounters. Typically they used condoms during their first one or two sexual encounters with a new partner, but condoms were abandoned if the relationship continued beyond that point. Condoms usually were no longer used at that stage because the man found them unsatisfying, neither partner wanted to prevent pregnancy (whether they actively sought pregnancy or not), and the partners trusted one another.

Many young men stopped using condoms because they felt it was not as pleasurable as unprotected intercourse. Specifically, they said that using condoms negatively delayed the onset of intercourse, changed friction, reduced sensation, and (most commonly) delayed ejaculation. As noted in chapter

3, achievement of multiple ejaculations within one sexual rendezvous was generally considered ideal for young men in the study area, both maximizing their pleasure and demonstrating their prowess. Men may thus have viewed prolonged intercourse with a condom negatively, because they believed it reduced the number of times they ejaculated during one sexual rendezvous.

However, a couple's trust in one another often was also an important issue in their decision to stop using condoms. Trust in this instance meant the partners had become more familiar with each other, each had stated or implied that they would not have other partners, they did not see any evidence of ill health, and they were open to the possibility of pregnancy and the more serious, long-term relationship that might result from it.

For example, a twenty-year-old man (Sababu) said that he had had many sexual partners and he had used condoms with most of them, if condoms were available and his partners did not refuse to use them. However, Sababu explained that he and his current partner had stopped using condoms after their first sexual encounter because of their commitment to each other:

R: On the first day [we had sex], I used condoms, but the second time I didn't, and not the third time either. . . . Because, you see, I informed her, "I am going to marry you." . . . Since we had already agreed that I was going to marry her, why would I use them? (II-02-I-316-m)

Sababu tested negative for all infections measured in early *MEMA kwa Vijana* surveys, but he tested positive for HIV in the 2001–2002 survey.

When a person insisted on continuing to use condoms in an extended premarital relationship, his partner sometimes resented it, believing that he was being distrustful or disrespectful, and that he was not interested in a more committed relationship. For example, a seventeen-year-old woman who had recently completed Year 7 in a *MEMA kwa Vijana* control school complained that her former lover of many months, a twenty-two-year-old Year 7 pupil, had used condoms with her:

She said the reason she broke up with him is that he got another girlfriend, and he stopped giving her money for expenses. Also, she said, "He used to have sex with me while wearing a condom. He didn't want me to have a child with him, or maybe he didn't trust me and thought that I had diseases." She said that he also used to have sex with [another Year 7 pupil] but they also broke up, and even that girl still complains that he used to wear a condom while having sex with her, because it meant he didn't want to have a baby with her. (PO-02-C-2-5f)

Young people were often concerned about a current partner's fidelity and trust, but rarely were concerned that a partner who appeared healthy and faithful could infect them with an infection contracted in a prior relationship. For example, an eighteen-year-old *MEMA kwa Vijana* intervention participant (Mhoja) said she used condoms to prevent pregnancy and infection the three times she had sex with her first sexual partner, a fellow pupil in an intervention school. However, once she left school she did not use condoms with her second partner, because she perceived herself and that relationship differently:

> *R*: They taught us about protection against diseases at the hospital. . . . All of us pupils in Years 5–7 went there one time. We were given condoms. . . . Later I told [my first partner] we should use condoms to protect ourselves against diseases.
>
> *I*: What did he say?
>
> *R*: He agreed. . . .
>
> *I*: So why are you not using them nowadays?
>
> *R*: [Long pause] . . . Perhaps because at that time I was still a pupil. Or I finished school, but I was waiting for my examination results so I still considered myself to be a pupil. . . . Now I have finished school, and that second man . . . we just trust each other. (II-02-I-294-f)

During a *MEMA kwa Vijana* survey two months before the interview above, Mhoja was one of 27 percent of female participants who tested positive for the sexually transmitted infection trichomonas (Ross et al., 2007).

Another example of an unmarried couple no longer using condoms because they trusted one another was provided by a twenty-one-year-old man (Fikiri) who had been a *MEMA kwa Vijana* peer educator when he was eighteen years old and in Year 7 at an intervention school. After Fikiri left school, he moved to urban Mwanza to work in a fish factory for one year before moving to a different village to work in a gold mine for two years. When Fikiri was interviewed at that time, he reported he had had a total of six sexual partners, and he had sometimes used condoms with the last three of them—a market worker, a beer seller, and a farmer:

> *I*: Do young men who use condoms use them every time they have sex, or just occasionally?
>
> *R*: It depends on whether you trust your lover. If you don't, then you decide to use protection. But if you trust her then you can't use protection. . . .
>
> *I*: And have you ever made a girl pregnant?
>
> *R*: I have. My girlfriend [of six to seven months] is pregnant. She will deliver in two months. I only used condoms with her at the beginning [of the relationship]. (II-02-I-243-m)

Fikiri tested negative for sexually transmitted infections in the first *MEMA kwa Vijana* survey that took place while he was still in school. He did not participate in any later surveys, so no subsequent biological data were available for him.

As noted earlier, very few young married couples ever reported using condoms because few wanted to prevent pregnancy. In addition, however, the widespread association of condom use with mistrust, infidelity, and lack of commitment made it unacceptable for many married individuals. For example, a randomly selected, twenty-one-year-old in-depth interview respondent, Restuta, explained that she had learned about condoms when she saw a male peer educator do a condom demonstration at her school, and she subsequently used condoms with her second sexual partner, with whom she had sex two times. However, she said had never used condoms with her husband, who was her third partner and with whom she had a one-year-old child. Restuta explained:

I: And how did you and your [second] lover come to an agreement to use a condom?

R: [Laughter]. We just agreed with each other.

I: Who started by saying, "Shall we use a condom?"

R: It was me. . . .

I: And did you use a condom the last time you had sex?

R: No. . . . You mean the last time I had sex with my husband?

I: Yes.

R: So long as he is my husband, we don't use condoms. . . . We have not planned to use condoms, or even talked about it. . . . If I have sex outside [of marriage] without using a condom, I can get AIDS.

I: Mm, but now that you are only with your husband?

R: I cannot. (II-02-I-334-f)

Six months before the interview above, Restuta had participated in the 2001–2002 *MEMA kwa Vijana* trial survey. At that time she tested positive for herpes and trichomonas, like 21 percent and 27 percent of all female participants, respectively (Ross et al., 2007).

Similarly, another young mother explained that she would not mind if her husband used condoms in an extramarital sexual relationship, but it would be unacceptable for him to use them with her:

I: If you agreed to have sex with a man but he wants to use condoms, what would you think of him?

R: I would think that he may not be safe. Yes, and maybe that he doesn't trust me. . . . I wouldn't feel good, because perhaps he doesn't trust me, that I'm safe.

I: Do you think you might ever use condoms with your husband?

R: No . . . to use condoms with my husband?! Maybe if he goes out—if he wants to go [have sex] with someone else out there besides me, let him use condoms. But he can't use condoms with me, no.

I: So does your husband go out?

R: He goes out, yes.

I: And how do you feel when you learn that he has gone out?

R: Me? [Laughter]. I just feel fine, because that is normal. [Laughter]. That is normal. (II-02-I-331-f)

This young woman tested negative for all infections measured for females in the three trial surveys.

DISCUSSION

The HALIRA study's findings on condom use were not very promising. Few sexually active young people in rural Mwanza had ever used a condom, and those who had typically had only used them once or a few times. Frequent condom use was rare, and consistent condom use with all partners was very rare. Even in the best case scenario—when a couple was motivated to use condoms at the beginning of a sexual relationship—condoms were usually abandoned after a few sexual encounters.

The vast majority of adults in rural Mwanza had misconceptions and negative attitudes toward condoms, and in such a context it is unlikely that an intervention that promotes condoms for sexually active adolescents will succeed. Indeed, while most *MEMA kwa Vijana* intervention participants came to perceive condom use in a neutral or positive light, their parents, neighbors, out-of-school peers, and sexual partners often continued to perceive condoms with hostility and suspicion, undermining any potential for intervention participants to adopt condom use. This was particularly a concern for school girls whose out-of-school sexual partners were five to ten years older than them, which was not uncommon.

The discussion below considers the implications of these findings for general condom promotion in rural Africa before specifically focusing on condom promotion with adolescents.

General Condom Promotion in Rural Africa

Twenty years into the AIDS epidemic in sub-Saharan Africa, the HALIRA study found condom promotion in Mwanza villages to be extremely limited, mainly consisting of general radio campaigns and isolated, vague posters where condoms were available at hospitals and kiosks. More recent research suggests this situation has only marginally improved in the last decade, and conditions are similar in many other parts of rural sub-Saharan Africa today (TACAIDS, 2008; Remes et al., 2010; Seidenfeld, 2010).

To increase condom uptake in rural areas, a first, fundamental step is thus simply to implement existing "best practice" condom promotion and distribution campaigns, similar to multi-faceted, intensive, and culturally-specific social marketing programs which have been employed in some other parts of Africa, particularly in urban areas (e.g., Meekers, Agha, and Klein, 2005; Taylor et al., 2010). Ideally such efforts would address condom use in its complexity, not only by increasing access and teaching the technically correct way to use condoms during intercourse, but also by addressing more complicated and subtle issues, such as those relating to culture, pleasure, risk perception, trust, contraception, fertility, negotiation, and consistency of use. Each of these issues will be discussed more below.

Balancing Male Pleasure and Risk

Villagers' negative comments about condoms often focused on the strong belief that condoms reduce physical sensitivity and pleasure, particularly for men. Some of the other reported concerns about condoms (e.g., that they might be contaminated, old, ineffective, or prohibited) may have been secondary rationalizations fueled by this fundamental male concern. Many rural men expressed this concern about condoms whether they had used condoms or not. However, men who had used condoms varied in the extent to which they felt condom use affected their sexual pleasure, ranging from those who said it did not, to those who said it did but they were willing to tolerate it to avoid infection (at least with certain partners), to those who said it reduced their pleasure to an unacceptable degree. In addition, as noted in chapter 3, a small minority of villagers reported that blocking a man's semen from entering a woman during intercourse was unnatural and dissatisfying, because semen was believed to enhance a woman's beauty and health, and/or it symbolized the man's sexual conquest of her, however temporary. Other studies in eastern and southern Africa have also found people may be opposed to condoms because they block the natural exchange of body fluids (Taylor, 1990; Collins and Stadler, 2000; Coast, 2007; Stadler and Saethre, 2011).

Condoms do change physical sensation during intercourse, and they do prevent the exchange of fluids which some people believe to be natural, healthy, and satisfying. If local people's values run counter to a particular element of an intervention, it is critical for intervention implementers to candidly acknowledge and engage with participants about those issues. Such a forthright approach will help gain participants' trust and confidence (Undie, Crichton, and Zulu, 2007). At a minimum, sexual health interventions with adult villagers could engage with this by explaining correct condom use in detail, ways to eroticize it, and how pleasure may increase with experience, even if such material is considered too controversial for adolescent interventions (Philpott, Knerr, and Boydell, 2006; Joshi, 2010).

Acknowledging possibly negative short-term consequences of condom use must be accompanied by in-depth and realistic evaluation of the potential long-term consequences of unprotected sex. In this study, young people and adults typically had very poor understandings of infectious disease transmission, often falsely believing, for example, that a healthy-appearing person could not infect others with HIV or other sexually transmitted diseases. In contrast, young men who were motivated to use condoms often had an unusually good understanding of their risk of sexually transmitted infection, either from prior experience of infection or intensive intervention participation. This highlights the importance of interventions targeting men's understanding of disease transmission, their perception of personal risk, and their desire for self-preservation, since men largely control condom use and may be most likely to use condoms when they have a heightened understanding of their own risk (Prata et al., 2006). Women ideally should have an equal role in deciding to use condoms within sexual relationships, and it is important to empower girls and women and to promote their ability to negotiate condom use, as will be discussed more below. Nonetheless, findings in this study and elsewhere in sub-Saharan Africa indicate it is overwhelmingly men who determine whether condoms are used within relationships, so the most successful condom promotion efforts will likely be those which convince men it is in their own best interest to use them.

A recent campaign in eastern and southern Africa provides one example of an intervention focusing on improved personal risk assessment. That intervention used mass media to profile appealing young men and women who were attractive, trustworthy, and responsible, but who were revealed at the end of the advertisement to be HIV-positive (Hattori, Richter, and Greene,

2008). The campaign resulted in a positive trend in reported condom use with regular partners for youth in Mozambique and young women in Zambia.

Addressing the Issue of Trust

Young people in this study often associated condoms negatively with sexually transmitted infections, so that suggesting condom use raised questions about disease and fidelity, either one's own or one's partner's. Similar strong negative associations have been found elsewhere in sub-Saharan Africa (e.g., Campbell, 2003; Montgomery et al., 2008; Collins and Stadler, 2000; Shai et al., 2010; Stadler and Saethre, 2011). As Tavory and Swidler (2009, 171) comment based on their research in rural Malawi, "Condom use signifies a risky, less serious, and less intimate partner. Even when people believe that condom use is appropriate, wise, or even a matter of life and death, the statement that condom use makes about a relationship usually trumps all other meanings."

In rural Mwanza, the association of condoms with mistrust not only inhibited people from initiating condom use, it also affected their ability to continue using condoms once initiated. One of the most common patterns was for a couple to use condoms during their first few encounters and then to abandon them if their sexual relationship continued. Sometimes this decision was based on a dislike of the physical experience, or the belief that a partner's apparent good health proved condoms were not necessary, as previously discussed. In addition, however, condoms typically were abandoned at that stage of a relationship as a way to reduce tension and distrust and to demonstrate interest and possible long-term commitment to a partner. Some individuals—particularly young women—specifically perceived pregnancy prevention in a premarital relationship as devaluing the relationship, because it eliminated the possibility of a long-term, serious relationship that could result from pregnancy.

Condom promotion campaigns may be more successful if they directly engage with and challenge this perceived association between condoms and mistrust. The issues of trust and respect can be re-framed by arguing that individuals who suggest condom use are demonstrating their caring and valuing of a partner, specifically because they are trying to protect and promote the partner's health and future fertility, an issue that will be discussed more in the next section. This could be represented as an issue of esteem and respect for one's self as well as one's partner. For example, just as no self-respecting girl in rural Mwanza would have sex without receiving something in exchange for it, no self-respecting girl should have sex with a partner who does not want to protect her health and fertility.

Pregnancy Prevention and Fertility Promotion

The small minority of young women in this study who initiated condom use almost always told their partners that they were afraid of getting pregnant. Even when they equally feared infection, they usually did not mention this to avoid offending their partner. Research elsewhere in sub-Saharan Africa similarly suggests that people may be more willing to use condoms when condoms are promoted for contraception rather than infection prevention (Cleland and Ali, 2006). Campaigns to promote condoms for contraception could also highlight the advantages of condoms relative to other contraceptive methods. In rural Mwanza and elsewhere in sub-Saharan Africa, for example, young women were often wary of the possible side effects of hormonal contraception, such as weight change, irregular menstrual bleeding, or delayed return to fertility once an injectable contraceptive is discontinued (e.g., Rutenberg and Watkins, 1997; Allen, 2002; Castle, 2003; Wood and Jewkes, 2006; Williamson et al., 2009). This suggests that condoms could be positively promoted as a contraceptive method that does not have such side effects.

In addition to promoting condoms as a short-term contraceptive, programs may be more effective if they highlight the long-term benefit condoms can have in protecting lifetime fertility. Such a campaign would need to clearly explain the diversity and prevalence of sexually transmitted infections, and that some infections may have no overt symptoms but nonetheless cause internal damage that reduces later fertility (Cleland and Ali, 2006; Pellati et al., 2008). In the HALIRA study, rural men typically aspired to have many children in their lifetimes, so the potential impact of infections on male fertility should be emphasized, in keeping with the broader promotion of condoms by appealing to men's self-preservation and masculinity (Pellati et al., 2008). However, the promotion of condoms as fertility protectors may be most important with young women, as the study found many single young women were not concerned about sexually transmitted infections per se, but they strongly wished to prevent pregnancy in the short-term and to have many children in the long-term.

Consistency and Selectivity of Condom Use

Of the small minority of young people in this study who had used condoms, very few had used them many times or consistently over an extended period of time, even after intervention participation. Clearly programs must not only help young people initiate condom use within a relationship, but also help them understand the importance of consistently using condoms over time. Most villagers in rural Mwanza had very little formal education, and in such settings it is critical for interventions to devote sufficient time to teaching basic, relevant biological and mathematical concepts, without which people cannot fully understand how harmful infections may have no overt symptoms for long periods, how diseases spread within sexual networks, and how condoms' protective potential directly relates to the consistency of their use.

In addition, one of the most commonly reported patterns in this study was for young men to only use condoms with women who they considered to be high risk, such as guesthouse workers or bar staff, but not with their wives or main partners. Such selective condom use relies on subjective judgment about other people's risk and may create a false sense of safety. Nonetheless, using condoms with partners who are perceived to be high risk is more protective than not using condoms at all, and some individuals may indeed make reasonable guesses about other people's risk of infection. Moreover, selective condom use with partners suspected of being high risk may be a much more feasible goal than consistent condom use with all partners. In contexts where pregnancy prevention is rare within regular partnerships, and occasional sex with other partners is common, consistent condom use with non-regular partners may be one of the most realistic ways for individuals to substantially reduce risk to themselves and their partners. Research elsewhere in sub-Saharan Africa has also found that condoms are most often used with non-regular partners or those perceived to be high risk (e.g., Adetunji, 2000; Tassiopoulos et al., 2006; Hendriksen et al., 2007; Wechsberg et al., 2010). Importantly, however, programs promoting condom use with non-regular partners still need to emphasize the importance of consistency of use with those partners, as in this study even in such relationships condoms often were abandoned after the first few sexual encounters.

Condom Promotion with Adolescents

Many adults in sub-Saharan Africa recognize that young people face serious risks when they have unprotected sex, but they do not want to promote condom use because they are concerned that it might lead to increased adolescent sexual activity. To date, however, strong evidence suggests condom promotion programs do not hasten or increase sexual behavior amongst young people (Kirby, Laris, and Rolleri, 2007). To the contrary, reviews of research suggest that teaching about and establishing low-risk behaviors prior to sexual debut is more effective than changing high-risk behaviors once youth become sexually active, so interventions might be more effective if they target younger adolescents (Gallant and Maticka-Tyndale, 2004).

Importantly, a recent review of Demographic and Health Surveys found that the majority of adults in eastern and southern African countries supported condom education for twelve- to fourteen-year-olds (Doyle et al., 2012). Indeed, support for this seems to be increasing, as in five of the seven countries where these questions were asked in successive surveys, men and/or women were significantly more favorable toward it in the later surveys.

Detailed and Comprehensive Information

As noted earlier in the book, controversy about condom promotion for adolescents has led to abstinence-only programs, but even abstinence-plus and comprehensive interventions have had highly variable content related to condoms (Gallant and Maticka-Tyndale, 2004; Dworkin and Santelli, 2007; Nixon et al., 2011). Within interventions, condom promotion information can range from brief and vague slogans (e.g., "Condoms protect"); to verbal descriptions of what a condom looks like and how it is used; to participants having opportunities to see condom demonstrations and to practice the correct steps themselves by putting a condom on an object such as a banana. The extent to which interventions repeat or reinforce such information, and the extent to which they develop participants' skills related to condom use (e.g., assertiveness, communication, and negotiation skills), can also vary widely.

Chapters 4 and 5 explained how *MEMA kwa Vijana* intervention developers negotiated an agreement with local educational authorities that increasing information and detail about condom use could be provided with each upper primary school year. However, educational authorities did not allow condoms to be shown or otherwise visually depicted at any point in the in-school curriculum. Therefore the only pupils who actually saw condoms and a condom demonstration were those whose class visited a health facility where an intervention health worker explained condom use.

The extent to which *MEMA kwa Vijana* intervention participants experienced condom promotion influenced the extent to which they perceived condoms positively, understood how to access and use them, and took the initiative to do so. This is not to say that all sexually active adolescents who received clear and comprehensive information about condoms then went on to use them, but rather that this was common for those few who did. For example, some sexually active adolescents in control communities had heard of condoms, but they typically did not know what condoms looked like or how they were used, and they often were confused about whether condoms were safe or protective against pregnancy and sexually transmitted infections. *MEMA kwa Vijana* intervention participants who dropped out of school or were frequently absent—so that they missed the detailed description of condom use in Year 7, or a condom demonstration at a health facility—tended to have positive attitudes toward condoms but only a vague understanding of what condoms looked like or how they were used. Intervention participants who instead had participated in the full program and had seen a condom demonstration—and particularly those who had participated in the intensive peer educator training—typically demonstrated the most positive, complex, and subtle understanding of condom use and its benefits, although even they sometimes still expressed confusion and uncertainty about specific aspects of condom use. Nonetheless, these individuals were the adolescents most likely to have initiated condom use in their sexual relationships.

Some other intervention evaluations also have found that the relatively intensive training peer educators receive can result in greater intervention impact on them than their peers, in terms of cognitive understanding, communication and social skills, self-esteem, and risk behaviors (Bastien, Flisher et al., 2008). However, it is difficult to isolate the effect of peer educator experience from a broader program, because peer educators are selected for specific characteristics and thus are different from their peers at the onset, and they may also have different reporting biases within intervention evaluations.

Other studies also have found that the content, quality, and detail of condom promotion information, and the extent to which it is repeated and reinforced, makes a difference to participant understanding, confidence, and use of condoms (e.g., Meekers, Agha, and Klein, 2005; Van Rossem and Meekers, 2007; Taylor et al., 2010). In Burkina Faso, Ghana, and Uganda, for example, Bankole, Ahmed, and colleagues (2007) found that adolescents who had seen a condom demonstration were two to five times more likely than others to know correct condom use. Similarly, a South African study found that urban and rural young women who had been exposed to more sources of AIDS information were more likely than others to report condom use (Katz, 2006). The author argued that exposure to numerous sources of information was more effective in promoting condom use because repetition improved message retention, and the different strengths of different sources of information complemented each other. Explicit discussion of the steps involved in correct condom use also may be important to ensure they are being used correctly. For example, in a study of Australian tertiary students who completed condom use diaries over a six-month period, de Visser and Smith (2000) found that 13 percent of the condoms used were put on incorrectly—after initial penetration—and 38 percent of condom users reported at least one such instance of late condom application.

These findings suggest that condom promotion for adolescents should be detailed, comprehensive, and reinforced in multiple ways. Where local policy imposes restrictions on such promotion, intervention developers should explore as many creative strategies and collaborations as possible to compensate for it. The *MEMA kwa Vijana* facilitation of condom demonstrations for pupils at health facilities provides one example of this. Importantly, recent research in Tanzania suggests that adolescents there continue to have substantial misconceptions about condom use. For example, in a 2007 study of 715 primary and secondary school students in Mwanza and Dar es Salaam, Mkumbo (2010) found it was common for respondents to ask whether it was necessary to use condoms with a loved partner, and whether new condoms contain HIV or allow HIV to pass through them.

Girls' Confidence and Negotiation Skills

In rural Mwanza, a few female intervention participants were extraordinarily assertive in initiating and negotiating condom use, including leaving sexual encounters when a partner did not produce them. Unmarried girls and women almost always negotiated money or gifts prior to sexual encounters, suggesting there may be potential to more broadly orient such skills toward condom negotiation as well. Nonetheless, given the social norms of female passivity and subservience, any program seeking to promote young women's confidence, assertiveness, and negotiation skills related to condom use would need to engage with these issues in depth. To date this has most often taken place within interventions with high-risk women (e.g., Wechsberg et al., 2010), but similarly intensive approaches should be developed with girls and young women in general populations.

Although some girls in this study successfully negotiated condom use, even they did not consider the possibility of obtaining condoms and bringing them to sexual encounters themselves. It was very challenging for a young woman to obtain condoms from a village kiosk or health facility without drawing unwanted attention. Clearly, there is a thus a need to improve young women's discreet access to condoms in rural areas. Nonetheless, even when condoms were more accessible young women who used them felt it would be inappropriate to secure them themselves. Instead they relied on their partners to bring condoms to encounters, and their partners typically did not do so consistently, so that the couple began to have unprotected sex.

As noted above, men may be more responsive to a young woman's request to use condoms if she emphasizes her desire to prevent pregnancy or protect her fertility, rather than directly referring to infection prevention. Similarly, in a study with workers in recreational venues elsewhere in Mwanza Region, Lees and colleagues (2009) found that women were most successful using condoms if they addressed condom use during the negotiation of material exchange; if they were insistent even if a man changed his mind once the sexual encounter began; and if they claimed that their priority was to prevent pregnancy. Importantly, like some other qualitative studies in the region, the authors found that girls' and women's ability to negotiate condom use was linked to their economic self-sufficiency (e.g., Gysels, Pool, and Nnalusiba, 2002). Poorer women's greater dependence on sex for material exchange probably makes it more difficult for them to refuse to have unprotected sexual encounters. This highlights the importance of alternative sources of income for girls and women, a topic that will be discussed more in the next chapter.

Condom Use at Different Stages of Life

Condom use, like all of the low-risk sexual behaviors discussed in this book, can be practiced in varying ways by the same individual at different stages of life. In this study, the few school girls who initiated condom use were perceived as very desirable partners and could use that to insist upon condoms if they felt confident and determined enough. In contrast, there was very little evidence of single women in their late teens and twenties initiating and insisting upon condom use, with the exception of third-hand reports about some female bar workers and guesthouse workers. The lack of such reports may have been due to the study's focus on school pupils. In addition, however, single young women may not have been as invested in preventing pregnancy as school girls, and/or they may have felt they did not have enough bargaining power to persuade their partners to use condoms.

This finding was supported by those of the fourth series of in-depth interviews conducted with randomly selected *MEMA kwa Vijana* intervention participants in 2009, which was described in chapter 2 (table 2.2). At that time, four of the twelve interviewed women (aged twenty-four to thirty years) reported having used condoms at some point in their lives, but said that they had used them infrequently because condom use depended on their partners' interest and cooperation, which usually did not continue beyond a first sexual encounter (Wamoyi and Mshana, 2010). In contrast, all of the eleven male respondents (aged twenty-four to twenty-nine years) reported having tried condoms. These young men reported a similar pattern of condom use to that of the young men in their twenties in HALIRA participant observation villages, that is, only using condoms with casual partners, such as bar workers or women met while traveling (Wamoyi and Mshana, 2010). This again suggests that condom use with extramarital partners can be a feasible goal within condom promotion campaigns, which will be discussed more in the next chapter.

This chapter completes the in-depth examination of each of the three ABC behaviors: abstinence, being faithful, and condom use. In concluding this book, the next chapter will discuss broad principles to better promote low-risk sexual behaviors with young people, and then review promising interventions which could complement and improve the effectiveness of school and health facility programs.

Part IV

INTERVENTION RECOMMENDATIONS

Chapter Eleven

Intervention Recommendations

Mary Louisa Plummer and Daniel Wight

Three decades into the AIDS epidemic, the high rates of new HIV infections among young people in sub-Saharan Africa raise profound questions about the effectiveness of sexual health interventions to date. Community activists, program developers, researchers, and others have gone to great effort to promote low-risk sexual behaviors, but the impact of those interventions has been limited. Many people working in these fields have become discouraged. As Ali and Cleland (2006, 23) note, "An aura of despondency and frustration hangs over the arena of HIV prevention." The promotion of the "ABCs"—abstinence, being faithful, and condom use—at the individual level has been the subject of particularly great criticism, with some describing this approach as fossilized, infantilizing, or over-simplistic (Thornton, 2008; Collins, Coates, and Curran, 2008). Many now argue, with good reason, that HIV prevention efforts at the individual level are unlikely to result in behavior change without intensive interpersonal, community, and structural interventions as well (e.g., Coates, Richter, and Caceres, 2008; Gupta et al., 2008; Hankins and Zalduondo, 2010; McCoy, Watts, and Padian, 2010; Padian et al., 2011).

Nonetheless, abstaining, having few partners, selecting low-risk partners, being faithful, and/or using condoms remain fundamental and complementary ways to reduce sexual health risk, and these behaviors take place at the individual level. Taking the example of condom use: while interpersonal and structural factors may contribute to low rates of condom use in sub-Saharan Africa (e.g., difficulty negotiating condom use, or limited condom supply), another important factor is simply that condom use can affect male pleasure, and pleasure is one of the main and overriding reasons why boys or men have sex. If instead condoms were widely perceived to enhance male sexual pleasure, it is likely that many of the broader barriers to condom use would greatly diminish.

Promoting low-risk sexual behaviors is a long-term, repetitive process that does not often show dramatic results. It also is a core component of HIV prevention, and one that we must continue striving to improve. As Cooper and Mills (2010, e357) note in a discussion of abstinence, partner number limitation, and condom use within HIV prevention in Africa:

> None of these interventions alone are likely to meet with large-scale success, but in combination they represent a pragmatic, common sense-based, and relatively inexpensive collection of preventive measures that can be broadly implemented, do not require high level technology, and are not dependant on antiretroviral availability. These measures are sustainable despite predicted future fluctuations in international funding.

The question then becomes: how can we better promote low-risk sexual behaviors with young people in sub-Saharan Africa? This chapter will address this question by considering this book's findings and those of its companion volume (Plummer and Wight, 2011) within the context of the broader research literature. The chapter begins with a review of factors which contributed to low-risk sexual practices within the *MEMA kwa Vijana* trial population. That is followed by a summary of the *MEMA kwa Vijana* intervention's process and impact findings. The chapter continues with a discussion of broad principles to better promote low-risk sexual behaviors with young people. It then reviews promising interventions which could complement and improve the effectiveness of school and health facility programs, including interventions that work at individual, interpersonal, community, and structural levels. Finally, the chapter concludes with a discussion of the importance of intervention transparency and evaluation.

FACTORS CONTRIBUTING TO
LOW-RISK SEXUAL BEHAVIORS

Adolescents who practiced low-risk sexual behaviors in rural Mwanza were in a minority, and for some behaviors (e.g., secondary abstinence or condom use) a very small minority. Nonetheless, this study found that—for each of the low-risk behaviors—at least a small proportion of adolescents found that particular practice desirable and feasible. Chapters 8–10 and their accompanying case study series examined the motivations and experiences of young people who provided some of the most detailed, plausible, and consistent reports of trying to abstain, reduce partner number, select low-risk partners, be faithful, and/or use condoms, whether or not they had participated in the *MEMA kwa Vijana* intervention. Those findings illustrate how sexual risk reduction is an ongoing process, as even those who were most motivated to reduce their risk had shifting priorities, strategies, and success in achieving their behavioral goals over time. The section below will review the main factors which seemed to help such young people adopt and maintain low-risk practices.

Social ideals about abstinence and fidelity (especially for girls) sometimes influenced young people to practice those behaviors. Other social factors which encouraged low-risk behaviors included close parental monitoring and communication, and having a close same-sex friend with similar values and practices, as seen in case studies 1.2, 1.3, and 2.2. Having a strict parent or a strong religious community sometimes also contributed to low-risk sexual behaviors. However, if a young person did not personally subscribe to those authorities' beliefs, he or she might simply pretend to do so while being very secretive in their sexual behaviors, as seen in case study 3.2.

Economic circumstances could also play a role in reducing sexual risk behavior. Relatively poor young men tended to have fewer partners and/or encounters than other young men, because they had little to offer in exchange for sex, as seen when the young man in case study 1.4 was in early adolescence. In contrast, relatively affluent young women were not dependent on sex to obtain basic supplies, and thus could choose to abstain, to be selective of partners, or to insist on condom use if they desired. As case studies 1.1 and 3.2 illustrate, however, poor girls who intentionally practiced low-risk behaviors sometimes did so by depending on the generosity of other girls, who were probably only able to assist them with what they received from transactional sex.

School experiences sometimes also promoted sexual risk reduction, including positive and mutually respectful relationships with teachers (e.g., case study 1.2), and experience of teachers who intervened in a concerned but non-abusive and non-punitive way when they suspected a pupil was engaged in risky activities (e.g., case studies 1.3 and 3.2). Having future aspirations and goals, such as education beyond primary school, getting a salaried job, or building an independent small business, also sometimes motivated young people to practice low-risk behaviors, as seen in case studies 1.2, 1.3, 2.2, and 3.1.

In addition, some young people who practiced low-risk sexual behaviors specifically attributed this to their participation in an HIV prevention program. As discussed in chapter 7, some intervention participants falsely reported low-risk behaviors, probably because they knew that those were promoted behaviors. However, a small proportion of intervention participants gave very consistent, detailed, and plausible reports of trying to reduce their sexual risk behaviors after intervention participation, arguing for the validity of their reports. This included some general primary school pupils within the *MEMA kwa Vijana* intervention, as well as peer educators who received more intensive training and who were more likely than others to report condom use (e.g., case studies 3.1 and 3.2). It is also noteworthy that two of the young people who gave some of the most plausible accounts of practicing low-risk sexual behaviors in control communities (case studies 1.3 and 2.2) had both participated in an HIV prevention program, unlike most control participants.

Some young people who intentionally tried to reduce their risk were highly motivated and reported that, for them, the potential negative outcomes of risky sexual behavior outweighed any possible benefits. For example, some individuals were faithful to one partner because they were emotionally attached to that partner and satisfied in the relationship, and they either did not desire another partner or did not want to risk losing their main partner through infidelity. Personal experience of negative consequences of unprotected sex—whether for one's self or a loved one—was also sometimes a strong motivator to reduce risk, as seen in case studies 1.4 and 3.3. Some young people who had had such experiences reported a great fear of dropping out of school and experiencing punishment or hardship due to unwanted pregnancy; of painful sexually transmitted infections; and/or of AIDS-related illness and death.

Sometimes young people, and especially young women, who practiced low-risk behaviors were extraordinarily independent, confident, and assertive (e.g., case studies 1.1 and 3.2). This enabled them to resist frequent pressure to have sex, or to insist upon condom use. However, while some young people actively and strategically tried to avoid pregnancy or sexually transmitted infections, others passively practiced low-risk behaviors due to external influences or constraints. For example, some obedient young women seemed to be abstinent or to have few partners mainly because their parents and/or sexual partners expected this (e.g., case study 2.1).

Sexual risk reduction can be complex, challenging, and variable at both an individual and a societal level, but these findings offer insight into how it nonetheless occurs, with or without intervention. None of the factors described above were prescriptive and ensured that young people practiced low-risk behaviors. Many adolescents and young adults had more than one of these factors influencing their lives, but nonetheless engaged in high-risk behaviors. However, the young people who actively attempted to reduce risk to their sexual health typically were influenced by several of these factors in combination. Many of these factors have similarly been associated with low-risk sexual behavior in other research in eastern and southern Africa (e.g., Babalola, Ouedraogo, and Vondrasek, 2006; Steele et al., 2006; Hendrikson et al., 2007; Sauvain-Dugerdil et al., 2008; Dlamini et al., 2009; Tenkorang, Rajulton, and Maticka-Tyndale, 2009; Clark, 2010; Helleve, Flisher, Onya, Mũkoma et al., 2011). Different intervention approaches to promoting or reinforcing these factors will be discussed later in this chapter, such as programs to promote parenting skills or alternative sources of income for girls.

Only one of these factors will be discussed in more depth here, namely the finding that some young people were highly motivated to change their sexual behavior due to a strong fear of AIDS, because the role of fear in HIV prevention and sexual risk reduction has been the subject of some controversy (e.g., Albarracín et al., 2005; Green and Witte, 2006; Halperin, 2006; Kirby, 2006; O'Grady, 2006; Slavin, Batrouney, and Murphy, 2007). This controversy partly relates to the different forms the epidemic has taken in different parts of the world. Specifically, in North America and Europe in the 1980s and 1990s the AIDS epidemic was mainly concentrated in marginalized groups, such as men who have sex with men, sex workers, and intravenous drug users. In that context, HIV educators generally discouraged strongly "fear-based" approaches, as they were reputed to be ineffective and potentially harmful (Green and Witte, 2006; Kirby, 2006). Some were concerned that such approaches might back-fire and make participants feel unduly frightened, overwhelmed, or hopeless; that they might not contribute to behavior change, or only to brief behavior change; and that they might stigmatize people living with HIV/AIDS who were already greatly marginalized (e.g., Sherr, 1990; van der Velde and van der Pligt, 1991).

During the same period in eastern and southern Africa, the HIV epidemic was generalized or even hypergeneralized. In the absence of antiretroviral therapy and adequate health facilities and social services, many people in the general population became the primary caregivers of family members with AIDS, tending, feeding, and bathing them as they experienced painful, drawn out illnesses and died. In such contexts, it was not unusual for people to develop a strong personal fear of AIDS, and some national HIV prevention programs also promoted risk reduction with simple and strong fear-based messages, such as posters depicting skulls and coffins, and slogans like, "Beware of AIDS: AIDS Kills" (Green and Witte, 2006; Pool, Kamali, and Whitworth, 2006). Green and Witte (2006) argue that fear of AIDS resulting from such personal experience and national fear appeals—combined with clear information about what one can do to avoid HIV infection—contributed to sexual behavior change and the reduction in HIV incidence observed in Uganda from 1992 to 2002.

The debate about whether "high" or "low" fear arousal is most effective and appropriate in interventions has existed in the fields of psychology and public

health at least since the mid-twentieth century (e.g., Higbee, 1969). In a more
recent meta-analysis by Witte and Allen (2000, 604), the authors found:

> . . . fear appeals appear to be effective when they depict a significant and rel-
> evant threat (to increase perceptions of severity and susceptibility) and when
> they outline effective responses that appear easy to accomplish (to increase per-
> ceptions of response efficacy and self-efficacy). Low-threat fear appeals appear
> to produce little, if any, persuasive effects. Thus . . . a persuader should promote
> high levels of threat and high levels of efficacy to promote attitude, intention,
> and behavior change.

The HALIRA study also found that some young people who gave very
plausible reports of low-risk sexual practices had both participated in an
HIV prevention intervention and also had a heightened personal fear of HIV,
other sexually transmitted infections, or unwanted pregnancies. In contrast to
those personal experiences of high fear arousal and behavior change, however, there were incidents when *MEMA kwa Vijana* intervention participants
rejected messages for which they perceived the risk to be overstated or, alternatively, to be so great that risk was unavoidable, so they resigned themselves
to it and did not try to change their behaviors. One example is the oft-repeated
slogan "even one time," as described in chapter 5, because this phrase was
sometimes misinterpreted to mean that if a person has vaginal intercourse
once that person *will* (not *could*) cause a pregnancy or contract an infection.
This reinforced some young people's fatalism that they could not avoid risk,
while others who had not experienced such consequences perceived the warn-
ing to be invalid.

These findings highlight how effective and appropriate fear arousal involves a very delicate balance, especially in a low-literate environment where
both simple and complex messages may be easily misconstrued. The discussion of promising intervention approaches later in this chapter will include
some programs which have focused on improving participants' understanding of HIV susceptibility and severity, for example, by involving people
living with HIV/AIDS as public speakers. Before that broader discussion of
intervention strategies, however, the next section will review the *MEMA kwa
Vijana* intervention process and impact evaluation findings.

THE *MEMA KWA VIJANA* INTERVENTION

One of the most important lessons of the *MEMA kwa Vijana* trial is that
implementation of a low-cost, large-scale adolescent sexual health program
in a rural African context is likely to involve great compromises. These in-

clude compromise between national policies and international "best practice" recommendations; between the most desirable intervention design and one that is affordable and sustainable at a large scale; between optimal teaching methods and real-world teaching capacity; between ideal curriculum content and what is acceptable to the local community; and between adults' values and youths' realities.

Despite such compromises, *MEMA kwa Vijana* produced a carefully designed intervention that addressed some relevant cultural practices (e.g., material exchange for sex) and followed local guidelines and international "best practice" recommendations when it was developed (Kirby et al., 1994; WHO, 1997). Chapters 4–7 described how the four intervention components were implemented largely as intended, but their potential effectiveness was reduced by gaps in their design and external challenges encountered during the trial. Those process and impact findings are summarized below.

Process Evaluation

The *MEMA kwa Vijana* community mobilization component (chapter 4) was intentionally limited to minimize costs. It mainly was designed to reduce opposition to the program. Few parents or children refused to participate in the intervention, but the HALIRA study found that many adults knew little about the purpose and the content of the intervention, and some topics remained controversial in the broader community during the trial, particularly adolescent sexual education and condom use.

Within the school component of the intervention (chapter 5), almost all teachers delivered most of the sessions (Appendices 1–3), some teachers adopted novel interactive teaching techniques, and corporal punishment decreased, especially during intervention sessions. *MEMA kwa Vijana* peer educators performed the drama serial well and generally understood the intervention content better than their classmates. However, they often had difficulty answering complex questions or being behavioral role models, and other pupils sometimes ignored or rejected their opinions. In addition, the lack of recognition of pupil sexual activity meant that the sexual behaviors and particularly the low-risk ABC behaviors were only addressed superficially within the school curriculum and peer educator training. This contributed to some pupils being confused about how to practice low-risk behaviors and some pupils feeling an unwarranted sense of safety when engaged in high-risk behaviors.

Unlike teachers, health workers in rural Mwanza had a unique authority and legitimacy that enabled them to teach intervention participants fairly explicit sexual information without invoking controversy. Within the health services component (chapter 6), class visits to health facilities were critical in ensuring that many pupils saw condoms, observed a condom demonstration, and understood that they could be obtained there for free. In clinical consultations, intervention health workers also were generally less judgmental, more respectful, and more likely to promote condoms with adolescents than control health workers. However, this component was unable to overcome critical barriers to clinical service, such as distance from homes and fear of stigma, and very few trial participants ever attended intervention or control health facilities for sexual health services. In addition, some undesirable practices which preceded the trial continued during it in intervention facilities, including poor privacy and inappropriate personal questions during clinical consultations, and forced pregnancy examinations of groups of school girls.

Finally, during the trial four young adults in each village were trained to distribute subsidized condoms (chapter 6), and most succeeded in establishing small clienteles of customers. However, very few pupils or other villagers were aware of this intervention component or ever obtained condoms from a distributor. In addition, the distributors themselves had difficulty using condoms consistently, so they were not effective role models. Due to the very low demand for condoms and challenges related to this component's cost and sustainability, it was discontinued at the end of the trial.

Importantly, with the exception of the condom distribution component, the *MEMA kwa Vijana* intervention was affordable, sustainable, and replicable on a large scale within a resource-poor African setting. Indeed, when the *MEMA kwa Vijana* intervention was expanded after the trial from 62 to 649 primary schools, and from 18 to 177 health facilities, there was some dilution of quality as anticipated, but overall implementation was good (Renju, Andrew, Medard et al., 2010; Renju, Andrew, Nyalali et al., 2010; Renju, Makokha et al., 2010). Meeting such criteria is essential, because expensive and difficult-to-replicate behavioral interventions are unlikely to have an impact on the HIV epidemic among young Africans, even if they genuinely improve sexual health on a small scale.

Impact Evaluation

At the end of the *MEMA kwa Vijana* trial, all of the research methods found that intervention participants had a better basic knowledge of sexual health, and of low- and high-risk behaviors, than their control counterparts (e.g., table 7.1). This is not a minor achievement, given understanding of biology, mathematics, and HIV/AIDS are still very limited in many parts of sub-Saharan Africa today (e.g., Chacko et al., 2007; Bastien, Flisher et al., 2008; Dixon-Mueller, 2009; Robins, 2009; Mkumbo, 2010; UNAIDS, 2010;

Dimbuene and Defo, 2011). Importantly, the *MEMA kwa Vijana* intervention participants who demonstrated the best knowledge were those who had relatively intensive intervention experiences, that is, peer educators who received training and an information booklet, and/or pupils who received two or three years of the intervention, rather than only one (Ross et al., 2007; Doyle, Weiss et al., 2011). As noted earlier, however, even those individuals often lacked a full understanding of each of the ABC behaviors.

In addition, the intervention only had a limited impact on other theoretical determinants of low-risk sexual behaviors, including personal risk perception, anticipated outcomes, behavioral goals, sense of self-efficacy, observational learning, and contextual facilitators and impediments. Overall the qualitative evaluation suggests that the intervention *did* have an impact on many of those determinants, but that this was only to a mild extent for most intervention participants, and/or to a great extent for a few, and this was insufficient to result in a significant and sustained impact on the trial population's behavior, unintended pregnancy, or sexually transmitted infections. Indeed, the *MEMA kwa Vijana* biomedical surveys found that the intervention did not have any significant, positive effects on pregnancy or sexually transmitted infections (table 7.1) (Ross et al., 2007; Doyle et al., 2010).

The next section will now draw on the book's main findings to outline broad principles for the promotion of low-risk sexual behaviors with young rural Africans. These are relevant to school and health facility programs for adolescents, as well as many other types of intervention programs.

GENERAL PRINCIPLES FOR ABC PROMOTION WITH YOUNG PEOPLE

Chapters 8–10 discussed ways to improve the promotion of each ABC within adolescent sexual health programs. General recommendations relevant to the promotion of all of these behaviors are summarized in table 11.1. Additional, specific recommendations for abstinence promotion are summarized in table 11.2, including reducing pressures and incentives for girls to have sex; clarifying safe ways to manage sexual desire, including masturbation; and promoting positive male attitudes and strategies related to abstinence. Further recommendations specific to the promotion of low partner number and fidelity are summarized in table 11.3, including: acknowledging youth sexual activity; strengthening young people's premarital and marital relationships; examining the risks related to multiple partnerships; promoting HIV testing; and encouraging alternative forms of masculinity. Finally, additional recommendations for condom promotion are summarized in table 11.4, including: providing

Table 11.1. General Recommendations for Promoting Abstinence, Low Partner Number, Partner Selectivity, Fidelity, and Condom Use with Young Rural Africans

Tables 11.2, 11.3, and 11.4 provide additional recommendations for specific behaviors.

1. Intervene at individual, interpersonal, community, and structural levels.
2. Train teachers in college to use participatory teaching methods and to teach adolescent sexual and reproductive health curricula.
3. Implement intensive sexual and reproductive health curricula in schools.
4. Promote each of the "ABCs"—that is, abstinence, low partner number, partner selectivity, mutual fidelity, and condom use—in depth and complexity.
5. Begin teaching about each low-risk sexual behavior in the preadolescent and early adolescent years, so young people understand the risks and their options before they become sexually active.
6. Implement interactive skills-based programs which promote adolescents' decision-making, communication, and relationship skills.
7. Engage adolescents about their future goals and specific strategies to achieve them, for example, saving money for financial independence; maximizing formal education by avoiding pregnancy; and protecting fertility by avoiding infections.
8. Promote supportive teacher-pupil relationships which boost pupils' confidence, encourage their critical thinking skills, and challenge dominant gender norms.
9. Improve the general education system in other ways, for example, increase youth access to quality primary and secondary education, and monitor and reduce male teacher sexual abuse of female pupils.
10. Promote youth-friendly health services, for example, provide pre-service and in-service training for all health facility staff.
11. Maximize the involvement of health workers in HIV prevention outreach and education with both youth and adults.
12. Combine intensive school-based and health facility interventions with broader community interventions, for example, programs with out-of-school youth, women, men, couples, parents, and the general population.
13. Improve parenting skills and parents' awareness of young people's premarital sexual relationships; the increased risks involved in secretive relationships; and the consequences of expecting adolescent girls to provide for their own material needs.
14. Facilitate financial alternatives for girls (e.g., increased parental support, or income-generating activities), so girls do not need to have sex (or to change partners, or to agree to unprotected sex) in order to obtain money or materials.
15. Use the mass media, youth leaders, and role models to target and promote each low-risk behavior as "smart," "cool," modern, and/or (for boys) "masculine," e.g., smart because the individual does not foolishly risk exposure to disease.
16. Promote alternatives to sexual pursuit to occupy boys' free time and encourage their sense of masculine accomplishment, for example, participating in sports competitions or building small businesses.
17. Make use of preexisting and culturally compelling motivations in promoting low-risk behaviors, for example, concerns about future fertility.
18. Provide education by people living with HIV to personalize HIV infection for young people and to promote their understanding of HIV susceptibility and severity.
19. Promote mutual HIV testing before couples have unprotected sex, and possibly at intervals during their relationship.
20. Provide culturally compelling edutainment (e.g., story serials, songs).
21. Explore the potential of limited and well monitored peer education (e.g., scripted dramas).

Table 11.2.   Additional Recommendations for Promoting Abstinence with Young Rural Africans

1. Engage with girls about positive social influences and outcomes which encourage abstinence, for example, parental attitudes.
2. Develop girls' skills to resist boys, men, and female peers who pressure them to be sexually active.
3. Challenge communities to not tolerate boys and men pressuring girls for sex, and develop strategies to reduce this.
4. Promote boys' positive attitudes towards abstinence, including ways it may reflect masculine traits, for example, financial independence or physical self-control.
5. Develop boys' skills to resist peer pressure to have sex.
6. Clarify safe ways to manage sexual desire, including masturbation.
7. Promote abstinence as a positive, short-term strategy for married or unmarried couples during the postpartum period or when separated due to travel.

Table 11.3.   Additional Recommendations for Promoting Low Partner Number and Fidelity with Young Rural Africans

1. Use interactive exercises to clearly convey the prevalence of HIV and other sexually transmitted infections; the nature of their transmission within networks; and the specific risks involved in multiple partnerships, concurrency, serial monogamy, and having short gaps between partners.
2. Emphasize how unprotected sex with one partner allows for both pleasure and reproduction but is not safe unless (a) neither partner is infected at the onset of the relationship, and (b) both are faithful during it.
3. Address how similar principles apply to fidelity within polygynous marriages, as a polygynous marriage can be safe if (a) no spouses have sexually transmitted infections when they enter the marriage, and (b) all are faithful during it.
4. Discuss the potential value of the "one-one-one" approach to sexual risk reduction, that is, one partner at a time; at least one month between partners; and in one locale or community only (Thornton, 2008).
5. Avoid vague slogans (e.g., "be faithful") which may be interpreted in multiple ways with very different implications for risk. Develop clear and unambiguous messages, e.g., "test together before starting a new relationship," "be faithful to one tested partner," and "avoid overlapping relationships" (Baumgartner et al., 2010).
6. Appeal to male desire for self-preservation, and stress that a man's own fidelity protects himself as well as his partner(s).
7. Promote alternative forms of masculinity than sexual conquest of new partners, including responsibility and accountability to protect a partner as well as one's self.
8. Encourage potential partners to get to know one another well before having unprotected sex and/or marrying, to reduce conflict and quick partner change.
9. Seek greater openness about young people's premarital sexual relationships so that risks can be discussed with parents, mutually monogamous relationships can be strengthened through social endorsement, and partners can be held more accountable.
10. Work with individuals and couples to develop their relationship skills and strategies to practice long-term, mutual fidelity. Promote stronger and more enduring relationships, so couples work through and resolve problems rather than change partners.
11. Develop specific interventions to promote fidelity with different kinds of couples, for example, hidden or unacknowledged couples; couples planning to marry; and married partners (both monogamous and polygynous).

Table 11.4. Additional Recommendations for Promoting Condom Use with Young Rural Africans

1. Employ existing "best practice" condom distribution campaigns to improve condom availability for both youth and adults in rural areas.
2. Implement intensive interventions for parents and other adults to convey the value of condom use in general and specifically for sexually active young people. Explain that youth who are provided with comprehensive condom information and skills development are more likely to protect themselves than other sexually active youth.
3. Provide adolescents with detailed information about the steps involved in correct condom use, using clear visual aids.
4. Use creative collaborations (e.g., health worker-teacher) if necessary to provide adolescents with comprehensive condom information.
5. Develop young people's skills to access, carry, negotiate, and use condoms, particularly young women's.
6. Work with young people's preexisting skills (e.g., material exchange negotiation skills) and promote new skills related to condom use, including risk assessment, assertiveness, and communication skills.
7. Acknowledge and engage with participants' misgivings about condoms, particularly concerns about reduced pleasure and trust.
8. Stress that a trustworthy person may unknowingly bring HIV into a new relationship, so condoms ideally should be used for every sexual encounter until both partners have been tested.
9. Promote condoms for pregnancy prevention and fertility protection, highlighting that sexually transmitted infections can also reduce men's fertility.
10. Convince men it is in their personal interest to use condoms by improving their risk assessment skills and targeting their desire for self-preservation.
11. Stress that condom use is most important with high-risk partners, but given it is difficult to identify who is high risk, only consistent condom use is fully protective.
12. Promote selective or consistent condom use as appropriate and feasible at different life stages, for example, encourage married individuals to use condoms when they want to space children or engage in extramarital relationships.

adolescents with detailed and comprehensive information; developing girls' confidence and negotiation skills; acknowledging the possible trade-off of male pleasure and risk; addressing the issue of trust in condom use decision-making; highlighting condoms' potential in both pregnancy prevention and fertility protection; and promoting selective and/or consistent condom use as appropriate and feasible at different stages of life.

Some of the recommendations above will be addressed more in the following discussion. That section will consider four broad principles for the promotion of low-risk sexual behaviors with young people: first, acknowledge young people's sexual relationships; second, promote each low-risk behavior in complexity and depth; third, work with preexisting and culturally compelling motivations; and fourth, intervene at individual, interpersonal, community, and structural levels.

Acknowledge Young People's Sexual Relationships

The HALIRA study identified many contradictory sexual norms and expectations which influenced young people's risk behaviors in rural Mwanza, as detailed in chapter 3 and this book's companion volume (Plummer and Wight, 2011). One example is that it was not unusual for young children to witness older people having sex, either when they first shared a sleeping room with their parents, or later when they shared a room with older, same-sex siblings and cousins who invited partners in after dark. Such practices were common but secretive, and resulted in many children becoming sexually aware at very young ages, as evidenced in the sexually explicit nature of some small children's play. Nonetheless, parents often did not realize the extent of their children's early sexual knowledge, either because they did not realize their children were aware during their own sexual encounters, or because they did not know people were sneaking into their children's rooms at night for sex. Indeed, participant observation found that most fifteen-year-olds had had sex, but this was very carefully hidden from their parents.

As discussed in chapter 3, the secrecy of premarital sexual relationships was a fundamental barrier to risk perception and risk reduction in rural Mwanza. First, it meant that couples mainly had contact while negotiating sex or having sex, and there was little opportunity for them to get to know one another well or develop emotional intimacy or commitment. Second, it obscured a partner's past and concurrent sexual partners and thus facilitated multiple relationships. These findings suggest that increased acknowledgement of young people's sexual relationships could support partner reduction and fidelity. In addition, with greater openness, young people's sexual risks could be discussed with parents, monogamous relationships could be strengthened through social endorsement, and partners could be held more accountable (e.g., Kenyon et al., 2010). Critically, greater openness would not be intended to encourage or increase youth sexual activity, but rather to acknowledge and address what is already taking place in secrecy.

Interventions trying to promote such openness in a rural African setting would face many obstacles, as discussed in chapter 9. Despite these formidable challenges, it would be worthwhile to explore ways to encourage parents to acknowledge and accept if their unmarried children are sexually active, and to recognize their child's boyfriend or girlfriend. Given many cultures highly value discretion, interventions would need to explore how to promote greater openness and honesty as tactfully and considerately as possible. Importantly, more open acknowledgement, support, and advice for unmarried couples may not only reduce secretive concurrent relationships but also help prevent quick and unhappy marriages and divorces. Reducing marital dissolution may also protect young people's sexual health, as studies in rural Mwanza and elsewhere in sub-Saharan Africa have found that separated, divorced, and widowed individuals are more likely to be HIV-infected than their peers (e.g., Doyle, Changalucha et al., 2011; de Walque and Kline, 2012).

In the HALIRA study, approximately one-half of young women married within two years of leaving primary school, and one-half of young men within another few years. Young people married for a number of reasons, including desires for independence, security, status, comfort, and/or legitimate children. Some also married because they wanted an open and legitimate sexual relationship with a faithful partner, something that had not been an option for them when they were sexually active in school. Some married out of a desire for stability, and some to reduce their sexual risk.

Often, young people did not perceive it as important to know a potential spouse well, as the important factor in deciding to marry was instead that both individuals were ready to be married. Indeed, about half of young married people in the study had only known their spouse for about one month before marrying, whether they married by elopement or engagement. As discussed in chapter 3, some couples were satisfied in those marriages and stayed together long-term. However, it also was not unusual for such marriages to end quickly, usually because spouses were not personally compatible or the circumstances were not as they expected. With greater acknowledgement of unmarried youth's existing sexual relationships, there thus might be more potential for them to get to know one another well to make sure that they are compatible, and to receive advice and develop relationships skills, before marrying.

Promote Each ABC in Complexity and Depth

The ABC acronym can be useful in neatly summarizing abstinence, being faithful, and condom use as three important and complementary ways to reduce sexual risk. In its simplicity, however, this term can obscure the fact that each of these behaviors is open to multiple interpretations which may be difficult or complicated to adopt, especially long-term. Often designers of adolescent sexual health interventions would like to address sexual risk reduction in depth, to ensure participants are fully informed about their options. However, providing explicit information in adolescent sexual health programs is often controversial, because adults are concerned that it might promote youth sexual activity. As Stone and Ingham (2006, 195) note:

> . . . one of the main barriers to the promotion of sex and relationships work (including education) is the fear that talking to young people about sex related matters will encourage them to participate in it. Such anxieties can lead to, at the extreme, complete silence or, alternatively, they can—and generally do— encourage an over-emphasis on the negative (for example, unplanned pregnancy

and [sexually transmitted infections]) rather than the positive aspects of sex (such as intimacy and pleasure). Such imbalanced approaches run the risk that young people may reject much of what adults have to say on the area, thereby leading them to seek guidance from less reliable or credible sources instead, such as peers and the media.

Given this potential controversy, a common compromise is to provide adolescents with only very basic information about sexual risk behaviors. Intervention designers may also decide to use very simple messages if adolescent participants have very limited literacy and formal education, as is often the case in sub-Saharan Africa, in the hopes that this will promote message clarity (e.g., Carstens, Maes, and Gangla-Birir, 2006; Coates, Richter, and Caceres, 2008; Van Dyk, 2008; Tanser et al., 2011). For example, there has been substantial debate about the relative risks of concurrent and serially monogamous sexual relationships, and some authors have argued that distinguishing between the two within interventions obscures and undermines an overarching message to have few partners (UNAIDS, 2007; Research to Prevention, 2009; Lurie and Rosenthal, 2010; Harrison and O'Sullivan, 2010; Morris, 2010; Tanser et al., 2011).

The HALIRA study found, however, that if messages are phrased too simply they may also be too vague, leaving young people confused, misunderstanding correct practices, and/or feeling an unwarranted sense of safety. Some other studies in sub-Saharan Africa have had similar findings (e.g., Johns Hopkins University Center for Communication Programs, 2003; Painter et al., 2007; Leclerc-Madlala, 2009; Crichton, Ibisomi, and Gyimah, 2012). For instance, in a survey of 1,375 Kenyan students aged thirteen to nineteen years, researchers found that 85 to 93 percent had heard of the terms "abstinence," "being faithful," and "condom use" in English and/or Swahili, but the proportions who fully comprehended them were much lower, that is, 48 percent for abstinence, 20 percent for being faithful, and 7 percent for condom use (Lillie, Pulerwitz, and Curbow, 2009). In that study, many young people defined "being faithful" in terms of trust rather than partner loyalty and exclusivity, and almost one-half did not seem to have a general knowledge of condom use, let alone a more specific understanding of the importance of consistent condom use. *MEMA kwa Vijana* intervention participants sometimes expressed similar misunderstanding or confusion about how one can safely practice abstinence (e.g., believing masturbation is harmful), fidelity (e.g., believing that serial monogamy with frequent partner change is safe), or condom use (e.g., believing that condom use is not necessary once a couple promises to be faithful to one another).

Interventions also need to better address how risk reduction is an ongoing process and a matter of degree, acknowledging that individuals may change their protective strategies at different times of life depending on a myriad of factors (e.g., Steele et al., 2006). In rural Mwanza, few youths or adults completely abstained from sex, had one lifetime mutually monogamous sexual relationship, and/or used condoms every time they had intercourse. Case study 3.3, for example, describes a young man who over the course of a decade attempted to abstain, reduce his partner number, select low-risk partners, be faithful, and/or use condoms, in an ongoing effort to reduce his sexual health risk. He was not always successful in those efforts, and his approach was sometimes problematic in other ways, as when he assumed he could assess a person's risk by how long she had lived in his village. But by alternating between abstinence and condom use with women who probably were relatively high risk, and by trying to select a low-risk partner with whom he could practice long-term, mutual monogamy, this young man may indeed have lowered his sexual health risk. Critically, his approach to risk reduction also allowed for sexual pleasure and reproduction, both of which were fundamentally important to young adults in this study. Such findings suggest that the more low-risk options young people understand early in their sexual lives, the more able they will be to flexibly adapt and move between them as needed when their life circumstances change.

Finally, in promoting realistic and practical strategies to reduce young people's sexual health risk, the HALIRA findings suggest that interventions should also address sexual partner selectivity in depth, as this can relate to both fidelity and condom use. Clearly, as noted above, it is not possible to be certain of a person's HIV status based on superficial characteristics. Nonetheless, some types of individuals are more likely than others to be infected with HIV or other sexually transmitted infections in settings like rural Mwanza, including older men who seek to seduce adolescent girls, urban visitors, frequent travelers, and bar or guesthouse workers (Boerma et al., 2002; Clift et al., 2003; Desmond et al., 2005). In addition, it was not unusual for young villagers to have short-term sexual relationships with people they met when they themselves traveled to other villages, for example, to visit relatives or to attend special events. Indeed, as noted in chapter 3, in-depth interviews with six young women who became infected with HIV during the *MEMA kwa Vijana* trial suggest that they did not have unusually high numbers of sexual partners or experience of concurrent partnerships, but rather that they were exposed to HIV by unprotected sex with a relatively high-risk partner, such as a man who was likely to have had many partners (e.g., a truck driver or a cotton ginnery operator), or a man met while living in settings with relatively high HIV prevalences (e.g., Mwanza City, a district capital, or large villages on major truck routes).

Some young people did not want to use condoms with all partners but found it feasible to avoid partners who they believed to be high risk, or to use condoms with them or other casual partners. Again, such a strategy does not guarantee that an individual avoids infection, but it is likely to be more protective than simply having unprotected sex with those individuals. To maximize the effectiveness of such partner selectivity, however, intervention participants need to have a good understanding of which types of people are likely to be high risk in their communities, especially as individuals in such groups may be seen as particularly desirable sexual partners, because of their perceived wealth, worldliness, or style.

This discussion of partner selectivity relates to Thornton's (2008) analysis of sexual networks and the AIDS epidemics in Uganda and South Africa. He argues that the 1992–2002 decrease in HIV incidence in Uganda reflected a reduction in sexual network connectivity, and particularly in links between the general population and highly infected persons or groups, such as soldiers or transportation workers. In contrast, Thornton attributes the unrelenting nature of the South African epidemic to the population continuing to be highly mobile and closely interlinked in dense, overlapping sexual networks. This analysis led Thornton to propose a "one, one, one" approach to altering sexual networks that would complement ABC promotion at the individual level, that is: one partner at a time; at least one month between partners; and in one locale or community only. Specifically, he argues that having one partner at a time reduces the density of a sexual network, and thus the flow of infection; that waiting at least one month between partners reduces the possibility of passing on HIV during its initially brief, intense period of infectivity (Pilcher et al., 2004; Wawer et al., 2005); and that limiting oneself to local partners reduces long-distance links that are likely to connect infected and uninfected pools of people within the network.

Work with Preexisting and Culturally Compelling Motivations

Many of the best examples of substantial and sustained sexual behavior change have taken place in groups that acted on their own initiative, such as gay communities in the United States in the 1980s, and general populations in Uganda in the 1990s, rather than occurring in response to external projects (Wilson, 2004; Merson et al., 2008). A fundamental difference between widespread behavior changes which seem to occur of their own accord and behavioral interventions which fail is the role of preexisting motivation within a population. Most behavior change theories assume that motivation can be generated by an intervention itself, but if the intervention does not also make use of participants' preexisting motivations, it is less likely to result in long-term behavior change. This is recognized in the field of social marketing, which stipulates that a promoted product or behavior should be "appealing, accessible, available and appreciated" by the target group (Hastings, 2007, 78). For example, 1990s British anti-smoking campaigns for young people shifted their focus away from death by lung cancer to the side effect of unpleasant breath odor, because the latter was found to be a more immediate concern and deterrent for young people (Pechmann, 1997).

Where vulnerable groups are not acting of their own accord in response to a health threat, program developers can closely examine the target group's preexisting motivations and identify overlaps with the program's objectives that make it more culturally compelling. In the *MEMA kwa Vijana* trial, the limited nature of ethnographic research prior to intervention development meant that some of young people's preexisting motivations were not fully recognized or incorporated within it, such as their desire to make money, to be *kisasa* and cool, or to safeguard their future fertility. Taking the example of fertility, adolescent school pupils almost universally aspired to have several children during their lifetime, as did almost all villagers in rural Mwanza. However, condoms were not promoted within the intervention as a way to be sexually active while protecting future fertility. Such an approach may have been particularly effective if it appealed to male desire for self-preservation, and emphasized the impact that sexually transmitted infections can have on male fertility (Pellati et al., 2008).

Similarly, sexual desire motivated boys to have unprotected sex and to change partners, but relatively safe ways to manage such desire either were not discussed within the intervention (e.g., masturbation), or were only briefly acknowledged (e.g., long-term, mutual premarital monogamy). Importantly, this preexisting motivation amongst adolescents was controversial amongst adults, resulting in the kind of compromises in intervention development discussed earlier. It thus illustrates the importance of supporting adolescent sexual health programs with similarly in-depth and intensive programs for adults.

Intervene at Individual, Interpersonal, Community, and Structural Levels

Even with more in-depth attention to preexisting motivations and each of the ABCs within adolescent HIV prevention programs, the HALIRA findings suggest such programs will still have difficulty succeeding if they are not integrated with intensive interventions for out-of-school youth and adults in the broader community. At the onset of the *MEMA kwa Vijana* trial, intervention developers knew that intensive HIV prevention work with adult community members would be a valuable complement to the adolescent program, but resource limitations meant this was hardly pursued beyond brief community mobilization activities. The findings presented here suggest that this may have been too great of a compromise, particularly given the importance of structural barriers to individual behavior change, such as gender inequality and girls' poverty. Critically, rural Mwanza adolescents—particularly girls— had such low social status that they were unlikely to adopt low-risk practices on a large scale if their out-of-school peers, sexual partners, family members, and other adults did not understand or support such practices.

Structural influences on behavior can be defined in different ways. Here the term is used inclusively to describe many underlying patterns of social systems which are beyond an individual's control, including those related to social status, gender, economics, the environment, and culture. Although all of these factors operate at a macro level, they are often maintained by continual, collective social practices at a micro level, within families, workplaces, and communities (Giddens, 1979). Many of the barriers and facilitators of sexual risk reduction discussed in chapter 3 operate at a structural level. Structural factors are often interrelated; for example, most societies with systematic gender inequalities have elaborate cultural beliefs that perpetuate and justify them. "Culture" is also a term open to varying interpretations. However, two generally agreed upon features of culture are that a culture is a *shared* way of thinking, and that it is a *system* of beliefs (Wright, 1998; Douglas, 2004; Kuran, 2004). In recent decades, culture has been recognized as dynamic and subject to modification by interested parties, rather than as simply static and homogeneous.

The most successful HIV prevention strategies are likely to combine a range of interventions with different mechanisms (e.g., information provision, changing norms, financial incentives, or new legislation), which operate at multiple levels (e.g., from individual to community to nation) and in multiple sectors (e.g., education, health, or justice), and which integrate behavioral, biomedical, and structural strategies (Coates, Richter, and Caceres, 2008; Piot et al., 2008; Hankins and Zalduondo, 2010; Kurth et al., 2011). This approach does not mean that every kind of intervention should be combined indiscriminately. A UNAIDS expert consultation report on behavior change and HIV prevention specified three important caveats for such "combination prevention": that the activities must be tailored to the local epidemic, informed by the existing evidence, and guided by international standards of human rights (UNAIDS, 2007). Tailoring a combination of interventions to a local epidemic requires understanding the local epidemiology, the underlying drivers of the epidemic, and which of these are modifiable. Many other factors also need to be considered in tailoring a combination of HIV prevention interventions to a particular population and setting, including evidence of intervention impact, potential size of effect, feasibility, acceptability, cost, risk of adverse outcomes, and potential for other health or social benefits (Galárraga et al., 2009; Mavedzenge, Doyle, and Ross, 2011).

As discussed in chapters 4 and 7, the Social Cognitive Theory and Theory of Reasoned Action were used to develop the *MEMA kwa Vijana* intervention, and these primarily focus on individual-level behavioral determinants, such as knowledge, personal risk perception, anticipated outcomes, self-efficacy, goals, and modeled behavior (Ajzen and Fishbein, 1980; Fishbein, 2000; Bandura, 2004; Michie et al., 2005; Aarø, Schaalma, and Åstrøm, 2008). These theories also address broader social factors to a limited extent, but even then they mainly focus on subjective perceptions at the individual level (e.g., perceptions of a sexual partner's desires), rather than objective factors at interpersonal and structural levels (e.g., poor education, dependence on sex for money, condom inaccessibility, and the power differentials influencing negotiation with a sexual partner). While individual-level theories clearly can have value in identifying and targeting important personal influences on behavior, ultimately they are insufficient if broader cultural, socioeconomic, and environmental determinants of behavior are not targeted as well. However, interventions which work at interpersonal, community, and structural levels can pose great challenges and be costly. Such programs are generally less clearly defined than those operating in institutions such as schools or health facilities, and they thus can be more difficult to implement, evaluate, replicate, and take to a large scale (e.g., Maticka-Tyndale and Barnett, 2010).

This book has focused on the promotion of low-risk sexual behaviors with adolescents through schools and health facilities. The rest of this chapter will now consider promising community-based activities which may provide an essential complement to such programs. These include broader interventions with schools and the general population, and programs which specifically target out-of-school youth, women, men, couples, and parents. Many of these interventions are interrelated. Some are already widely recommended and implemented in many parts of Africa, but they warrant renewed, intensive approaches. Others are relatively novel and have hardly been evaluated, and thus should be further developed and tested before possible implementation on a larger scale.

The following discussion is not intended to be an exhaustive review addressing every possible intervention and the evidence of effectiveness for each. Nor will it address all possible target groups or sexual risk behaviors. For example, it is beyond the scope of this book to examine specialized programs for high-risk populations, such as commercial sex workers or men who have sex with men, or interventions focused on non-sexual risk behaviors (e.g., alcohol abuse) which may influence sexual risk behaviors. As noted in chapter 1, several biomedical methods also show great promise in HIV prevention, including HIV testing, antiretroviral therapy, treatment of sexually transmitted infections, and male circumcision. Some of these have implications for the practice and effectiveness of low-risk sexual behaviors, but given limited space they also will not be examined in depth below.

INTERVENTIONS TO COMPLEMENT SCHOOL-BASED SEXUAL HEALTH PROGRAMS

The Broader School Environment

Whole School Ethos and Teaching Styles

In the *MEMA kwa Vijana* trial, severe limitations within the existing educational system greatly limited the potential of the program's school curriculum. One of the challenges facing the intervention, for example, was that the target population—pupils in Years 5–7 of primary school—typically ranged in age from twelve to eighteen years, but they could be as young as nine or as old as twenty-two, an age range that is not unusual in upper primary school classes across Tanzania (e.g., Leshabari, Kaaya, and Tengia-Kessy, 2008). It is very difficult to design an intervention that is appropriate and meets the needs of pupils with such varied social and sexual experiences and at such different stages of neurocognitive and physical development (Wilson et al., 2010).

The overall features of schools in high income countries have been found to influence many aspects of adolescent health and behavior, such as smoking, drinking, illegal drug use, and mental health (e.g., West, Sweeting, and Leyland, 2004; Aveyard et al., 2004; Bond et al., 2007; Henderson et al., 2008). Research has found that the quality of teacher-pupil interactions plays an important role in this, so positive teacher-pupil relationships have been central to the "Health Promoting School" model advocated by the World Health Organization (WHO, 1993; Swart and Reddy, 1999; WHO, 2003a; WHO, 2003b). In contrast, curriculum-based school health education specifically focused on sex, smoking, or illegal drugs has shown much less evidence of impact on those behaviors. Such specialized programs usually do not last more than twenty hours, while young people are exposed to general relationships in school for an estimated fifteen thousand hours, which helps explain their relative impacts (Rutter et al., 1979).

There has only been limited research on the impact of the broader school environment on adolescent health and behavior in sub-Saharan Africa (e.g., Mensch et al., 2001). In one HIV prevention program in South Africa, high school teachers received a four-day training in knowledge, facilitation skills, participatory teaching methods, and creating a safe and non-judgmental environment for students, before they implemented a sixteen-session program for Year 8 students in thirty schools (Helleve, Flisher, Onya, Mathews et al., 2011). Researchers found that students who perceived their teachers to care for their health and well-being were significantly less likely to report having started sexual activity, and intervention participants perceived greater care from their teachers than control participants did. This supports the HALIRA study finding that *MEMA kwa Vijana* intervention and control teachers who intervened when they believed pupils might be engaged in risk activities, and who expressed concern rather than punishing those pupils, sometimes successfully discouraged pupils' sexual risk behaviors.

These findings illustrate the need for substantial reforms to modify the school environment as a way of tackling HIV "upstream." Teacher training should promote new styles of teaching which: encourage critical thinking and problem solving; develop more supportive and less authoritarian teacher-pupil relationships to boost pupils' self-esteem and engagement in school; stimulate school girls' aspirations; and change the dominant school norms relating to gender. A promising example of such an intervention was implemented from 2003 to 2008 in 172 primary schools in Shinyanga Region, immediately south of Mwanza Region (Sedere, Mengele, and Kajela, 2008). In that program, teachers were trained to practice child-centered pedagogy and then received school-based mentoring and support. In addition to training to improve the quality of teacher-pupil relationships, however, reform also needs to take place at management and policy levels, particularly to prohibit, identify, and punish physical and sexual abuse by teachers.

In settings like Tanzania, where the quality of teacher training and primary school education is extremely poor, substantial improvement in the quality of the broader education system will take time. In the interim, other relatively simple and cost-effective methods of standardizing and improving educational standards could be employed on a large scale, such as interactive radio instruction. This method combines radio broadcasts with active learning to improve educational quality and teaching practices. It requires teachers and students to react verbally and physically to questions and exercises posed by radio characters, and to participate in group work, experiments, and other activities suggested by the radio program. Interactive radio instruction has been found to be effective in teaching basic primary subjects as well as HIV-related information in many parts of rural Africa (World Bank, 2005b).

Helping Young People Stay in School

The HALIRA study found that most primary school pupils desired to go on to secondary school, but few had the opportunity to do so, especially girls. Secondary school enrollment is particularly low in Tanzania, but this general pattern is not unusual elsewhere in sub-Saharan Africa. In 2002–2003, for example, the average number of students enrolled in secondary education as a percentage of the population of official school age was 7 percent for Tanzania and 28 percent for sub-Saharan Africa overall (Palmer et al., 2007).

Importantly, young people and especially young women who complete secondary school are more likely to report low-risk sexual practices and less likely to be HIV infected than those who did not attend secondary school (e.g., Mmbaga et al., 2007; Bastien, 2008; Biddlecom et al., 2008; Hargreaves et al., 2008; Jukes, Simmons, and Bundy, 2008; Moyo et al., 2008; Pettifor et al., 2008; Hargreaves and Howe, 2010; Adamczyk and Greif, 2011; Stroeken et al., 2012). There are several reasons why prolonged schooling might make young women less vulnerable to HIV infection. These include greater knowledge and/or understanding of sexual risks; greater confidence to resist sex or to negotiate safer sex; the cultural norm that school pupils should not be sexually active; increased behavioral monitoring by parents who have invested a lot in their daughters' schooling; and greater motivation of young women who have much to lose if they drop out because of pregnancy. In addition, education may distance female students from dangerous social environments, either because they develop safer social networks, or simply because they have to be in school (Hargreaves and Boler, 2006).

In South Africa and Malawi, programs are being tested in which current school girls and recent dropouts are provided with school fees and cash transfers on the condition that they stay in, or return to, school (e.g., Baird et al., 2009). However, even if such programs prove effective they would probably be too costly to deliver on a large scale in much of sub-Saharan Africa, where currently there are insufficient resources to provide adequate education to the pupils already attending schools. School feeding programs offer a more modest intervention to encourage school attendance. Such programs often take the form of volunteers providing a low-cost, simple breakfast to pupils before school. They have been demonstrated to increase school attendance as well as to reduce nutritional deficiencies (Greenhalgh, Kristjansson, and Robinson, 2007). Providing free menstrual products for school girls may also encourage attendance, as recently demonstrated in Ghana (Saïd Business School, 2010), because African girls often miss school when menstruating, due to inadequate soap, water, sanitary products, and toilet facilities in schools (Abrahams, Mathews, and Ramela, 2006; Sommer, 2009; Sommer, 2010). Another approach would be to address parents' limited expectations for their daughters, which can be a great obstacle to girls moving from primary to secondary school in many parts of sub-Saharan Africa (e.g., Warrington and Kiragu, 2011).

Although there is strong evidence that extending girls' schooling is protective in many ways, possible unintended negative effects of such interventions also need to be thoroughly evaluated. An authoritarian educational system that perpetuates negative gender stereotypes might weaken girls' self-esteem and sense of control, undermining their confidence to resist sex or negotiate safer sex. In addition, being at school makes girls vulnerable to sexually abusive teachers, a problem that has been recognized in many African countries, as discussed in chapter 5. Finally, for the minority of girls who attend secondary school, the need to obtain school fees and/or reduced parental supervision while boarding may result in increased sexual activity (e.g., Luke, 2003).

Out-of-School Youth

Although there are many challenges in working within existing school systems in sub-Saharan Africa, that institutional setting offers many advantages as well. Some adolescent sexual health programs have attempted to combine the benefits of working within school systems with those of working outside of them, primarily by selecting participants from student populations and conducting sessions at schools after school hours using independent curricula and implementers. The South African Stepping Stones intervention described in chapter 7 provides one example of how this can be done on a fairly large scale (Jewkes et al., 2006).

Notably, however, such interventions primarily work with student populations, so like school-based programs they hardly reach the sizable proportion of African adolescents who either never went to school or stopped schooling by early to mid adolescence (Singh, Bankole, and Woog, 2005). As already noted, unmarried out-of-school youth generally have been found to have higher risk practices than their school-going peers (e.g., Bastien, 2008; Moyo et al., 2008; Stroeken et al., 2012). While they would clearly benefit from HIV prevention interventions as well, the mechanisms to best reach them on a large scale are not obvious. Out-of-school youth represent diverse populations that typically only gather together in small groups and are unlikely to have much free time. Many young women are married with children and domestic duties, or are working full-time in their parents' homes and agricultural plots, while most out-of-school young men are engaged in work, at least during the day.

Some African sexual health interventions have used peer education to try to reach out-of-school youth. In one example, Ghanaian and Nigerian young people were trained to conduct peer education either in schools or out of school, and the relative impacts of the different interventions were then assessed (Brieger et al., 2001). The authors found that out-of-school peer education only had limited reach with out-of-school youth, and there was no intervention impact on those participants' reported behavioral determinants or behavior. In contrast, the school-based peer educators reached many more youths in their activities and also had a significant impact on their peers' reported knowledge, contraceptive self-efficacy, willingness to buy condoms, and use of modern contraceptives. The authors concluded that peer education was more effective within schools, because the institutional setting created larger and denser social networks than existed informally in the general community.

A peer education program for out-of-school youth in Cameroon had more promising results (Speizer, Tambashe, and Tegang, 2001). In that study, forty-two volunteer peer educators were recruited from schools and youth associations to participate in an initial one-week training and subsequent quarterly trainings for two years. During that period, peer educators worked at sports events and community gatherings, ultimately holding 353 discussion groups with twelve thousand young people and having personal contact with more than five thousand adolescents. The program evaluation found that contact with a peer educator was associated with greater unprompted knowledge of contraception and symptoms of sexually transmitted infection, and greater reported use of condoms and other contraception. The authors noted, however, that it was unclear whether such a community-based intervention could be replicated on a large scale.

A recent review of peer-led, community-based HIV prevention interventions for youth in low and middle income countries found several factors were necessary for effective peer education. These included: a community needs assessment; well-thought out selection of peer educators; adequate peer educator training, monitoring, and supervision; involvement of youth and community stakeholders in program development and implementation; a structure for program delivery; efforts to retain peer educators; a system to locate and train replacement peer educators; and a system for sustainability (Maticka-Tyndale and Barnett, 2010). Most of these features would involve considerable resources.

Other programs have attempted to reach out-of-school youth through interventions in formal and informal community settings without necessarily using peer educators. A review of community HIV prevention programs by Maticka-Tyndale and Brouillard-Coyle (2006) found that the most promising programs engaged in HIV prevention work within existing community groups or youth-service organizations (e.g., Gregson et al., 2004). In a study of 4,800 randomly selected fourteen- to twenty-two-year-olds in South Africa, for example, Camlin and Snow (2008) found that reported condom use at last sex was positively associated with participation in community groups (e.g., sports clubs, music clubs, church groups, and community organizations); this latter effect was particularly pronounced for girls. The authors proposed that social organizations can have a critical role in helping youth resist social norms that reinforce young people's—and particularly young women's—vulnerability to HIV infection.

Some researchers have argued that intervening with out-of-school youth in popular informal gathering places could be valuable, if the protective features of such places were augmented and the risk-related features reduced (e.g., Singh et al., 2010; Yamanis et al., 2010). However, such programs would probably require the creation of new systems and structure for delivery, and logistical concerns could take up time and resources that would otherwise be focused on intervention quality. Indeed, the review by Maticka-Tyndale and Brouillard-Coyle (2006) found that youth programs in geographically bounded communities (e.g., rural villages or urban neighborhoods) which required the creation of a new organization, and/or those which were implemented for the whole community through traditional or family networks or community-wide events (e.g., theatrical performances, health fairs, and competitions), have relatively little evidence of effectiveness in comparison to geographically bounded youth programs delivered through existing organizations or centers.

A different approach to interventions with out-of-school youth, and particularly adolescent girls and young women, involves microcredit or cash transfers. One Tanzanian study involved 2,399 eighteen- to thirty-year-old men and women who had mean individual annual earnings of $250 (de Walque et al., 2012). In that trial, intervention participants were eligible to receive payments of $10–$20 if they tested negative for curable sexually transmitted infections every four months. After twelve months, the authors found a significant reduction in the combined point prevalence of four curable sexually transmitted infections in the group that was eligible for $20 payments.

Other interventions specifically targeting adolescent girls and women have involved income-generating schemes, microfinance, or job training intended to reduce poverty-related transactional sex. Such programs will be discussed in the next section.

Women

The HALIRA study found that gender and age-related hierarchies inhibited young women's abilities to practice low-risk sexual behaviors. This was most evident in the common practices of coercive sex, intergenerational sex, transactional sex, and men's multiple partnerships described in chapter 3, each of which has also been found to undermine young women's ability to protect themselves in other African settings as well (UNAIDS, 2007; Underwood et al., 2011). The goal of reducing gender and generational inequalities through intervention is ambitious, but several programs have been developed and tested primarily to address these issues in eastern and southern Africa, including the Stepping Stones program discussed in chapter 7 (e.g., Michau and Naker, 2003; Naker and Michau, 2004; Jewkes et al., 2006; Michau, 2007). Some of these interventions seek to promote women's financial independence in order to reduce transactional sex that is primarily motivated by poverty (e.g., Hunter, 2002; Leclerc-Madlala, 2003; Pronyk et al., 2006; Pronyk et al., 2008).

For example, the Intervention with Microfinance for AIDS and Gender Equity (IMAGE) in South Africa combined microfinance targeted at very poor women with a participatory curriculum on gender and HIV education that was delivered through loan meetings. A randomized trial found that IMAGE had no effect on unprotected sex or HIV incidence in the wider community, but there was a 55 percent reduction in intimate partner violence reported by intervention participants (Pronyk et al., 2006). In addition, a follow-up study found that, when compared with women who only had participated in a microfinance program, IMAGE participants reported significantly greater empowerment and less intimate partner violence and sexual risk behaviors (Kim et al., 2009). As in any intervention evaluation based on self-reported data, it is possible that these results were biased by participant knowledge of program goals. Nonetheless, it is promising that these results support the Stepping Stones trial findings described in chapter 7, that interventions can modify the social and cultural environment that influences sexual risk and health (Jewkes et al., 2008; Jewkes, Wood, and Duvvury, 2010).

While income-generating programs have shown promise with adult women, relatively few have targeted adolescent girls and young women, and those programs have not had desirable results (e.g., Gupta et al., 2008; Dunbar et al., 2010). For example, one feasibility study provided life skills training, small loans, and mentorship to fifty adolescent female orphans in urban and peri-urban Zimbabwe (Dunbar et al., 2010). To do so, researchers relaxed core rules of microcredit programs and did not require that participants had their own savings or businesses; the program also did not follow a group-lending model. The microcredit program failed, and the researchers attributed this to a combination of the extremely harsh economic environment in Zimbabwe at the time, and participants' lack of business experience, capital, and family support. In addition, the intervention had the unintended consequence of making participants vulnerable to theft and physical harm, illustrating the importance of carefully evaluating interventions when they are adapted in new settings or populations. Similarly, a microcredit program in urban Kenya was found to have put young women at greater sexual risk, because they sometimes relied on transactional sex to meet the conditions of their loans (Gupta et al., 2008).

Finally, it is important to consider that, while providing alternative economic opportunities to young women may be a very important way to reduce their dependence on transactional sex, it is unlikely to end the practice, given how embedded it is in sexual cultures in sub-Saharan Africa. Girls might continue to practice material exchange for sex because of the self-esteem associated with it, and the few other ways they have to distinguish themselves. In addition, greater choice about whether or not to be sexually active may not be beneficial if it means girls only agree to have sex with more affluent men, as such men may be more likely to be HIV-infected. However, for those intervention participants who continue to engage in material exchange for sex, having some alternative income might help them to negotiate higher amounts and fewer sexual encounters, and/or to avoid multiple partners, high-risk sexual partners, or unprotected sex, if those risks are salient to them (e.g., Camlin and Snow, 2008). Given the complex motivations involved in material exchange for sex, such a harm-reduction approach aimed at altering the balance of power in sexual relationships might be more realistic than ending material exchange for sex entirely (Swidler and Watkins, 2007). More generally, alternative sources of income might enable young women to have a stronger identity independent of their boyfriends, encourage them to develop aspirations for the future, and help them access sexual health services.

Men

To date, gender-specific interventions to reduce sexual risk in sub-Saharan Africa have largely focused on ways to empower women and promote their negotiation skills, because men tend to be the decision-makers within sexual relationships. However, if men are primarily identified as a problem within sexual behavior change, interventions risk alienating them and provoking negative reactions (Montgomery et al., 2006). An approach that accentuates men's positive behavior and tries to re-shape masculinity around constructive elements is likely to be more effective (e.g., MacPhail, 2003; Naker and Michau, 2004; Peacock et al., 2008; Groes-Green, 2009b; Thaler and Sunstein, 2009; Jewkes, Wood, and Duvvury, 2010; Pulerwitz et al., 2010). Interventions targeting men may also be important if new economic and other opportunities are promoted for women, as discussed in the last section, because such programs might undermine men's conventional concept of their masculinity. This could have a counter-productive effect, unless there are simultaneous attempts to modify perceptions of masculinity so that men can feel masculine in ways other than economic power and physical dominance.

In rural Mwanza, for example, young villagers often admired and sought after urban styles, which suggests that low-risk sexual behaviors could be promoted for young men as modern, urban, smart, and/or cool methods of avoiding disease. Youth leaders and role models who are admired for their masculinity could be recruited for this approach, and they may also provide a valuable role in discussing strategies and experiences of risk reduction with their peers. In the HALIRA study, for example, several of the young men who reported secondary abstinence said it was most physically difficult during the first weeks after abstaining, but that it became progressively easier over time.

The potential for young men's sense of masculinity to shift in such ways is illustrated by a study in Mozambique which found that male secondary school students who consistently reported condom use after a peer education program tended to express a new and "modern" kind of masculinity (Groes-Green, 2009b). To those youths, condom use reflected that they were strong, in control, responsible, intelligent, and sexually experienced. They instead perceived others who did not use condoms as "ignorant." Alternative forms of masculinity could also be addressed in the promotion of abstinence (e.g., demonstrating physical self-control, or saving money to become financially independent), and in the promotion of partner reduction and fidelity (e.g., demonstrating responsibility and protection of a partner).

A recent review of research and programs relating to masculinity in sub-Saharan Africa identified four key principles for working with young men: discuss masculinity explicitly in educational activities; support individual changes with broader changes in social norms; build alliances; and recognize the multiple needs of young men (Barker and Ricardo, 2005). That report also identified factors which promote gender equality, health-protective behaviors, and non-violence amongst young men, each of which could be targeted within sexual health interventions. Those factors include: self-reflection and scope to rehearse new behaviors; a sense of responsibility and positive engagement as fathers; rites of passage and traditions that constitute positive forms of social control; close relatives who model more equitable or non-violent behaviors; and community mobilization to address young men's vulnerabilities.

In addition, given sexual encounters largely are controlled by boys and men in sub-Saharan Africa, it is also critical that interventions address male motivation, and particularly male risk perception and desire for self-preservation.

Indeed, the HALIRA study found that these factors were some of the strongest motivators for young men who actively tried to practice low-risk behaviors. One intervention in Nigeria specifically tried to target men's sense of personal susceptibility, with promising results: after two five-hour workshops, intervention participants reported fewer risk behaviors and less male dominance in their primary partnerships than men in a control group (Exner et al., 2009).

It would also be useful to explore how other preexisting motivations for men may be exploited to reduce sexual risk, such as male bonding, marital harmony, protecting a partner, and maintaining good relationships with in-laws or respectability in the village. Research in rural Malawi found that men's current extramarital sexual behavior was closely correlated with their best friends', leading the author to propose that men's social networks be used to discourage extramarital sexual relationships (Clark, 2010). One possible model for such an intervention could involve anti-AIDS self-help groups, as a study with male workers in the informal sector in Kenya found that longer participation in such groups was associated with higher reports of consistent condom use with casual partners (Ferguson et al., 2004).

Similarly, in a male-initiated indigenous response to the AIDS epidemic in eastern Uganda, members of a town's taxi drivers' association recognized that extramarital relationships undermined household economic development and made them highly vulnerable to HIV infection (Parikh, 2007). They therefore initiated meetings where the men engaged in activities to discourage extramarital relationships and to reinforce marital bonds. For example, each member was required to bring his wife (or wives) to these meetings and to stand with her (or them) to recite her name (or their names) during the opening roll call. At each meeting, a randomly selected couple also received a monetary prize supplied from the membership dues, thereby encouraging ongoing participation. This occupational association attempted to compensate for the diminishing influence extended families have in regulating sexuality today. In addition, it introduced spouses to the culturally unfamiliar practices of socializing together and expressing affection in public, encouraging commitment and emotional intimacy.

Finally, one important avenue for sexual health interventions with young people, and especially young men, is HIV prevention programs integrated within sports activities (e.g., Molassiotis et al., 2004; Beutler, 2008; Delva et al., 2010; Mwaanga, 2010). In rural Mwanza, as in many parts of Africa, when male youth were not engaged in income-generating activities they often focused on seducing or pressuring girls and women to have sex (e.g., Beutler, 2008). However, male youth also greatly enjoyed playing and watching sports, particularly soccer, even when the only equipment available was a ball of rags tied together. The *MEMA kwa Vijana* intervention took advantage of this inclination by encouraging sports activities and competitions during the program's Youth Health Week. Nonetheless, this was an optional and relatively minor aspect of the broader intervention, and its practice varied widely from school to school.

As Khan (2010, 6) notes, many different HIV prevention initiatives in Africa have exploited "the competitive, team based, participatory and communicative aspects of [soccer] to facilitate both knowledge acquisition and the development of communication skills, leadership skills, and life skills." These programs sometimes use local coaches whose soccer skills and knowledge of their communities make them credible role models. The activities can attract large groups, providing excellent platforms to mobilize populations, promote HIV prevention messages, and deliver related interventions such as HIV counseling and testing services. Some programs have also drawn on the endorsement of soccer celebrities and mass media reinforcement.

One example of soccer-based HIV prevention is the Grassroot Soccer initiative that started in Zimbabwe and now has projects in 14 African countries (e.g., Fuller et al., 2010; Khan, 2010). The curriculum is led by trained volunteer community role models and consists of eight forty-five-minute sessions of soccer activities to deliver HIV prevention and life skills education. Evaluation of the program found it improved participants' knowledge, attitudes, and decision-making skills; reduced AIDS-related stigma; and reduced reported sexual risk behaviors. In a similar initiative in Dar es Salaam, Tanzania, peer coaches provided HIV education to early adolescent soccer teams over a two-month period, and this was found to improve participants' knowledge, attitudes, and perceived behavior control (Maro, Roberts, and Sørenson, 2009).

While sports-based interventions show substantial promise, they need further exploration and evaluation, particularly to establish how they can be delivered on a wide scale at low cost without losing their impact. They also need careful monitoring to prevent unintended consequences. The HALIRA study found, for example, that rural youth often used sports events as opportunities to negotiate and have sex, particularly with strangers, so programs would need to be carefully monitored to ensure that they did not inadvertently contribute to sexual risk behaviors.

Couples

HIV prevention programs which target both members of a couple may be very valuable, as both individuals need to cooperate for low-risk sexual behaviors to be most protective. Both need to be involved in mutual HIV testing and mutual fidelity, for example, and condom use also often involves the consent of both individuals in a couple, although in some circumstances the man alone may determine it. As Burton, Darbes, and Operario (2010, 2) note:

> ... couples-focused HIV prevention programs may differ from individual-focused HIV prevention programs by addressing the ongoing dynamic and interactional forces within dyads that contribute to sexual risk behavior, including gender roles, power imbalances, communication styles, child-bearing intentions, and quality of relationship issues (e.g., commitment, satisfaction, intimacy).

To date, most couple-oriented HIV prevention interventions in sub-Saharan Africa have targeted married couples and/or couples in which one partner is HIV-positive (e.g., Gregson et al., 1998; Painter, 2001; Zulu and Chepngeno, 2003; Watkins, 2004; Parikh, 2007; Montgomery et al., 2008; Miller et al., 2009; Burton, Darbes, and Operario, 2010; Njau et al., 2011; Venkatesh et al., 2012; Wall et al., 2012). It is likely that interventions for other kinds of couples have been more limited because of the challenges they pose. For example, it is difficult to design an intervention targeting couples in brief, casual relationships specifically because the relationships are transient and the individuals involved may not know one another well. Similarly, it would be challenging to develop a couple-oriented intervention for unmarried adolescents in ongoing relationships, because those relationships are likely to be hidden. Recognizing such limitations, the following section will none-theless consider the possibility of intervening with couples in three types of partnerships which may be common for young people in rural Africa: hidden and unacknowledged couples (e.g., unmarried adolescents); couples who are planning to marry; and married couples.

Hidden or Unacknowledged Couples

As noted earlier, the HALIRA study found that most fifteen-year-old boys and girls had had sex, and girls were especially likely to have ongoing rela-tionships, often with older youths and men. Given the hidden nature of such relationships, it would be difficult to tailor an intervention for such couples, but nonetheless the possibility should be explored rather than rejected out-right. One possibility, for instance, is to create programs with trusted com-munity confidants who make themselves available to give confidential advice to young couples. "Senga" interventions in southern Uganda provide one example of how this might be done (Muyinda et al., 2001; Muyinda et al., 2003; Tamale, 2006). Traditionally sengas, or paternal aunts, educated their nieces at marriage about sex, how to please their husbands, and how to be "good" subservient wives. The institution has been resilient and adaptable, with commercial sengas becoming popular on FM radio call-in programs and in newspapers today (Tamale, 2006). In the past, sengas reinforced wives' subordinate role but they also celebrated sexuality, and today commercial sengas often challenge gender roles and educate women about their bodies and female sexual pleasure (Tamale, 2006).

In one study in Uganda, female villagers elected adolescent girls and women to take on the role of sengas (Muyinda et al., 2003). These modern sengas were given seven days' training and then offered advice to thirteen- to nineteen-year-old females about sex, sexual health, and relationship problems. The researchers were surprised, however, by the high uptake of senga services by the broader community, with half of all visits from non-target groups, that is, adolescent boys, adult men, and adult women. A senga-like initiative could also be explored within African ethnic groups like the Sukuma, which do not have such a tradition, and confidential counseling of unmarried couples on HIV testing, fidelity, and condom use could be an objective of it.

Programs targeting young, unmarried couples would ideally focus on decision-making, communication, and relationship skills. The HALIRA study found, for example, that adolescent sexual relationships often developed very quickly, as young couples typically had sex soon after first expressing attraction for one another and negotiating the money or materials to be exchanged. While desire, possessiveness, and affection were not unusual in premarital sexual relationships, there was little evidence of emotional intimacy. In addition, although young people highly valued a partner's fidelity, they often did not feel conflicted about their own infidelity, even if they sought to hide it to avoid confrontation.

Other recent African studies have similarly found that unmarried adolescents often perceived sex as natural, utilitarian, pleasurable, and passionate, but there was little evidence that they experienced emotional intimacy within their sexual relationships (e.g., Balmer et al., 1997; Nzioka, 2004; Silberschmidt and Rasch, 2001; Undie, Crichton, and Zulu, 2007). Interventions for unmarried individuals and couples could thus promote more thoughtful partner selection prior to beginning relationships, as well as responsibility, skills, and strategies to help couples have stronger and more enduring relationships once they begin, so they can work through and resolve problems rather than simply change partners. The Stepping Stones intervention described in chapter 7 provides one example of how an in-depth, participatory intervention can help facilitate stronger and more gender-equitable relationships, although that intervention primarily worked with same sex groups rather than couples (Jewkes et al., 2008; Jewkes, Wood, and Duvvury, 2010).

Given few programs have attempted to promote fidelity with young, unmarried couples, and particularly adolescents, it would be important to closely evaluate new interventions to ensure that they do not have unintended consequences. For example, interventions should be careful in how they address romantic love, which has been described as an intense attraction involving idealization of a partner, with an erotic component and an expectation of a shared future (Jankowiak and Fischer, 1992; Giddens, 1992; Vaughan, 2009). Recently, there has been an increase in research on romantic love in sub-Saharan Africa, and this implicitly relates to the role it may have in mutual monogamy and sexual risk reduction (e.g., Samuelsen, 2006; Cole and Thomas, 2009). In the absence of a romantic belief that two individuals are uniquely suited to one another, it may be that each partner feels less desire or obligation to practice monogamy or to stay in a relationship if problems arise. However, a study in South Africa suggests that romantic ideals taken to an extreme may also involve higher risk (Harrison et al., 2006). That study found that young women who were "hyperromantic"—that is, who strongly expressed beliefs in an intimate relationship's importance, such as "I cannot live without my partner for even one day"—reported significantly more sexual partners in the last three months than other women. The authors postulated that young women with such extreme romantic beliefs had higher numbers of partners because they were desperate to experience an emotional connection within an intimate relationship at all times.

Couples Planning to Marry

Another key life stage that might be targeted in couple interventions is when young couples plan to marry. As noted earlier, in the HALIRA study half of randomly selected female in-depth interview respondents had married by the end of the trial; approximately half of those young women married by engagement, and the other half by elopement. Engagement usually involved a brief period of about one month between the couple first meeting and officially being married, and there were some formal steps during that period which could be exploited in HIV prevention work. One important step involved the man obtaining the permission of the young woman's parents or guardians, including an agreement of bridewealth conditions. In-depth interview respondents from different districts who were members of the Protestant African Inland Church additionally reported that, prior to marrying, they were required by their church to have medical tests to ensure they did not bring infections into the marriage; they did not specify HIV tests, but this was implied. Other churches elsewhere in Africa have also mandated HIV testing prior to marriage (e.g., Arulogun and Adefioye, 2010).

A similar, secular initiative could target communities, families, and couples to promote HIV testing as a routine step in the broader engagement process. If this were made into a widespread practice and presented as a recommended general health check at the time of an important life transition—conducted to promote the family's future health and fertility—it may reduce personalized questions about trust and prior sexual partners. Such an intervention could be tailored to accommodate polygynous unions as well, which in settings such as rural Mwanza constituted approximately one-quarter of marriages. In addition, if HIV testing and counseling became a widely accepted procedure for young engaged couples, testing services could also be discreetly promoted for couples planning to elope, or—if they have already eloped—who are new to marriage. Critically, such services would need to be affordable, accessible, and confidential.

Married Couples

Marriage frequently was believed to be protective for young adults in rural Mwanza, as elsewhere in Africa, on the assumption that faithful spouses would not introduce new infections into a marriage. Similarly, some African studies have found that people may strategically try to reduce their risk by marrying a low-risk partner, or communicating with a spouse to improve the spouse's risk perception and persuade them to be faithful (e.g., Gregson et al., 1998; Zulu and Chepngeno, 2003; Watkins, 2004; Reniers, 2008). Nonetheless, marriage may involve relatively high risk for some individuals, particularly for women, because older, higher risk men often marry younger, lower risk women, and because extramarital sexual relationships are not uncommon, especially for men (e.g., Caldwell, Caldwell, and Quiggin, 1989; Omorodian, 1993; Ferguson et al., 2004; Helle-Valle, 2004; Kimuna and Djamba, 2005; Clark, Bruce, and Dude, 2006; Parikh, 2007; Jana, Nkambule, and Tumbo, 2008; Smith, 2009; Hirsch et al., 2009; Hageman et al., 2010).

Interventions with married couples might engage with participants about how to address sensitive issues within their relationships. For example, a study of committed couples in Kenya identified several strategies couples used to address sensitive topics, including monitoring a spouse's mood, gradual or indirect revelation, and using select third-parties as intermediaries (Miller et al., 2009). In rural Mwanza, as in many other parts of Africa, neither abstinence nor condom use were considered an option for newly married couples, as they typically sought to have a child within a year of marrying (e.g., Chimbiri, 2007; Speizer and White, 2008). Strategies for practicing long-term, mutual fidelity thus should be intensively promoted with young married couples, taking advantage of the fact that fidelity is already supported by community ideals. Such ideals also can be carefully reinforced in interventions in the broader community. Given the scale-up of HIV-testing services in many African countries, behavioral interventions also increasingly can promote early and repeated testing at intervals throughout a marriage, involving couples learning their test results together or disclosing their status to each other soon after receiving results. As noted above, all efforts to promote mutual fidelity within a monogamous marriage could similarly be applied to polygynous marriages.

Finally, sexual risk reduction programs for young married individuals could promote abstinence and/or condom use in particular circumstances, for example, during the postpartum period, or when a couple are separated due to travel. In the 2010 Tanzanian Demographic and Health Survey, for instance, approximately half of women who gave birth in the three years prior to the survey reported they had abstained from sexual intercourse for four months after childbirth (National Bureau of Statistics and ORC Macro, 2011). Condom use by young married couples may also have more potential if promoted for pregnancy prevention and fertility protection after a couple has had one or more children, if they wish to space their remaining children. In a study of thirty-eight married Ugandan couples who reported consistent condom use, for example, women reported that they had convinced their husbands to use condoms by insistence, refusal to have sex, persuasion, and arguments in favor of condoms for family planning or, indirectly, to protect their children (Williamson et al., 2006). Finally, condom promotion for young married individuals and couples may have the most potential and importance if targeted toward extramarital relationships, as a way to demonstrate care for a spouse and to protect marital health, fertility, and harmony by avoiding unwanted pregnancy and infection (e.g., Adetunji, 2000; Chimbiri, 2007).

Parents

The HALIRA study found that parental supervision, connection, and positive communication influenced some adolescents who actively tried to practice low-risk sexual behaviors, as has similarly been found elsewhere in sub-Saharan Africa (e.g., Babalola, Tambashe, and Vondrasek, 2005; Kumi-Kyereme et al., 2007; Amoran and Fawole, 2008; Camlin and Snow, 2008; Biddlecom, Awusabo-Asare, and Bankole, 2009; Peltzer, 2009; Puffer et al., 2011; Wamoyi et al., 2011b; Wamoyi et al., 2011c; Crichton, Ibisomi, and Gyimah, 2012). Some African studies have found that the presence of a father in a household is protective for young people, and particularly girls (e.g., Ngom, Magadi, and Owuor, 2003; Babalola, Tambashe, and Vondrasek, 2005). In the HALIRA study, however, as well as a later qualitative study in Mwanza Region (Wamoyi et al., 2011b), the quality of parent-child relationships seemed to influence young people's low-risk behaviors more than the specific presence of a father in the household. The research in Mwanza suggests that many girls living with their fathers were simply more secretive about their sexual behavior than those living with their mothers only.

The World Health Organization has identified five dimensions of parenting which influence adolescent health outcomes: connection, behavior control, respect for individuality, modeling of appropriate behavior, and provision and protection (WHO, 2007a). Research projects and non-governmental organizations in sub-Saharan Africa have developed interventions to promote those parenting skills in general and also specifically as a way to facilitate adolescent sexual risk reduction (WHO, 2007b). Some research-led initiatives have adapted programs initially designed for African Americans in the United States, such as the Collaborative HIV Prevention and Adolescent Mental Health (CHAMP) Program in South Africa (Bhana et al., 2004; Paruk, Petersen, and Bhana, 2009; Bhana et al., 2010) and the Families Matter program in Kenya (Poulsen et al., 2010). A before-and-after study of the latter program found that it was highly acceptable to parents, it changed their initially negative views about parent-child communication about sex, and it increased such communication (Vandenhoudt et al., 2010). Similarly, a ten-session program for mothers was incorporated into the IMAGE trial in South Africa described above. An evaluation of that mothering program found it increased women's HIV knowledge and awareness, gave them a sense of responsibility to protect young people from sexual risks, and helped them challenge cultural norms and taboos around sexuality (Phetla et al., 2008).

The HALIRA study findings detailed in this book and its companion volume (Plummer and Wight, 2011) highlight several areas which could be addressed within parenting interventions to promote adolescent sexual health. Such interventions would ideally address the contradictory sexual norms and expectations that young people face in many African communities. For example, the HALIRA study found that men and boys frequently approached adolescent girls in public settings to negotiate sex, but other adults rarely questioned this. Parents and other villagers could consider how men approaching girls in this way could be held more accountable. Parents might also consider how the common expectation that adolescent daughters should provide for many of their own material needs contributes to transactional sex, as has also been found in some other African studies (e.g., Camlin and Snow, 2008). Parents could be involved in identifying alternative ways to meet girls' material needs, such as increasing parental support, or assisting girls to pursue money-earning activities which are typically only available to boys. The goal of greater recognition of young people's existing sexual relationships is particularly relevant to parenting programs, as parental acknowledgement would be important in strengthening their children's relationships through social endorsement and accountability. Parenting interventions might also address constructive ways to react to youth sexual activity when it is discovered after the fact.

Within parenting programs, focusing primarily on risks facing adolescents and young adults would be regarded as legitimate and would harness parents' preexisting motivation to protect them. Such interventions are thus likely to be well received from the start at all levels of society. For example, the 2008–2012 Tanzanian government policy on HIV/AIDS identified a need for parental involvement in youth HIV prevention (TACAIDS, 2007). However, a secondary parenting intervention objective could be to raise parents' awareness of their own sexual risks. The HALIRA study found, for example, that parents often said it was challenging to communicate with their children about HIV prevention, in part because they themselves understood too little about it and felt ill-prepared and uncomfortable with the topic. Similar findings have been documented elsewhere in sub-Saharan Africa (e.g., Paruk et al., 2005; Mbonile and Kayombo, 2008; Phetla et al., 2008; Remes et al., 2010; Bastien, Kajula, and Muhwezi, 2011).

After the *MEMA kwa Vijana* trial, needs assessment was conducted with parents in four Mwanza villages and the results were used to develop and pilot test a program for parents of ten- to fourteen-year-olds (Remes et al., 2010). This program, called *Mema kwa Jamii* (Good Things for the Community), aims to promote positive norms and behaviors around sexual health at a community level by raising awareness of the issues, addressing prevailing power relations between men and women, promoting parenting skills and knowledge, and strengthening community efficacy to influence children's futures. The intervention consists of five participatory sessions with formal and informal village opinion leaders, who then go on to facilitate similar sessions with other villagers, who then train groups of their own peers within a cascading design.

General Population

Finally, there are many different kinds of HIV prevention activities which can target general rural African populations in ways that reinforce and support adolescent sexual health programs, including condoms social marketing, outreach by health workers or people living with HIV/AIDS, and public broadcast campaigns. Each of these will be discussed briefly below.

Condom Distribution

Condom distribution was extremely low in rural Mwanza at the time of the *MEMA kwa Vijana* trial, and it remains very low in many parts of rural Africa today (e.g., Papo et al., 2011). As Price (2001, 234) notes in a review of condom social marketing for poor populations, "[Condom social marketing programs] tend to reach the non-poor first because formal distribution networks make sales of social marketing products easier in urban areas; it takes time and effort to develop informal distribution networks in peri-urban and rural areas." Indeed, the *MEMA kwa Vijana* condom distribution initiative described in chapter 6 illustrates how, in a context of extremely limited resources and infrastructure, condom distribution can be very challenging and costly.

Clearly, limited demand for condoms contributed to their limited supply in rural Mwanza. The negative attitudes toward condoms described in chapter 3 meant that many villagers would not have adopted condom use even if their misconceptions were addressed and condoms were made more accessible. Nonetheless, even in such a hostile environment a small minority of young people used condoms to prevent pregnancy (particularly school girls), and/or to reduce risk of infection (particularly men with casual partners). If condom promotion were optimized in rural areas—that is, if misconceptions about them were widely addressed, and if they were made much more accessible to youth and adults alike—it seems likely that more young people would adopt condom use for the same reasons. However, if condoms are to be promoted to their maximum potential in rural Africa, much more needs to be invested in "best practice" social marketing and distribution campaigns to substantially increase their availability, accessibility, and acceptability (Hattori, Richter, and Greene, 2008; Charania et al., 2011).

Health Worker Outreach

One of the more innovative and effective aspects of the *MEMA kwa Vijana* intervention was health worker outreach with young people, as discussed in chapter 6. Relatively few school and community-based interventions have involved local health workers, although they are often a respected community authority on sexual health issues (e.g., Agbemenu and Schlenk, 2011). In one promising example in Malawi, trained government health workers facilitated same-sex groups of villagers in six two-hour sessions (Kaponda et al., 2011). That intervention provided information about sexual health and safer sex and also focused on skills-building, using group feedback, support, and discussions to clarify values and change group norms. Over two thousand adults in one district participated in that program, and evaluators found it had a positive impact on knowledge and reported attitudes and behaviors.

There is a well documented health worker shortage in Tanzania and many other parts of Africa, and health services in rural areas are particularly poor (WHO, 2006). Large-scale adolescent sexual health interventions involving government health workers thus would need to consider the extent to which existing health worker productivity could be improved to accommodate additional responsibilities, and the extent to which the workforce would need to be expanded to accommodate them (Kurowski et al., 2003; Mc-Kinsey and Company, 2005; Mæstad, 2006; Kinfu et al., 2009). Importantly, while any large-scale intervention would require financial investment, those working with existing government health workers and facilities are likely to be more sustainable and cost-effective than those requiring substantially increased staff and infrastructure.

Outreach by People Living with HIV/AIDS

As noted earlier in the chapter, young people who had a realistic sense of their susceptibility to HIV and other sexually transmitted infections—and the potential severity of those conditions—were more likely to actively reduce their sexual risk behaviors. However, developing such an awareness can be difficult in settings where people believe that healthy-appearing people cannot be infected or infectious. As discussed in chapter 3, symptoms were very important in illness recognition, diagnosis, and treatment in rural Mwanza, and once symptoms resolved people were generally believed to have been cured of an illness. In such contexts promoting intervention participants' understanding of HIV susceptibility and severity is particularly challenging, because the majority of people living with HIV do not have symptoms, especially in the era of large-scale antiretroviral therapy services.

In both high income and low income countries, some interventions have responded to this challenge by involving people living with HIV and AIDS as public speakers. HIV-positive educators can play a valuable role by sharing their personal accounts of exposure, particularly if they come from similar backgrounds to the audience, as this can increase intervention participant identification with them. In addition, HIV-positive educators can convey the importance of testing and early treatment to stay healthy; illustrate how difficult it is to know someone's status (if they appear healthy), or how devastating AIDS itself can be (if they have full-blown AIDS); and explain that—even with the benefits of antiretroviral therapy—there can be many unpleasant side effects and other challenges related to living with HIV which make it critical to avoid infection, if possible. In South Africa, for example, a training course attached to a microfinance scheme incorporated HIV-positive guest speakers, and this was found to have a crucial role in motivating participants to take HIV seriously (Phetla et al., 2008).

Mass Media Interventions

Finally, mass media interventions can offer relatively simple and low-cost support to adolescent sexual health programs by improving knowledge and attitudes at a population level, especially when initial awareness levels are very low (e.g., Katz, 2006; Bertrand and Anhang, 2006; Bankole, Biddlecom et al., 2007; Van Rossem and Meekers, 2007; Bankole et al., 2009; Mitchell et al., 2011). Such programs seek to change knowledge, attitudes, and behaviors by disseminating messages to a broad audience through radio, television, video/DVD, print media, mobile phones, or the internet. Mass media interventions exist in most African settings, but they rarely have been optimized, so there remains potential to strengthen, diversify, and expand them. For example, while improved knowledge is usually considered the first and easiest step toward sexual behavior change, this fundamental step clearly had not been achieved in rural Mwanza at the time of the *MEMA kwa Vijana* trial, and basic knowledge of HIV and AIDS remains low in many parts of sub-Saharan Africa today. As Thornton (2008, 223) notes in his discussion of the epidemics in Uganda and South Africa: "While it is not enough simply to know more about HIV and AIDS, it is also clearly detrimental to personal and public health to know nothing at all, to know only a little, or to know the wrong things."

"Edutainment" programs which combine education with entertainment in health promotion have been found to improve knowledge, to create positive attitudes, to shift norms, and to change reported behaviors (e.g., Vaughan et al., 2000; Singhal et al., 2004; Bankole et al., 2009). Dramas such as soap operas can strengthen an audience's engagement with a topic through the relationships that they make with positive or negative characters (Papa et al., 2000). In rural sub-Saharan Africa, where electricity and television access is extremely low, mass media programs for youth have typically involved radio programs (such as advertisements, talk shows, and drama serials) and print materials (such as posters and leaflets) (e.g., Kim et al., 2001; Peltzer and Seoka, 2004; Fonseca-Becker, Bakadi, and Sow, 2005; Underwood et al., 2006).

In Tanzania, for example, the 2010 Demographic and Health Survey found that 55 percent of rural households owned a radio and 34 percent owned a mobile telephone, but only 3 percent owned a television (National Bureau of Statistics and ORC Macro, 2011). That survey found that the family planning radio dramas *Twende na Wakati* and *Zinduka* (Wake Up/Become Aware), which have aired twice per week since 1993, have had substantial reach in rural areas (Jato et al., 1999; Rogers et al., 1999). In the six months prior to the survey, 28 percent of rural men and 20 percent of rural women had listened to *Twende na Wakati*, while 24 percent and 17 percent had listened to *Zinduka*, respectively (National Bureau of Statistics and ORC Macro, 2011).

Edutainment programs are likely to be most effective when locally produced and complemented by community-based support activities (Bertrand

and Anhang, 2006). For example, the Tanzanian *Sikia Kengele* campaign has combined radio programming with "big bell" community mobilization and "bell ringer" interpersonal activities, to promote reduced partner number and fidelity from a secular perspective (Mahler and Ndegwa, 2008). In the last decade, other Tanzanian initiatives have used multimedia specifically to target youth in Swahili, including the *Pilika Pilika* (Busy Busy) radio soap opera; televised music competitions like "Bongo Star Search"; Fema and *Si Mchezo!* (No Joke!) magazines; special series of sexual and reproductive health information booklets; and the *"chezasalama"* (play safely) website (Görgen et al., 2002; Femina Health Information Project, 2008). These initiatives have made creative use of pop culture, music, and drama to produce appealing edutainment for youth. However, with the exception of the radio program, they primarily serve urban and/or relatively educated audiences due to poor rural education, infrastructure, and utilities.

Finally, music provides a very valuable opportunity to promote low-risk sexual behaviors with rural African youth in a culturally relevant and affordable way (Bastien, 2009). Since the 1990s, for example, local and national musicians in Tanzania have produced a multitude of AIDS-related songs which have been popularized through the media. Using AIDS metaphors and narratives, these songs often promote abstinence, partner number reduction, avoidance of high-risk partners, fidelity, and condom use in culturally compelling ways (Bastien, 2009). Such popular, indigenous HIV prevention efforts warrant much more exploration for their potential within systematic edutainment campaigns in rural Africa.

THE IMPORTANCE OF INTERVENTION EVALUATION

Across sub-Saharan Africa many millions of dollars are spent each year on a wide range of HIV prevention programs, yet very few are evaluated to assess their impact. The people delivering those interventions may have good intentions and may be convinced of their effectiveness, but policy makers need to allocate their resources on the basis of evidence. Impact data are essential in such considerations, and evidence of cost-effectiveness is ideal (Mavedzenge, Doyle, and Ross, 2011). However, it is additionally important to understand the processes leading to any impact, or lack thereof, so that effective programs can be sustained and scaled-up, while ineffective ones are improved or discontinued (Pawson and Tilley, 1997). For instance, some of the promising, innovative interventions discussed in this chapter are largely untested, so they would require careful piloting and evaluation before broader implementation.

Chapter 1 reviewed some of the main approaches to intervention evaluation. Three additional considerations will be highlighted here. First, while more evaluation of HIV prevention interventions would be valuable, this does not necessarily require highly complex and expensive study designs. As discussed in chapter 1, for example, a randomized controlled trial may be a rigorous way to assess the impact of certain kinds of interventions, but it is not always appropriate, affordable, or effective in assessing interventions which promote behavior change (Kippax, 2003; Kippax and Stephenson, 2005; Bonell et al., 2006; Pettifor et al., 2007; Bonell et al., 2011; Laga et al., 2012). The few randomized controlled trials of behavioral interventions in sub-Saharan Africa have found little robust evidence of effectiveness, particularly in terms of biological outcomes (Hayes et al., 2010). However, if other forms of careful evaluation are considered, there is reasonable evidence that behavior change has occurred to varying extents in response to HIV prevention efforts in different African countries (Ferguson, Dick, and Ross, 2006; Pettifor et al., 2007; The International Group on Analysis of Trends in HIV Prevalence and Behaviors in Young People in Countries Most Affected by HIV, 2010; Michielsen et al., 2010; UNAIDS, 2010; Katsidzira and Hakim, 2011; Mavedzenge, Doyle, and Ross, 2011). Triangulation of multiple sources of quantitative and qualitative data can be particularly useful, and indeed may be critical in measuring and interpreting complex behavioral outcomes (Kippax and Stephenson, 2005; Bonell et al., 2011).

The second factor to take in consideration in evaluating behavioral programs is timescale. It is often hoped that behavioral programs will benefit health in the way that a vaccination or inoculation does, through a one-off, brief intervention with a demonstrable and immediate outcome. However, long-term behavior change can be a complex, subtle, and variable process, so behavioral programs are more likely to protect or improve health in the way that good nutrition does, through continuous practice over a very long period (Kippax and Stephenson, 2005; Eccles, 2008). Furthermore, with some behavioral programs the effect may not be linear but may instead involve a tipping point, before which there is little detectable impact and after which there is a major impact (Ross, 2010). This has profound implications both for interventions and their evaluation, suggesting that both need to be carried out over much longer time periods than are generally practiced at present.

Finally, the third consideration related to intervention evaluation is the need to improve program transparency and the availability of evaluation findings. Historically, detailed descriptions of programs have been difficult to access, and few interventions published their process and impact evaluation findings. Today the internet provides an unprecedented opportunity to share experiences with other program developers, and thus to improve "best practice" interventions globally. Ideally, leaders of carefully designed and implemented sexual health projects in sub-Saharan Africa would make their detailed curricula, training manuals, and process and impact evaluation reports available online, in all languages in which they are drafted. Given many program managers have limited time, funding, and technological expertise to achieve this—and in order to make the materials easier to locate—it may be most practical for an international body such as the World Health Organization to sponsor a central website where such materials are organized.

CONCLUSION

The HALIRA study found that many adolescents in rural Mwanza began engaging in unprotected sexual intercourse at a young age; studies elsewhere in sub-Saharan Africa have had similar findings (e.g., Doyle et al., 2012). Effective adolescent sexual health interventions are urgently needed in rural Africa, and school systems offer the most feasible and sustainable way to reach rural adolescents on a large scale. However, the *MEMA kwa Vijana* trial found that the fairly simple promotion of different low-risk sexual behaviors within an "abstinence-plus" school program did not have the desired impact on behaviors, unintended pregnancy, or sexually transmitted infections. The HALIRA findings suggest that school-based programs are more likely to be effective if they comprehensively address each potential low-risk sexual behavior with explicit information and skills development, including abstinence, selecting low-risk partners, limiting partner number, avoiding overlapping partners or short gaps between partners, being faithful, and using condoms.

The findings presented here further suggest that it may not be feasible to implement a high quality, comprehensive, and effective intervention at a low cost in a setting where infrastructure and capacity are extremely limited. Instead, the most successful school-based programs are likely to be intensive, in-depth, and integrated with similarly intensive and in-depth programs which target out-of-school youth and adults in the broader community. Implementing such complex, combined interventions is likely to be substantially more challenging and costly than simple, individual-level interventions. The increased funding involved in developing, implementing, and evaluating such programs may seem like a luxury, given limited resources and the urgency of the AIDS epidemic in sub-Saharan Africa. However, such an expanded approach may be essential if programs are to have a genuine and sustained impact on adolescent sexual risk behaviors and health.

APPENDICES

Appendix 1. Outline of the Teacher's Guide for Year 5 in the Final MEMA kwa Vijana School Curriculum[a]

Box 5.1 describes the content of the drama, story, and letter serial used in Year 5 sessions 7–10.

Session No.	Title o Teaching Methods	Objectives	Key Points
1	What is reproductive health and why is it important? o Group discussion	1. Outline the topics that will be addressed in reproductive health education. 2. Explain why it is important to learn about reproductive health. 3. Agree to ground rules for participating in these lessons.	1. Do not feel shy or embarrassed during these lessons. Feel free to share what you know so that it can be discussed. 2. Pay careful attention to what you learn here so you can do well in exams and, more importantly, make wise decisions in your life.
2	Leaving childhood: Puberty o Group discussion o Flipchart	1. Explain what puberty is and the changes that take place during puberty. 2. Explain the relationship between puberty and pregnancy.	1. Once a girl enters puberty she can become pregnant even if she only has sex one time. 2. Once a boy enters puberty he can make a girl pregnant even if he only has sex one time.
3	What are HIV and AIDS? o Group discussion o Flipchart o Personalization exercise	1. Explain the difference between HIV and AIDS. 2. Clarify the different ways in which HIV can be transmitted. 3. State the common symptoms of AIDS.	1. You cannot get infected with HIV through everyday contact with someone who has HIV. 2. The main way to become infected with HIV is through sex with someone who has HIV. 3. In many cases, those who are infected with HIV mistakenly believed they were not in danger of becoming infected, so they did not take precautions. 4. Everyone has the ability to protect themselves from HIV. 5. A person can have HIV for many years without having symptoms. You cannot know whether a person is infected simply by looking at them. 6. It is difficult to know whether a person has AIDS because their symptoms can be caused by other illnesses. To be certain, a person has to have a special blood test for HIV.

			7. Having HIV is like having any other disease, although there is no vaccine or cure for HIV and AIDS. 8. People living with HIV and AIDS deserve our compassion and care.
4	Facts about AIDS o *Flipchart* o *Story*	1. Clarify sex is the main way HIV is transmitted. 2. State other ways that HIV can be transmitted. 3. Explain the different ways of protecting oneself from HIV infection.	1. HIV cannot be transmitted by casual contact or caring for someone who is ill with AIDS. 2. Sex is the main way to become infected with HIV. 3. Limiting yourself to only one lover is not enough to protect yourself from HIV, because your lover may have been infected by other people before having sex with you. 4. The safest approach is to not have sex until you marry, and then to have sex with your spouse only. 5. People who are infected with HIV who take care of their health, eat balanced diets, get all infections treated early and properly, and have caring and supportive environments can live for many years.
5	Facts about sexually transmitted infections o *Network simulation game* o *Group competition* o *Group discussion*	1. Explain what sexually transmitted diseases are. 2. Demonstrate how sexually transmitted diseases spread within networks. 3. State the key symptoms of sexually transmitted diseases. 4. Explain the dangers of not treating sexually transmitted diseases as quickly as possible.	1. A person can become infected with sexually transmitted diseases even if they only have sex one time. 2. Many sexually transmitted diseases have symptoms, but often there are no symptoms, especially for girls and women. 3. If you think you may have symptoms of a sexually transmitted disease, or you are worried that you may have been infected, go to a health facility for advice and treatment.

(continued)

Session No.	Title / Teaching Methods	Objectives	Key Points
6	Girls and boys have equal abilities ○ Group competition ○ Role play	1. Explain that girls and boys have equal abilities.	1. Mental ability does not depend on the sex of a person. 2. Girls and boys have the same mental ability. 3. The differences between women and men are only in their bodies and their physical strengths and abilities. 4. It is good for girls to be assertive and firm, so that their bodies and thoughts are respected and valued.
7	Misconceptions about sex ○ Drama ○ Group discussion ○ Personalization exercise	1. Explain the importance of believing in themselves. 2. Explain the importance of avoiding groups that will encourage sexual activity. 3. Demonstrate the importance of avoiding peer pressure to do things that may be harmful to themselves and others.	1. It is not necessary for a boy and girl who are friends to have sex. 2. Everyone can refuse to be persuaded to do something they think is bad. 3. There is always a risk of creating a pregnancy or getting HIV or other sexually transmitted diseases if you have sex, even once. 4. Condoms can prevent all of these risks if they are used correctly, every time you have sex. 5. However, the best way to avoid sexually transmitted diseases, HIV, or pregnancy is not to have sex at all.
8	Refusing temptations ○ Drama ○ Group discussion	1. Outline reasons for rejecting sexual temptations. 2. Demonstrate how to refuse sex.	1. You are not obliged to have sex with someone just because they are your friend. 2. A friend who tries to force you to have sex is not a good friend. It is better to lose a friendship than to suffer the negative consequences of having sex. 3. A girl can become pregnant even if she only has sex once, so it is important to reject pressure or temptation to have sex.

9	Saying no to sex o *Story* o *Role play* o *Group competition*	1. Explain the possible negative consequences of having sex. 2. Practice different ways of refusing temptations.	1. Every person has the ability to refuse to have sex. 2. It is not necessary to give a specific reason for refusing sex. Not wanting to have sex is reason enough. 3. When you say no, your voice and actions should be saying the same thing.
10	Sexually transmitted infections: Going to the clinic o *Story* o *Group competition*	1. Explain the importance of treating sexually transmitted diseases immediately. 2. Explain why it is best to get treatment at a health facility.	1. You can have more than one sexually transmitted disease at a time. 2. Common symptoms for sexually transmitted diseases include watery discharge or sores on your genitals, but sometimes there may be no visible symptoms. 3. Girls especially may only experience symptoms long after infection, or no symptoms at all. 4. Once infected with a sexually transmitted disease, it is important to get treatment quickly to avoid long-term dangers. 5. Everything that happens in a health facility should be kept secret, so you should not be afraid to go there for treatment. 6. Make sure that all your lovers are also treated.
11	Revision o *Letter* o *Group competition* o *Personalization exercise*	1. Review everything learned in these lessons this year.	

Appendix 2. Outline of the Teacher's Guide for Year 6 in the Final _MEMA kwa Vijana_ School Curriculum[a]

Box 4.1 describes the network simulation game used in Year 6 session 3.

Session No.	Title o _Teaching Methods_	Objectives	Key Points
1	Review of last year o _Group discussion_ o _Letter_ o _Group competition_	1. Review key issues taught the year before. 2. Review the agreed ground rules for participating in these lessons.	1. When refusing to have sex: have a clear intention; look directly into the eyes of the other person; talk clearly and with certainty; repeat your refusal as many times as you think is necessary; both your voice and your body should show refusal; and if all this fails, then walk away.
2	How HIV infection causes AIDS o _Group discussion_ o _Personalization exercise_	1. Explain the difference between HIV and AIDS. 2. Explain what HIV does to the body's defense system. 3. List the fluids that transmit HIV.	1. AIDS is caused by tiny viruses (HIV) which enter the body, primarily through having sex with someone who is HIV-infected. 2. These viruses destroy the body's defense (immune) system. 3. Body fluids which transmit HIV are blood, vaginal fluids, semen, and breast milk. 4. It is possible to avoid HIV infection by not having sex or by always using a condom correctly when having sex. 5. You cannot get infected with HIV through everyday contact with someone who has HIV. 6. Having HIV is like having any other disease, although there is no vaccine or cure for HIV and AIDS. 7. People living with HIV and AIDS need our compassion and care.

| 3 | How sexually transmitted infections are spread

o *Network simulation game*
o *Group discussion* | 1. Demonstrate how sexually transmitted diseases spread within networks.
2. Explain the risks involved in having unprotected sex with youth of the same age.
3. Explain the risks involved in having unprotected sex with adults. | 1. Even if someone had sex once only, they can become infected with sexually transmitted diseases.
2. A sexually transmitted disease can easily pass within a group, even if only one person had it at the beginning and each person only has two partners.
3. A person of any age can be infected with a sexually transmitted disease if he/she has sex without using a condom.
4. Condoms prevent pregnancy and infection with HIV and sexually transmitted diseases during sex, but the only way to protect yourself completely is to not have sex at all.
5. If sexually transmitted diseases are not treated early, they can have serious, long-term consequences.
6. Having sex with adults puts young people in greater danger of being infected with a sexually transmitted disease. |
| 4 | Relationship between HIV and sexually transmitted infections

o *Story*
o *Flipchart* | 1. Explain the negative consequences of being infected with sexually transmitted diseases.
2. Identify the main risks involved in infidelity.
3. Explain how a mother can infect her child with HIV and/or sexually transmitted diseases. | 1. You cannot tell whether a person has HIV by their appearance.
2. A woman who is infected with HIV can infect her child in the womb, while giving birth, or while breast-feeding.
3. Sexually transmitted diseases are like a key that opens the door for easier HIV transmission.
4. Having HIV is like having any other disease, although there is no vaccine or cure for HIV and AIDS.
5. You cannot get infected with HIV through everyday contact with someone who has HIV.
6. People living with HIV and AIDS deserve our compassion and care. |

(*continued*)

Appendix 2. (continued)

Session No.	Title / Teaching Methods	Objectives	Key Points
5	Reproductive organs and their functions ○ Flipchart ○ Group discussion ○ Group work	1. Name the male and female reproductive organs. 2. Explain the functions of each of the male and female reproductive organs.	1. Sperm are produced by males and eggs are produced by females. The sperm and egg meet inside a woman through sexual intercourse. That is how babies are created. 2. Even before a man ejaculates, small amounts of semen leak out of the penis. That fluid contains enough sperm to make a woman pregnant, even without ejaculation. 3. Millions of sperm are produced any time a man ejaculates. That is why you can get pregnant, even if you only have sex once.
6	Pregnancy and menstruation ○ Group competition ○ Group work ○ Flipchart	1. Explain what menstruation is and why it occurs. 2. Explain how pregnancy occurs.	1. The duration of menstrual cycles vary from girl to girl. Some cycles are short and some are long, but the most common duration is 28 days. 2. Many things can affect menstrual cycles and their symptoms, for example, physical exercise, stress, travel, and losing or gaining weight. 3. Once a girl starts to menstruate, she can become pregnant even if she only has sex one time.
7	Respecting the decisions of others ○ Letter ○ Flipchart ○ Group discussion	1. Explain that boys and girls have equal rights. 2. Explain the importance of respecting the opposite sex when making decisions.	1. Both girls and boys have the ability and the right to refuse to have sex. 2. These decisions must be valued and respected. 3. Girls and boys must respect themselves in order to have their decisions respected by others.

		4. Many men take advantage of their wealth or position to pressure girls to have sex with them. Having sex with older men increases girls' risk of infection with HIV and other sexually transmitted diseases.
		5. If anybody is putting you under such pressure, you should seek help from an adult whom you trust.
8	Recognizing and avoiding temptations ○ *Drama* ○ *Story* ○ *Group discussion*	1. Identify the possible negative consequences of sexual temptation. 2. Identify the possible negative consequences of having many lovers.
		1. Someone may tempt you to have sex by offering you gifts, but the danger of AIDS far outweighs the benefit of gifts.
		2. Many men take advantage of their wealth or position to pressure girls to have sex with them. Having sex with older men increases girls' risk of infection with HIV and other sexually transmitted diseases.
		3. If anybody is putting you under such pressure, you should seek help from an adult whom you can trust.
		4. Changing lovers increases risk of becoming infected with HIV, other sexually transmitted diseases, and unintended pregnancies. This is true even if you only change lovers once or twice per year.
		5. If you have sex, the best way to avoid infection is by using a condom every time.
		6. You cannot get infected with HIV through everyday contact with someone who has HIV.
		7. Having HIV is like having any other disease, although there is no vaccine or cure for HIV and AIDS.
		8. People living with HIV and AIDS deserve our compassion and care.

(continued)

Appendix 2. (*continued*)

Session No.	Title ○ *Teaching Methods*	Objectives	Key Points
9	Protecting yourself: What are condoms? ○ *Group work* ○ *Role play* ○ *Group competition*	1. Explain what condoms are. 2. Explain the benefits of using condoms. 3. State where condoms are available locally.	1. The safest way to protect your health and future is to not have sex at a young age. 2. Some young people will still decide to have sex. If you have sex, the safest way to avoid HIV, other sexually transmitted diseases, and unintended pregnancy is to use condoms every time.
10	Revision ○ *Letter* ○ *Role play* ○ *Group competition* ○ *Personalization exercise*	1. Review everything learned in these lessons this year.	

[a]Obasi, Chima, Cleophas-Frisch et al., 2002c; Obasi, Chima, Cleophas-Frisch et al., 2002d.

Appendix 3. Outline of the Teacher's Guide for Year 7 in the Final *MEMA kwa Vijana* School Curriculum[a]

Box 4.2 describes the correct condom use game recommended for the group competition activity in Year 7 session 9.

Session No.	Title / Teaching Methods	Objectives	Key Points
1	Review of last year o *Group discussion* o *Story* o *Group competition*	1. Review key issues taught during the previous two years. 2. Review the agreed ground rules for participating in these lessons.	1. When refusing to have sex: have a clear intention; look directly into the eyes of the other person; talk clearly and with certainty; repeat your refusal as many times as you think is necessary; both your voice and your body should show refusal; and if all this fails, then walk away.
2	How to avoid HIV infection and AIDS o *Drama* o *Group competition* o *Personalization exercise*	1. Explain the difference between HIV and AIDS. 2. State the main ways of being infected with HIV.	1. You cannot get infected with HIV through everyday contact with someone who has HIV. 2. You cannot know if a person has HIV by looking at them. 3. A mother who has been infected with HIV can give birth to a child who is not infected with HIV. However, often the child is also infected. 4. Having HIV is like having any other disease, although there is no vaccine or cure for HIV and AIDS. 5. People living with HIV and AIDS deserve our compassion and care.
3	Sexually transmitted infections and their consequences o *Group competition* o *Story* o *Flipchart* o *Personalization exercise*	1. List the various sexually transmitted diseases. 2. Describe the common symptoms of sexually transmitted diseases. 3. Explain the negative effects of sexually transmitted diseases.	1. Sexually transmitted diseases have different signs and symptoms, such as pain while urinating, an unusual genital discharge, and sores on the genitals. 2. Sometimes sexually transmitted diseases do not have any visible symptoms, especially for girls and women. 3. Long-term negative consequences of having sexually transmitted diseases include infertility and infecting an infant while giving birth.

(continued)

Appendix 3. *(continued)*

Session No.	Title / Teaching Methods	Objectives	Key Points
4	Making good decisions ○ Story ○ Flipchart ○ Group discussion	1. Explain the importance of refusing to have sex at a young age.	1. Our decisions can have good or bad consequences. 2. Before we make decisions it is important to think about the potential consequences and how we can avoid danger. 3. Many men take advantage of their wealth or position to pressure girls to have sex with them. Having sex with older men increases girls' risk of infection with HIV and other sexually transmitted diseases. 4. If anybody is putting you under such pressure, you should seek help from an adult whom you trust. 5. Everyone has the ability to refuse temptation or persuasion. 6. It is important to respect ourselves and our health. If we lose our sense of self worth or health, it can be difficult to regain it. So we must respect ourselves and make wise decisions.
5	Practicing saying no ○ Group discussion ○ Role play ○ Group competition	1. Practice the key points to make when refusing to have sex.	1. Each of us has the ability to reject pressure or temptation. 2. Words alone are not enough. When you refuse to have sex, it is essential that your words and actions say the same thing. 3. Having sex to get money or things is not a good reason to have sex, even if you are poor, because of the risks involved. 4. Many men take advantage of their wealth or position to pressure girls to have sex with them. Having sex with older men increases girls' risk of infection with HIV and other sexually transmitted diseases. 5. If anybody is putting you under such pressure, you should seek help from an adult whom you trust.

6	Being faithful ○ Story ○ Flipchart ○ Group competition	1. Explain the importance of being faithful to one lover. 2. Explain the risks of having many lovers. 3. Describe the symptoms of sexually transmitted diseases.	1. When you have sex with a person, the risk of being infected with HIV is like having sex with all of that person's previous lovers, because your partner may have been infected by any previous lovers. 2. Therefore it is very important to use a condom every time you have sex. 3. Having unprotected sex with even one lover puts you in danger of being infected with HIV and other sexually transmitted diseases. 4. Risk also increases if you change lovers frequently.
7	Achieving your future expectations ○ Group competition ○ Drama	1. Explain the importance of planning for the future. 2. Explain the importance of using one's knowledge and striving to achieve one's goals.	1. Abstaining from sex is the only way to be absolutely sure that you will avoid HIV, other sexually transmitted diseases, and unintended pregnancies. 2. Abstaining now will help you meet your life expectations in the future. 3. Many things in our lives are under our control. It is our responsibility to avoid those things that could have a negative impact on our lives. 4. Remember it sometimes takes 10 years or more before someone who is infected with HIV develops AIDS. 5. People who are infected with HIV who take care of their health, eat balanced diets, get all infections treated early and properly, and have caring and supportive environments can live for many years.
8	Planning for your future ○ Group competition	1. Explain the benefits of family planning. 2. Describe the various family planning methods.	1. It is wise to plan the size of your future family, because your ability to meet your family's needs will depend on the number of children you have. 2. It is important for both women and men to think about the number of children they would like to have. 3. The condom is the only family planning method that helps you avoid HIV and other sexually transmitted diseases as well as unintended pregnancies.

(continued)

Appendix 3. *(continued)*

Session No.	Title ○ *Teaching Methods*	Objectives	Key Points
9	Protecting yourself: Correct use of condoms ○ *Drama* ○ *Group competition* ○ *Flipchart*	1. Explain the importance of using condoms if sexually active. 2. Explain how to use condoms properly. 3. Explain where condoms are available.	1. Experts, including the Ministry of Health of Tanzania, certify that condoms offer effective protection against HIV, other sexually transmitted diseases, and unintended pregnancies. 2. For condoms to work well, you must use them properly every time you have sex. 3. Using condoms when having sex shows you care about yourself and your lover. 4. If you use condoms, follow the instructions you learned today, which are also explained in condom packets.
10	Revision ○ *Drama* ○ *Group competition* ○ *Personalization exercise*	1. Review all the things learned during these lessons this year.	

[a]Obasi, Chima, Cleophas-Frisch et al., 2002e; Obasi, Chima, Cleophas-Frisch et al., 2002f.

Swahili and Sukuma Glossary

SWAHILI

chezasalama literally "play safely" (truncated as one word); a website for Tanzanian young people that has addressed sexual health issues since 2004

dagaa small fish similar to whitebait

hata mara moja literally "even one time," this was a *MEMA kwa Vijana* intervention slogan used to emphasize that a person could cause a pregnancy or contract an infection from just one sexual encounter

jamii community or society

kanga rectangle of colored patterned cotton cloth with a border and message, typically sold in pairs, one of which a woman wears wrapped around her waist like a skirt

kisasa modern

kuacha kufanya mapenzi kabisa literally "to completely stop making love," meaning secondary abstinence

kupenda to like or to love

kupunguza idadi ya wapenzi to reduce one's number of lovers

kusubiri kufanya mapenzi hadi hapo utakapokua zaidi literally "to wait to make love when one is older/physically mature," meaning delay of sexual debut and/or primary abstinence

kutokufanya mapenzi kabisa literally "to not make love at all," meaning abstinence

kutumia kondom to use a condom

kuwa mwaminifu   to be faithful/trustworthy
kuwa na mpenzi   literally "to have one lover," meaning to be
  mmoja   monogamous
kwa   for
mabaya   evils
magonjwa ya zinaa   literally "illnesses of fornication/adultery,"
                    meaning sexually transmitted infections
mawakala wa   literally "condom distribution agents," this was the
  usambazaji kondom   term used for *MEMA kwa Vijana* out-of-school
                    youth condom distributors
mema   good things
MEMA kwa Vijana   literally "Good Things for Youth," also the acronym
                    for *Mpango wa Elimu na Maadili ya Afya kwa*
                    Vijana (Health Education and Ethics/Morals
                    Program for Youth), an adolescent sexual health
                    intervention and trial in Mwanza, Tanzania
mhuni   (pl. *wahuni*) badly behaved person, such as a thief,
                    vagabond, or sexually promiscuous person
ngoma   traditional drumming-dancing events
ngonjera   traditional poetry recitation
Pilika Pilika   literally "Busy Busy," a Tanzanian radio soap
                    opera set in a rural village that has addressed
                    sexual health issues since 2004
rika   literally "peers of the same age," in this context
                    a youth peer group that shares farming
                    responsibilities and sometimes other activities
                    such as *ngoma* competitions
Saba saba   July 7th, a Tanzanian national holiday; formerly
                    Farmer's Day or Peasant's Day, currently
                    International Trade Fair Day
Salama   literally "safety" or "peace," also the main brand
                    name for condoms in Tanzania
Si Mchezo!   literally "No Joke!" a bi-monthly magazine for
                    rural out-of-school youth addressing sexual
                    health issues since 2003
Sikia Kengele: Tulia   literally, "Listen to the Bell: Stick to Your
  Na Wako   Partner(s)," an initiative that has promoted
                    partner reduction and fidelity with high-risk
                    individuals along transport corridors in Tanzania
                    since 2007
tamaa   literally desire, longing, greed, or lust; colloquially
                    often used to describe male sexual desire and
                    female desire for nice commodities

Twende na Wakati	literally "Let's Go with the Times," a Tanzanian radio soap opera that has addressed sexual health issues since 1993
ugali	stiff porridge staple made of maize, millet, or maize and cassava mixed
uhuni	socially disapproved of behavior, such as theft, vagrancy and sexual promiscuity
uji	maize- or millet-based porridge
UKIMWI	acronym for "*Upungufu/Ukosefu wa Kinga ya Mwili*," meaning AIDS
Upungufu/Ukosefu wa Kinga ya Mwili	literally "reduction/lack of protection for the body," meaning Acquired Immunodeficiency Syndrome (AIDS)
vijana	youths or young people
virusi vya UKIMWI	literally "the AIDS virus," meaning Human Immunodeficiency Virus (HIV)
vitenge	large rectangles of colored patterned cotton cloth similar to a *kanga* but without a border or message and of higher quality and cost
waelimishaji wa rika	literally "peer educators," this was the term used for pupils who were trained to assist teachers in teaching *MEMA kwa Vijana* sessions
wazee	elders
Zinduka	literally "Wake Up/Become Aware," a Tanzanian radio soap opera that has addressed sexual health issues since 1993

SUKUMA

bukwilima	traditional Sukuma wedding
Bulabo	the Christian Eucharist holiday
Kabambalu	a symptomatic form of chlamydia
kutogwa	to like or to love
luhya	sexual desire
nzoka	literally "snake," also a variety of illnesses believed to have supernatural causes and to be treated effectively with traditional medicine
nzoka ja buhale	a female condition typically characterized by severe menstrual pain and, if not treated with traditional medicine, perceived infertility
wasimbe	unmarried women of reproductive age, such as single mothers, divorced or widowed women, and most never-married women who have been out of school for two or more years. Also referred to as **bashimbe**

Bibliography

Aarø, Leif A., Herman Schaalma, and Anne Nordrehaug Åstrøm. 2008. Social Cognition Models and Social Cognitive Theory: Predicting sexual and reproductive behaviour among adolescents in sub-Saharan Africa. In *Promoting adolescent sexual and reproductive health in east and southern Africa*, ed. Knut-Inge Klepp, Alan J. Flisher, and Sylvia F. Kaaya, 37–55. Capetown: HSRC Press.

Abrahams, N., S. Mathews, and P. Ramela. 2006. Intersections of sanitation, sexual coercion and girls' safety in schools. *Tropical Medicine and International Health* 11(5): 751-56.

Abrahams, Ray G. 1967. *The peoples of Greater Unyamwezi, Tanzania (Nyamwezi, Sukuma Sumbwa, Kimbu, Konongo).* London: International African Institute.

Adamczyk, Amy, and Meredith Greif. 2011. Education and risky sex in Africa: Unraveling the link between women's education and reproductive health behaviors in Kenya. *Social Science Research* 40: 654–66.

Adelore, O. O., M. G. Olujide, and R. A. Popoola. 2006. Impact of HIV/AIDS prevention promotion programs on behavioral patterns among rural dwellers in south western Nigeria. *Journal of Human Ecology* 20(1): 53–58.

Adetunji, Jacob. 2000. Condom use in marital and nonmarital relationships in Zimbabwe. *International Family Planning Perspectives* 26(4): 196–200.

Agadjanian, Victor. 2005. Fraught with ambivalence: Reproductive intentions and contraceptive choices in a sub-Saharan fertility transition. *Population Research and Policy Review* 24: 617–45.

Agbemenu, Kafuli, and Elizabeth A. Schlenk. 2011. An integrative review of comprehensive sex education for adolescent girls in Kenya. *Journal of Nursing Scholarship* 43(1): 54–63.

Agha, Sohail, and Dominique Meekers. 2004. The availability of socially marketed condoms in urban Tanzania, 1997–99. *Journal of Biosocial Science* 36: 127–40.

Agha, Sohail, and Ronan Van Rossem. 2004. Impact of a school-based peer sexual health intervention on normative beliefs, risk perceptions, and sexual behavior of Zambian adolescents. *Journal of Adolescent Health* 34: 441–52.

Agha, Sohail, Paul Hutchinson, and Thankian Kusanthan. 2006. The effects of religious affiliation on sexual initiation and condom use in Zambia. *Journal of Adolescent Health* 38: 550–55.

Agha, Sohail. 2002a. An evaluation of the effectiveness of a peer sexual health intervention among secondary-school students in Zambia. *AIDS Education and Prevention* 14(4): 269–81.

Agha, Sohail. 2002b. A quasi-experimental study to assess the impact of four adolescent sexual health interventions in sub-Saharan Africa. *International Family Planning Perspectives* 28(2): 67–70 and 113–18.

Agnew, Christopher R., and Timothy J. Loving. 1998. The role of social desirability in self-reported condom use attitudes and intentions. *AIDS and Behavior* 2(3): 229–39.

Ahlberg, Beth Maina. 1994. Is there a distinct African sexuality? A critical response to Caldwell. *Africa* 64(2): 220–42.

Ahmed, Nazeema, Alan J. Flisher, Catherine Mathews, Shahieda Jansen, Wanjiru Mukoma, and Herman Schaalma. 2006. Process evaluation of the teacher training for an AIDS prevention programme. *Health Education Research* 21(5): 621–32.

Ahmed, Nazeema, Alan J. Flisher, Catherine Mathews, Wanjiru Mukoma, and Shahieda Jansen. 2009. HIV education in South African schools: The dilemma and conflicts of educators. *Scandinavian Journal of Public Health* 37: 48–54.

Airhihenbuwa, Collins O., and Rafael Obregon. 2000. A critical assessment of theories/models used in health communication for HIV/AIDS. *Journal of Health Communication* 5(Supplement): 5–15.

Albarracín, Dolores, Jeffrey C. Gillette, Allison N. Earl, Laura R. Glasman, Marta R. Durantini, and Moon-Ho Ho. 2005. A test of major assumptions about behavior change: A comprehensive look at the effects of passive and active HIV-prevention interventions since the beginning of the epidemic. *Psychological Bulletin* 131(6): 856–97.

Ali, Mohamed, and John Cleland. 2006. Uses and abuses of surveys on the sexual behaviour of young people. In *Promoting young people's sexual health: International perspectives*, ed. Roger Ingham and Peter Aggleton, 9–26. Oxon, UK: Routledge.

Allen, Denise Roth. 2002. *Managing motherhood, managing risk: Fertility and danger in west central Tanzania.* Ann Arbor: University of Michigan.

Allen, Susan, Etienne Karita, Elwyn Chomba, David L. Roth, Joseph Telfair, Isaac Zulu, Leslie Clark, et al. 2007. Promotion of couples' voluntary counselling and testing for HIV through influential networks in two African capital cities. *BMC Public Health* 7: 349.

Altman, David G. 2009. Challenges in sustaining public health interventions. *Health Education and Behavior* 36(1): 24–28.

Amoran, O. E., and O. Fawole. 2008. Parental influence on reproductive health behavior of youths in Ibadan, Nigeria. *African Journal of Medicine and Medical Sciences* 37(1): 21–27.

Amuyunzu-Nyamongo, Mary, Ann E. Biddlecom, Christine Ouedraogo, and Vanessa Woog. 2005. *Qualitative evidence on adolescents' views on sexual and reproduc-*

tive health in sub-Saharan Africa. Occasional Report No. 16. New York: The Alan Guttmacher Institute.

Andersson, Neil, and Ari Ho-Foster. 2008. 13,915 reasons for equity in sexual offences legislation: A national school-based survey in South Africa. *International Journal for Equity in Health* 7: 20.

Angotti, Nicole, Agatha Bula, Lauren Gaydosh, Eitan Zeev Kimchi, Rebecca L. Thornton, and Sara E. Yeatman. 2009. Increasing the acceptability of HIV counseling and testing with three C's: Convenience, confidentiality and credibility. *Social Science and Medicine* 68: 2263–70.

Angotti, Nicole. 2010. Working outside of the box: How HIV counselors in sub-Saharan Africa adapt Western HIV testing norms. *Social Science and Medicine* 71: 986–93.

Ankrah, E. Maxine. 1989. AIDS: Methodological problems in studying its prevention and spread. *Social Science and Medicine* 29(3): 265–76.

Aral, Sevgi O., and Betsy Foxman. 2003. Spatial mixing and bridging: Risk factors for what? *Sexually Transmitted Diseases* 30(10): 750–51.

Aral, Sevgi O., and Mead Over, with Lisa Manhart and King K. Holmes. 2006. Sexually transmitted infections. In *Disease control priorities in developing countries, 2nd edition,* ed. Dean T. Jamison, Joel G. Breman, Anthony R. Measham, George Alleyne, Mariam Claeson, David B. Evans, Prabhat Jha, Anne Mills, and Philip Musgrove, 311–30. New York: The World Bank and Oxford University Press.

Aral, Sevgi, and Thomas A. Peterman. 2002. A stratified approach to untangling the behavioral/biomedical outcomes conundrum. *Sexually Transmitted Diseases* 29(9): 530–32.

Arnfred, Signe. 2004. "African sexuality"/sexuality in Africa: Tales and silences. In *Re-thinking sexualities in Africa,* ed. Signe Arnfred, 59–78. Uppsala, Sweden: Nordiska Afrikainstitutet.

Arthur, Jo. 2001. Perspectives on educational language policy and its implementation in African classrooms: A comparative study of Botswana and Tanzania. *Compare* 31: 347–62.

Arube-Wani, John, Jessica Jitta, and Lillian Mpabulungi Ssengooba. 2008. Adolescent-friendly health services in Uganda. In *Promoting adolescent sexual and reproductive health in east and southern Africa,* ed. Knut-Inge Klepp, Alan J. Flisher, and Sylvia F. Kaaya, 214–33. Capetown: HSRC Press.

Arulogun, Oyedunni S., and Olumide A. Adefioye. 2010. Attitude towards mandatory pre-marital HIV testing among unmarried youths in Ibadan Northwest Local Government Area, Nigeria. *African Journal of Reproductive Health* 14(1): 83–94.

Attia, Suzanna, Matthias Egger, Monika Müller, Marcel Zwahlena, and Nicola Low. 2009. Sexual transmission of HIV according to viral load and antiretroviral therapy: Systematic review and meta-analysis. *AIDS* 23: 1397–404.

Auerbach, Judith D., Richard J. Hayes, and Sonia M. Kandathil. 2006. Overview of effective and promising interventions to prevent HIV infection. In *Preventing HIV/ AIDS in young people: A systematic review of the evidence from developing countries,* ed. David A. Ross, Bruce Dick, and Jane Ferguson, 43–78. Geneva: WHO.

Aveyard, P., W. A. Markham, E. Lancashire, A. Bullock, C. Macarthur, K. K. Cheng, and H. Daniels. 2004. The influence of school culture on smoking among pupils. *Social Science and Medicine* 58: 1767–80.

Babalola, Stella, B. Oleko Tambashe, and Claudia Vondrasek. 2005. Parental factors and sexual risk-taking among young people in Côte d'Ivoire. *African Journal of Reproductive Health* 9(1): 49–65.

Babalola, Stella, Dieneba Ouedraogo, and Claudia Vondrasek. 2006. Motivation for late sexual debut in Côte d'Ivoire and Burkina Faso: A positive deviance inquiry. *Journal of HIV/AIDS Prevention in Children and Youth* 7(2): 65–87.

Babbie, Earl. 1986. *The practice of social research.* Belmont, California: Wadsworth.

Baddeley, Alan. 1979. The limitations of human memory: Implications for the design of retrospective surveys. In *The recall method of social surveys*, ed. Louis Moss and Harvey Goldstein, 13–27. London: University of London Institute of Education.

Bagamoyo College of Arts, Tanzania Theatre Centre, Richard Mabala, and Karen B. Allen. 2002. Participatory action research on HIV/AIDS through a popular theatre approach in Tanzania. *Evaluation and Program Planning* 25: 333–39.

Baird, Sarah, Ephraim Chirwa, Craig Mcintosh, and Berk Özler. 2009. The short-term impacts of a schooling conditional cash transfer program on the sexual behavior of young women. *Health Economics* 19: 55–68.

Balmer, D. H., E. Gikundi, M. C. Billingsley, F. G. Kihuho, M. Kimani, J. Wang'ondu, and H. Njoroge. 1997. Adolescent knowledge, values, and coping strategies: Implications for health in sub-Saharan Africa. *Journal of Adolescent Health* 21: 33–38.

Bandura, Albert. 2004. Health promotion by social cognitive means. *Health Education and Behavior* 31: 143–64.

Bankole, Akinrinola, Ann Biddlecom, Georges Guiella, Susheela Singh, and Eliya Zulu. 2007. Sexual behavior, knowledge and information sources of very young adolescents in four sub-Saharan African countries. *African Journal of Reproductive Health* 11(3): 28–43.

Bankole, Akinrinola, Fatima H. Ahmed, Stella Neema, Christine Ouedraogo, and Sidon Konyani. 2007. Knowledge of correct condom use and consistency of use among adolescents in four countries in Sub-Saharan Africa. *African Journal of Reproductive Health* 11(3): 197–220.

Bankole, Akinrinola, Susheela Singh, Rubina Hussain, and Gabrielle Oestreicher. 2009. Condom use for preventing STI/HIV and unintended pregnancy among young men in sub-Saharan Africa. *American Journal of Men's Health* 3(1): 60–78.

Barker, David, and Christine Ricardo. 2005. *Young men and the construction of masculinity in sub-Saharan Africa: Implications for HIV/AIDS, conflict, and violence. Social Development Papers: Conflict Prevention and Reconstruction, No. 26.* Washington, DC: World Bank. Downloaded from www.eldis.org/vfile/upload/1/document/0708/DOC21154.pdf on February 27, 2012.

Barrett, Angeline M. 2007. Beyond the polarization of pedagogy: Models of classroom practice in Tanzanian primary schools. *Comparative Education* 43(2): 273–94.

Bastien, S., L. J. Kajula, and W. W. Muhwezi. 2011. A review of studies of parent-child communication about sexuality and HIV/AIDS in sub-Saharan Africa. *Reproductive Health* 8: 25.

Bastien, S., W. Sango, K. S. Mnyika, M. C. Masatu, and K. I. Klepp. 2008. Changes in exposure to information, communication and knowledge about AIDS among school children in Northern Tanzania, 1992–2005. *AIDS Care* 20(3): 382–87.

Bastien, Sheri. 2008. Out-of-school and at risk? Socio-demographic characteristics, AIDS knowledge and risk perception among young people in northern Tanzania. *International Journal of Educational Development* 28: 393–404.

Bastien, Sheri. 2009. Reflecting and shaping the discourse: The role of music in AIDS communication in Tanzania. *Social Science and Medicine* 68(7): 1357–60.

Bastien, Sherri, Alan J. Flisher, Catherine Mathews, and Knut-Inge Klepp. 2008. Peer education for adolescent reproductive health: An effective method for program delivery, a powerful empowerment strategy, or neither? In *Promoting adolescent sexual and reproductive health in east and southern Africa*, ed. Knut-Inge Klepp, Alan J. Flisher, and Sylvia Kaaya, 185–213. Capetown: HSRC Press.

Baumgartner, Joy Noel, Helen Lugina, Laura Johnson, and Tumaini Nyamhanga. 2010. "Being faithful" in a sexual relationship: Perceptions of Tanzanian adolescents in the context of HIV and pregnancy prevention. *AIDS Care* 22(9): 1153–58.

Beegle, Kathleen, Deon Filmer, Andrew Stokes, and Lucia Tiererova. 2010. Orphanhood and the living arrangements of children in sub-Saharan Africa. *World Development* 38(12): 1727–46.

Beguy, Donatien, Caroline W. Kabiru, Evangeline N. Nderu, and Moses W. Ngware. 2009. Inconsistencies in self-reporting of sexual activity among young people in Nairobi, Kenya. *Journal of Adolescent Health* 45: 595–601.

Bell, Stephanie G., Susan F. Newcomer, Christine Bachrach, Elaine Borawski, John B. Jemmott, Diane Morrison, Bonita Stanton, Susan Tortolero, and Richard Zimmerman. 2007. Challenges in replicating interventions. *Journal of Adolescent Health* 40: 514–20.

Béné, Christophe, and Sonja Merten. 2008. Women and fish-for-sex: Transactional sex, HIV/AIDS and gender in African fisheries. *World Development* 36(5): 875–99.

Benefo, Kofi D. 2008. Determinants of Zambian men's extra-marital sex: A multilevel analysis. *Archives of Sexual Behavior* 37: 517–29.

Bennell, Paul, and Faustin Mukyanuzi. 2005. *Is there a teacher motivation crisis in Tanzania?* Brighton, UK: Knowledge and Skills for Development. Downloaded from www.eldis.org/vfile/upload/1/document/0709/Teacher_motivation_Tanzania .pdf on August 6, 2010.

Benson, John. 2006. *"A complete education?" Observations about the state of primary education in Tanzania in 2005. HakiElimu Working paper no. 06.1.* Dar es Salaam: HakiElimu. Downloaded from www.hakielimu.org on August 6, 2010.

Berege, Zachariah, and Arnoud Klokke. 1997. Reducing HIV transmission via blood transfusion: A district strategy. In *HIV prevention and AIDS care in Africa: A district level approach,* ed. Japhet Ng'weshemi, Ties Boerma, John Bennett, and Dick Schapink, 292–304. Amsterdam: Royal Tropical Institute.

Bernard, H. Russell. 1995. *Research methods in anthropology: Qualitative and quantitative approaches.* Walnut Creek, California: AltaMira Press.

Bertozzi, Stefano M., Marie Laga, Sergio Bautista-Arredondo, and Alex Coutinho. 2008. Making HIV prevention programmes work. *Lancet* 372: 831–44.

Bertrand, Jane T., and Rebecca Anhang. 2006. The effectiveness of mass media in changing HIV/AIDS related behavior among young people in developing countries. In *Preventing HIV/AIDS in young people: A systematic review of the evidence from developing countries. World Health Organization Technical Report Series 938*, ed. David A. Ross, Bruce Dick, and Jane Ferguson, 205–41. Geneva: WHO.

Bessire, Aimée, and Mark Bessire. 1997. *Sukuma.* New York: Rosen.

Beutler, Ingrid. 2008. Sport serving development and peace: Achieving the goals of the United Nations through sport. *Sport in Society* 11(4): 359–69.

Bhana, A., I. Petersen, A. Mason, Z. Mahintsho, C. Bell, and M. McKay. 2004. Children and youth at risk: Adaptation and pilot study of the CHAMP (Amaqhawe) programme in South Africa. *African Journal of AIDS Research* 3(1): 33–41.

Bhana, Arvin, Mary M. McKay, Claude Mellins, Inge Petersen, and Carl Bell. 2010. Family-based HIV prevention and intervention services for youth living in poverty-affected contexts: The CHAMP model of collaborative, evidence-informed programme development. *Journal of the International AIDS Society* 13(Supplement 2): S8.

Biddlecom, Ann, Kofi Awusabo-Asare, and Akinrinola Bankole. 2009. Role of parents in adolescent sexual activity and contraceptive use in four African countries. *International Perspectives on Sexual and Reproductive Health* 35(2): 72–81.

Biddlecom, Ann, Richard Gregory, Cynthia B. Lloyd, and Barbara S. Mensch. 2008. Associations between premarital sex and leaving school in four sub-Saharan African countries. *Studies in Family Planning* 39(4): 337–50.

Bingenheimer, Jeffrey B. 2010. Men's multiple sexual partnerships in 15 sub-Saharan African countries: Sociodemographic patterns and implications. *Studies in Family Planning* 41(1): 1–17.

Bloor, Michael, Jane Frankland, Michelle Thomas, and Kate Robson. 2001. *Focus groups in social research.* London: Sage.

Boerma, J. T., M. Urassa, S. Nnko, J. Ng'weshemi, R. Isingo, B. Zaba, and G. Mwaluko. 2002. Sociodemographic context of the AIDS epidemic in a rural area in Tanzania with a focus on people's mobility and marriage. *Sexually Transmitted Infections* 78(Supplement 1): i97–105.

Bogale, G. W., H. Boer, and E. R. Seydel. 2010. Condom use among low-literate, rural females in Ethiopia: The role of vulnerability to HIV infection, condom attitude, and self-efficacy. *AIDS Care* 22(7): 851–57.

Bommier, Antoine, and Sylvie Lambert. 2000. Education demand and age at school enrollment in Tanzania. *Journal of Human Resources* 35: 177–203.

Bond, L., H. Butler, L. Thomas, J. B. Carlin, S. Glover, G. Bowes, and G. Patton. 2007. Social and school connectedness in early secondary school as predictors of late teenage substance use, mental health and academic outcomes. *Journal of Adolescent Health* 40(4): 357e9–18.

Bond, Virginia, and Paul Dover. 1997. Men, women and the trouble with condoms: Problems associated with condom use by migrant workers in rural Zambia. *Health Transition Review* 7(Supplement): 377–91.

Bonell, C. P., J. R. Hargreaves, S. N. Cousens, D. A. Ross, R. J. Hayes, M. Petticrew, and B. Kirkwood. 2011. Alternatives to randomisation in the evaluation of public-health interventions: Design challenges and solutions. *Journal of Epidemiology and Community Health* 65: 582–87.

Bonell, Chris, Rebecca Bennett, and Ann Oakley. 2003. Sexual health interventions should be subject to experimental evaluation. In *Effective sexual health interventions: Issues in experimental evaluation*, ed. Judith M. Stephenson, John Imrie, and Chris Bonell, 4–16. Oxford: Oxford University Press.

Bonell, Christopher, James Hargreaves, Vicki Strange, Paul Pronyk, and John Porter. 2006. Should structural interventions be evaluated using RCTs? The case of HIV prevention. *Social Science and Medicine* 63: 1135–42.

Bornemisza, Olga. 2001. *ASRH policy study interim summary.* Unpublished report.

Bosmans, Marleen, Marie Noël Cikuru, Patricia Claeys, and Marleen Temmerman. 2006. Where have all the condoms gone in adolescent programmes in the Democratic Republic of Congo. *Reproductive Health Matters* 14(28): 80–88.

Bove, Riley, and Claudia Valeggia. 2009. Polygyny and women's health in sub-Saharan Africa. *Social Science and Medicine* 68: 21–29.

Boyce, Carolyn, and Palena Neale. 2006. *Using mystery clients: A guide to using mystery clients for evaluation input. Pathfinder International Tool Series: Monitoring and Evaluation–3.* Downloaded on August 21, 2010 from www.pathfind.org/site/DocServer/m_e_tool_series_mystery_clients.pdf?docID=6303.

Bratholm, Clara, Asgeir Johannessen, Ezra Naman, Svein G. Gundersen, Sokoine L. Kivuyo, Mona Holberg-Petersen, Vidar Ormaasen, and Johan N. Bruun. 2010. Drug resistance is widespread among children who receive long-term antiretroviral treatment at a rural Tanzanian hospital. *Journal of Antimicrobial Chemotherapy* 65: 1996–2000.

Breinbauer, Cecilia, and Matilde Maddaleno. 2005. *Youth: Choices and change: Promoting healthy behaviors in adolescents.* Washington, DC: PAHO.

Brent, Robert J. 2010. Why countries have both subsidized and free condoms to prevent HIV/AIDS: The role of stigma mitigation. *Journal of African Development* 12(2): 61–72.

Brewer, Devon D., Sharon B. Garrett, and Shalini Kulasingam. 1999. Forgetting as a cause of incomplete reporting of sexual and drug injection partners. *Sexually Transmitted Diseases* 26(3): 166–76.

Brieger, William R., Grace E. Delano, Catherine G. Lane, Oladimeji Oladepo, and Kola A. Oyediran. 2001. West African Youth Initiative: Outcome of a reproductive health education program. *Journal of Adolescent Health* 29: 436–46.

British Broadcasting Corporation. 2010. *Hundreds of Kenyan teachers sacked over sex abuse.* Downloaded from www.bbc.co.uk/news/world-africa-11492499 on November 23, 2010.

Brock-Utne, Birgit, and Halla B. Holmarsdottir. 2004. Language policies and practices in Tanzania and South Africa: Problems and challenges. *International Journal of Educational Development* 24: 67–83.

Brock-Utne, Birgit. 2007. Learning through a familiar language versus learning through a foreign language: A look into some secondary school classrooms in Tanzania. *International Journal of Educational Development* 27(5): 487–98.

Brouillard-Coyle, Chris, Eleanor Maticka-Tyndale, Karen Metcalfe, Dan Holland, Janet Wildish, and Mary Gichuru. 2005. The inclusion of condoms in a school-based HIV prevention intervention in Kenya. 17th World Congress of Sexology, Montreal, Canada. July 10–15, 2005. Abstract no. 810.3.

Bulmer, Martin, and Donald P. Warwick. 2000. *Social research in developing countries: Surveys and censuses in the Third World*. London: University College London.

Burton, Jennifer, Lynae A. Darbes, and Don Operario. 2010. Couples-focused behavioral interventions for prevention of HIV: Systematic review of the state of evidence. *AIDS and Behavior* 14: 1–10.

Buvé, Anne, Kizito Bishikwabo-Nsarhaza, and Gladys Mutangadura. 2002. The spread and effect of HIV-1 infection in sub-Saharan Africa. *Lancet* 359: 2011–17.

Buvé, Anne. 2006. The HIV epidemics in sub-Saharan Africa: Why so severe? Why so heterogenous? An epidemiological perspective. In *The HIV/AIDS epidemic in sub-Saharan Africa in a historical perspective: Online edition*, ed. Philippe Denis and Charles Becker, 41–55. Downloaded on November 7, 2006 from www.refer.sn/rds/IMG/pdf/AIDSHISTORYALL.pdf.

Caldwell, John C., and Pat Caldwell. 1987. The cultural context of high fertility in sub-Saharan Africa. *Population and Development Review* 13(3): 409–37.

Caldwell, John C., Pat Caldwell, and Pat Quiggin. 1989. The social context of AIDS in sub-Saharan Africa. *Population and Development Review* 15(2): 185–234.

Caldwell, John C., Pat Caldwell, Bruce K. Caldwell, and Indrani Pieris. 1998. The construction of adolescence in a changing world: Implications for sexuality, reproduction, and marriage. *Studies in Family Planning* 29(2): 137–53.

Camlin, Carol S., and Rachel C. Snow. 2008. Parental investment, club membership and youth sexual risk behavior in Cape Town. *Health Education and Behavior* 35: 522–40.

Campbell, C., and B. Williams. 1999. Beyond the biomedical and behavioral: Towards an integrated approach to HIV prevention in the South African mining industry. *Social Science and Medicine* 48: 1625–39.

Campbell, Catherine. 2003. *"Letting them die": Why HIV/AIDS prevention programs fail*. Oxford: James Currey.

Caraël, Michel. 2006. Twenty years of intervention and controversy. In *The HIV/AIDS epidemic in sub-Saharan Africa in a historical perspective: Online edition*, ed. Philippe Denis and Charles Becker, 29–40. Downloaded on November 7, 2006 from www.refer.sn/rds/IMG/pdf/AIDSHISTORYALL.pdf.

Carstens, Adelia, Alfons Maes, and Lilian Gangla-Birir. 2006. Understanding visuals in HIV/AIDS education in South Africa: Differences between literate and low-literate audiences. *African Journal of AIDS Research* 5(3): 221–32.

Carter, Marion W., Joan Marie Kraft, Todd Koppenhaver, Christine Galavotti, Thierry H. Roels, Peter H. Kilmarx, and Boga Fidzani. 2007. "A bull cannot be contained in a single kraal": Concurrent sexual partnerships in Botswana. *AIDS and Behavior* 11: 822–30.

Castle, Sarah. 2003. Factors influencing young Malians' reluctance to use hormonal contraceptives. *Studies in Family Planning* 34(3): 186–99.

Catania, Joseph A., David R. Gibson, Dale D. Chitwood, and Thomas J. Coates. 1990. Methodological problems in AIDS behavioral research: Influences on measurement error and participation bias in studies of sexual behavior. *Psychological Bulletin* 108(3): 339–62.

Catania, Joseph A., Heather Turner, Robert C. Pierce, Eve Golden, Carol Stocking, Diane Binson, and Karen Mast. 1993. Response bias in surveys of AIDS related sexual behavior. In *Methodological issues in AIDS behavioral research*, ed. D. G. Ostrow and R. C. Kessler, 133–62. New York: Plenum Press.

Chacko, Sunita, Walter Kipp, Lory Laing, and Geoffrey Kabagambe. 2007. Knowledge of and perceptions about sexually transmitted diseases and pregnancy: A qualitative study among adolescent students in Uganda. *Journal of Health, Population, and Nutrition* 25(3): 319–27.

Chalamilla, Guerino, Judica Mbwana, Fred Mhalu, Eunice Mmari, Mtebe Majigo, Andrew Swai, Willy Urassa, and Eric Sandstrom. 2006. Patterns of sexually transmitted infections in adolescents and youth in Dar es Salaam, Tanzania. *BMC Infectious Diseases* 6: 22.

Changalucha, J., A. Gavyole, H. Grosskurth, R. Hayes, and D. Mabey. 2002. STD/HIV intervention and research programme Mwanza Region, NW Tanzania. *Sexually Transmitted Infections* 78(Supplement 1): i91–6.

Charania, Mahnaz R., Nicole Crepaz, Carolyn Guenther-Gray, Kirk Henny, Adrian Liau, Leigh A. Willis, and Cynthia M. Lyles. 2011. Efficacy of structural-level condom distribution interventions: A meta-analysis of U.S. and international studies, 1998–2007. *AIDS and Behavior* 15: 1283–97.

Chen, Li, Prabhat Jha, Bridget Stirling, Sema K. Sgaier, Tina Daid, Rupert Kaul, Nico Nagelkerke, for the International Studies of HIV/AIDS Investigators. 2007. Sexual risk factors for HIV infection in early and advanced HIV epidemics in Sub-Saharan Africa: Systematic overview of 68 epidemiological studies. *PLoS ONE* 10: e1001.

Chiao, Chi, and Vinod Mishra. 2009. Trends in primary and secondary abstinence among Kenyan youth. *AIDS Care* 21(7): 881–92.

Chimbiri, Agnes M. 2007. The condom is an 'intruder' in marriage: Evidence from rural Malawi. *Social Science and Medicine* 64: 1102–15.

Clark, Shelley, Judith Bruce, and Annie Dude. 2006. Protecting young women from HIV/AIDS: The case against child and adolescent marriage. *International Family Planning Perspectives* 32(2): 79–88.

Clark, Shelley. 2010. Extra-marital sexual partnerships and male friendships in rural Malawi. *Demographic Research* 22: 1–28.

Cleland, John, and Mohamed M. Ali. 2006. Sexual abstinence, contraception, and condom use by young African women: A secondary analysis of survey data. *Lancet* 368: 1788–93.

Cleophas-Frisch, B., A. Obasi, M. Rwakatare, A. Magadulla, R. Alex, J. Charles, R. Balira, J. Tudo, and D. Ross. 2000. Condom accessibility and attitudes to condom use amongst adolescents in rural Mwanza region, Tanzania. 13th International AIDS Conference, Durban, South Africa. 9–14 July, 2000. Abstract no. ThPpC1498.

Cleophas-Frisch, B., A. Obasi, M. Rwakatare, R. Alex, A. Magadula, J. Charles, F. Kabumbire, D. Ross, R. Hayes, and A. Gavyole. 2002. Community condom promotion and distribution among adolescents in rural Mwanza, Tanzania. 14th International AIDS Conference, Barcelona, Spain. 7–12 July, 2002. Abstract no. MoPeF4034.

Cleophas-Frisch, B., A. Obasi, T. Manchester, M. Rwakatare, R. Alex, J. Charles, D. Ross, and R. Hayes. 2000. Pilot study of a village-based peer condom social marketing initiative in rural Mwanza region, Tanzania. 13th International AIDS Conference, Durban, South Africa. 9–14 July, 2000. Abstract no. ThPeC5356.

Clift, S., A. Anemona, D. Watson-Jones, Z. Kanga, L. Ndeki, J. Changalucha, A. Gavyole, and D. A. Ross. 2003. Variations of HIV and STI prevalences within communities neighbouring new goldmines in Tanzania: Importance for intervention design. *Sexually Transmitted Infections* 79: 307–12.

Coast, Ernestina. 2007. Wasting semen: Context and condom use among the Maasai. *Culture, Health and Sexuality* 9(4): 387–401.

Coates, Thomas J., Linda Richter, and Carlos Caceres. 2008. Behavioural strategies to reduce HIV transmission: How to make them work better. *Lancet* 372: 669–84.

Coffee, Megan P., Geoffrey P. Garnett, Makalima Mlilo, Hélène A. C. M. Voeten, Stephen Chandiwana, and Simon Gregson. 2005. Patterns of movement and risk of HIV infection in rural Zimbabwe. *Journal of Infectious Diseases* 191(Supplement 1): S159–67.

Cohen, Barney. 1998. The emerging fertility transition in sub-Saharan Africa. *World Development* 26(8): 1431–61.

Cole, Jennifer, and Lynn M. Thomas, ed. 2009. *Love in Africa.* Chicago: University of Chicago Press.

Collins, Chris, Thomas J. Coates, and James Curran. 2008. Moving beyond the alphabet soup of HIV prevention. *AIDS* 22(Supplement 2): S5–8.

Collins, Terri, and Jonathan Stadler. 2000. Love, passion and play: Sexual meaning among youth in the northern province of South Africa. *Journal des Anthropologues* 82–83: 325–37.

Colvin, M., M. O. Bachmann, R. K. Homan, D. Nsibande, N. M. Nkwanyana, C. Connolly, and E. B. Reuben. 2006. Effectiveness and cost effectiveness of syndromic sexually transmitted infection packages in South African primary care: Cluster randomised trial. *Sexually Transmitted Infections* 82: 290–94.

Cooksey, Brian, and Sibylle Riedmiller. 1997. Tanzanian education in the nineties: Beyond the diploma disease. *Assessment in Education* 4: 121–35.

Cooper, Curtis L., and Edward J. Mills. 2010. Successes in the HIV epidemic response in Africa: Maintaining momentum in uncertain times. *International Journal of Infectious Diseases* 14S: e357–58.

Cory, Hans. 1953. *Sukuma law and custom.* London: Oxford University Press.

Cowan, Frances M., and Mary Plummer. 2003. What are the relative advantages of biological, behavioral, and psychosocial outcome measures? In *Effective sexual health interventions: Issues in experimental evaluation*, ed. Judith M. Stephenson, John Imrie, and Chris Bonell, 111–35. Oxford: Oxford University Press.

Cowan, Frances M., Lisa F. Langhaug, George P. Mashungupa, Tellington Nyamurera, John Hargrove, Shabbar Jaffar, Rosanna W. Peeling et al. 2002. School based HIV prevention in Zimbabwe: Feasibility and acceptability of evaluation trials using biological outcomes. *AIDS* 16: 1673–78.

Cowan, Frances M., Lisa F. Langhaug, John W. Hargrove, Shabbar Jaffar, Lovemore Mhuriyengwe, Todd D. Swarthout, Rosanna Peeling et al. 2005. Is sexual contact with sex workers important in driving the HIV epidemic among men in rural Zimbabwe? *Journal of Acquired Immune Deficiency Syndromes* 40(3): 371–76.

Cowan, Frances M., Sophie J. S. Pascoe, Lisa F. Langhaug, Webster Mavhu, Samson Chidiya, Shabbar Jaffar, Michael T. Mbizvo et al. 2010. The Regai Dzive Shiri project: Results of a randomized trial of an HIV prevention intervention for youth. *AIDS* 24: 2541–52.

Cremin, I., P. Mushati, T. Hallett, Z. Mupambireyi, C. Nyamukapa, G. P. Garnett, and S. Gregson. 2009. Measuring trends in age at first sex and age at marriage in Manicaland, Zimbabwe. *Sexually Transmitted Infections* 85(Supplement 1): i34–40.

Crichton, Joanna, Latifat Ibisomi, and Stephen Obeng Gyimah. 2012. Mother–daughter communication about sexual maturation, abstinence and unintended pregnancy: Experiences from an informal settlement in Nairobi, Kenya. *Journal of Adolescence* 35(1): 21–30.

Dane, Andrew V., and Barry H. Schneider. 1998. Program integrity in primary and early secondary prevention: Are implementation effects out of control? *Clinical Psychology Review* 18(1): 23–45.

Davis, Karen R., and Susan C. Weller. 1999. The effectiveness of condoms in reducing heterosexual transmission of HIV. *Family Planning Perspectives* 31(6): 272–79.

de Visser, R. O., and A. M. A. Smith. 2000. When always isn't enough: Implications of the late application of condoms for the validity and reliability of self-reported condom use. *AIDS Care* 12(2): 221–24.

de Walque, Damien, and Rachel Kline. 2012. The association between remarriage and HIV infection in 13 sub-Saharan African countries. *Studies in Family Planning* 43(1): 1–10.

de Walque, Damien, William H. Dow, Rose Nathan, Ramadhani Abdul, Faraji Abilahi, Erick Gong, Zachary Isdahl et al. 2012. Incentivising safe sex: A randomised trial of conditional cash transfers for HIV and sexually transmitted infection prevention in rural Tanzania. *BMJ Open* 2: e000747.

Delva, Wim, Kristien Michielsen, Bert Meulders, Sandy Groeninck, Edwin Wasonga, Pauline Ajwang, Marleen Temmerman, and Bart Vanreusel. 2010. HIV prevention through sport: The case of the Mathare Youth Sport Association in Kenya. *AIDS Care* 22(8): 1012–20.

Desmond, Nicola, Caroline F. Allen, Simon Clift, Butolwa Justine, Joseph Mzugu, Mary L. Plummer, Deborah Watson-Jones, and David A. Ross. 2005. A typology of groups at risk of HIV/STI in a gold mining town in north-western Tanzania. *Social Science and Medicine* 60(8): 1739–49.

Devine, Owen J., and Sevgi O. Aral. 2004. The impact of inaccurate reporting of condom use and imperfect diagnosis of sexually transmitted disease infection in studies of condom effectiveness. *Sexually Transmitted Diseases* 31(10): 588–95.

Dick, Bruce, Jane Ferguson, Venkatraman Chandra-Mouli, Loretta Brabin, Subidita Chatterjee, and David A. Ross. 2006. Review of the evidence for interventions to increase young people's use of health services in developing countries. In *Preventing HIV/AIDS in young people: A systematic review of the evidence from developing countries,* ed. David A. Ross, Bruce Dick, and Jane Ferguson, 151–204. Geneva: WHO.

Dickson, Kim Eva, Joanne Ashton, and Judy-Marie Smith. 2007. Does setting adolescent-friendly standards improve the quality of care in clinics? Evidence from South Africa. *International Journal for Quality in Health Care* 19(2): 80–89.

DiClemente, Ralph J., and Gina M. Wingood. 2003. Human Immunodeficiency Virus prevention for adolescents: Windows of opportunity for optimizing intervention effectiveness. *Archives of Pediatrics and Adolescent Medicine* 157: 319–20.

Dimbuene, Zacharie Tsala, and Barthelemy Kuate Defo. 2011. Fostering accurate HIV/AIDS knowledge among unmarried youths in Cameroon: Do family environment and peers matter? *BMC Public Health* 11: 348.

Dixon-Mueller, Ruth. 2009. Starting young: Sexual initiation and HIV prevention in early adolescence. *AIDS and Behavior* 13: 100–109.

Dlamini, Siyabonga, Myra Taylor, Nosipho Mkhize, Rosemarie Huver, Reshma Sathiparsad, Hein de Vries, Kala Naidoo, and Champak Jinabhai. 2009. Gender factors associated with sexual abstinent behavior of rural South African high school going youth in KwaZulu-Natal, South Africa. *Health Education Research* 24(3): 450–60.

Doherty, Irene A., Stephen Shiboski, Jonathan M. Ellen, Adaora A. Adimora, and Nancy S. Padian. 2006. Sexual bridging socially and over time: A simulation model exploring the relative effects of mixing and concurrency on viral sexually transmitted infection transmission. *Sexually Transmitted Diseases* 33(6): 368–73.

Douglas, M. 2004. Traditional culture—Let's hear no more about it. In *Culture and public action,* ed. V. Rao and M. Walton, 85–109. Palo Alto, California: Stanford University Press.

Doyle, A. M., H. A. Weiss, K. Maganja, S. McCormack, D. Watson-Jones, J. Changalucha, R. J. Hayes, and D. A. Ross. 2011. The long-term impact of the MEMA kwa Vijana adolescent sexual and reproductive health intervention: Effects of dose and time since exposure to intervention. *Sexually Transmitted Infections* 87(Supplement 1): A215.

Doyle, A. M., J. Changalucha, H. A. Weiss, D. Watson-Jones, S. Kapiga, R. J. Hayes, B. Zaba, and D. A. Ross. 2011. The association between marital transition and HIV seroconversion in a cohort of young people in rural Tanzania. *Sexually Transmitted Infections* 87(Supplement 1): A181.

Doyle, Aoife M., David A. Ross, Kaballa Maganja, Kathy Baisley, Clemens Masesa, Aura Andreasen, Mary L. Plummer et al. 2010. Long-term biological and behavioural impact of an adolescent sexual health intervention in Tanzania: Follow-up survey of the community-based MEMA kwa Vijana Trial. *PLoS Medicine* 7(6): e1000287.

Doyle, Aoife M., Sue Napierala Mavedzenge, Mary L. Plummer, and David A. Ross. 2012. The sexual behaviour of adolescents in sub-Saharan Africa: Patterns and trends from national surveys. *Tropical Medicine and International Health* 17(7): 796–807.

Drumright, Lydia N., Pamina M. Gorbach, and King K. Holmes. 2004. Do people really know their sex partners? Concurrency, knowledge of partner behavior, and sexually transmitted infections within partnerships. *Sexually Transmitted Diseases* 31(7): 437–42.

Dunbar, Megan S. M., Catherine Maternowska, Mi-Suk J. Kang, Susan M. Laver, Imelda Mudekunye-Mahaka, and Nancy S. Padian. 2010. Findings from SHAZ!: A feasibility study of a microcredit and life-skills HIV prevention intervention to reduce risk among adolescent female orphans in Zimbabwe. *Journal of Prevention and Intervention in the Community* 38: 147–61.

Dunkle, K., R. Jewkes, H. Brown, G. Gray, J. Mcintyre, and S. Harlow. 2004. Transactional sex among women in Soweto, South Africa: Prevalence, risk factors and association with HIV. *Social Science and Medicine* 59: 1581–92.

Dworkin, Shari L., and Kim Blankenship. 2009. Microfinance and HIV/AIDS prevention: Assessing its promise and limitations. *AIDS and Behavior* 13: 462–69.

Dworkin, Shari L., and John Santelli. 2007. Do abstinence-plus interventions reduce sexual risk behavior among youth? *PLoS Medicine* 4(9): e276.

Dyson, Tim. 2003. HIV/AIDS and urbanization. *Population and Development Review* 29(3): 427–42.

Eaton, Liberty, Alan J. Flisher, and Leif E. Aarø. 2003. Unsafe sexual behavior in South African youth. *Social Science and Medicine* 56: 149–65.

Eccles, J. 2008. The value of an off-diagonal approach. *Journal of Social Issues* 64(1): 227–32.

Eloundou-Enyegue, Parfait M., Dominique Meekers, and Anne Emmanuèle Calvès. 2005. From awareness to adoption: The effect of AIDS education and condom social marketing on condom use in Tanzania (1993–1996). *Journal of Biosocial Science* 37: 257–68.

Etienne, Lucie, Eric Delaporte, and Martine Peeters. 2011. Origin and emergence of HIV/AIDS. In *Genetics and evolution of infectious diseases*, ed. Michel Tibayrenc, 689–710. London: Elsevier.

Exner, Theresa M., J. E. Mantell, L. A. Adeokun, I. A. Udoh, O. A. Ladipo, G. E. Delano, J. Faleye, and K. Akinpelu. 2009. Mobilizing men as partners: The results of an intervention to increase dual protection among Nigerian men. *Health Education Research* 24(5): 846–54.

Eyawo, Oghenowede, Damien de Walque, Nathan Ford, Gloria Gakii, Richard T. Lester, and Edward J. Mills. 2010. HIV status in discordant couples in sub-Saharan Africa: A systematic review and meta-analysis. *Lancet Infectious Diseases* 10: 770–77.

Ezekiel, Mangi Job, Aud Talle, James M. Juma, and Knut-Inge Klepp. 2009. "When in the body, it makes you look fat and HIV negative": The constitution of antiretroviral therapy in local discourse among youth in Kahe, Tanzania. *Social Science and Medicine* 68: 957–64.

Femina Health Information Project. 2008. *Femina HIP annual report 2008*. Dar es salaam, Tanzania: Femina HIP. Downloaded on April 11, 2011 from http: //www .feminahip.or.tz/fileadmin/pics/research/Femina_HIP_Annual_Report_2008_for _web.pdf.

Fenton, K. A., A. M. Johnson, S. McManus, and B. Erens. 2001. Measuring sexual behavior: Methodological challenges in survey research. *Sexually Transmitted Infections* 77: 84–92.

Ferguson, A., M. Pere, C. Morris, E. Ngugi, and S. Moses. 2004. Sexual patterning and condom use among a group of HIV vulnerable men in Thika, Kenya. *Sexually Transmitted Infections* 80: 435–39.

Ferguson, Alan G., and Chester N. Morris. 2007. Mapping transactional sex on the Northern Corridor highway in Kenya. *Health and Place* 13(2): 504–19.

Ferguson, Jane, Bruce Dick, and David A Ross. 2006. Conclusions and recommendations. In *Preventing HIV/AIDS in young people: A systematic review of the evidence from developing countries,* ed. David A. Ross, Bruce Dick, and Jane Ferguson, 317–41. Geneva: WHO.

Fishbein, M. 2000. The role of theory in HIV prevention. *AIDS Care* 12(3): 273–8.

Fishbein, Martin, and Blair Jarvis. 2000. Failure to find a behavioral surrogate for STD incidence: What does it really mean? *Sexually Transmitted Diseases* 27(8): 452–55.

Fishbein, Martin, and Willo Pequegnat. 2000. Evaluating AIDS prevention interventions using behavioral and biological outcome measures. *Sexually Transmitted Diseases* 27(2): 101–10.

Fonseca-Becker F., G. Bakadi, and A. Sow. 2005. *Mobilizing communities for behavior change: HIV/AIDS and pregnancy prevention among youth in upper Guinea.* Baltimore, Maryland: Johns Hopkins Bloomberg School of Public Health, Center for Communication Programs.

Forrest, S. 2004. They treated us like one of them really: Peer education as an approach to sexual health promotion with young people. In *Young people and sexual health: Individual, social and policy contexts*, ed. E. Burtney and M. Duffy, 202–16. Basingstoke: Palgrave Macmillan.

Foss, A. M., M. Hossain, P. T. Vickerman, and C. H. Watts. 2007. A systematic review of published evidence on intervention impact on condom use in sub-Saharan Africa and Asia. *Sexually Transmitted Infections* 83: 510–16.

Fox, Matthew P., Kelly McCoy, Bruce A. Larson, Sydney Rosen, Margaret Bii, Carolyne Sigei, Douglas Shaffer, Fred Sawe, Monique Wasunna, and Jonathon L. Simon. 2010. Improvements in physical wellbeing over the first two years on antiretroviral therapy in western Kenya. *AIDS Care* 22(2): 137–45.

Francis, Dennis A. 2010. Sexuality education in South Africa: Three essential questions. *International Journal of Educational Development* 30: 314–19.

Frumence, Gasto, Japhet Killewo, Gideon Kwesigabo, Lennarth Nyström, Malin Eriksson, and Maria Emmelin. 2010. Social capital and the decline in HIV transmission—A case study in three villages in the Kagera region of Tanzania. *Journal of Social Aspects of HIV/AIDS* 7(3): 9–20.

Fuglesang, Minou. 1997. Lessons for life: Past and present modes of sexuality education in Tanzanian society. *Social Science and Medicine* 44(8): 1245–54.

Fuller, Colin W., Astrid Junge, Jeff DeCelles, James Donald, Ryan Jankelowitz, and Jiri Dvorak. 2010. Football for Health: A football-based health-promotion programme for children in South Africa: A parallel cohort study. *British Journal of Sports Medicine* 44: 546–54.

Gage-Brandon, Anastasia J., and Dominique Meekers. 1993. Sex, contraception and childbearing before marriage in sub-Saharan Africa. *International Family Planning Perspectives* 19: 14–18.

Galárraga, Omar, M. Arantxa Colchero, Richard G. Wamai, and Stefano M. Bertozzi. 2009. HIV prevention cost-effectiveness: A systematic review. *BMC Public Health* 9(Supplement 1): S5.

Gallant, Melanie, and Eleanor Maticka-Tyndale. 2004. School-based HIV prevention programmes for African youth. *Social Science and Medicine* 58(7): 1337–51.

Geary, Cynthia Waszak, Jean-Paul Tchupo, Laura Johnson, Claude Cheta, and Tiburce Nyama. 2003. Respondent perspectives on self-report measures of condom use. *AIDS Education and Prevention* 15(6): 499–515.

Gerbase, A. C., J. T. Rowley, D. H. L. Heymann, S. F. B. Berkley, and P. Piot. 1998. Global prevalence and incidence estimates of selected curable STDs. *Sexually Transmitted Infections* 74(Supplement 1): S12–16.

Gersovitz, M. 2007. HIV, ABC and DHS: Age at first sex in Uganda. *Sexually Transmitted Infections* 83: 165–68.

Gersovitz, M., J. Jacoby, F. Dedy, and A. G. Tape. 1998. The balance of self-reported heterosexual activity in KAP surveys and the AIDS epidemic in Africa. *Journal of the American Statistical Association* 93(443): 875–83.

Giddens, A. 1979. *Central problems in sociological theory: Structure and contradiction in social analysis.* London: MacMillan.

Giddens, A. 1992. *The transformation of intimacy.* California: Stanford University Press.

Gleason, H. A. 1961. The role of tone in the structure of Sųkúma [Book Review]. *Language* 37: 294–308.

Goodrich, J., K. Wellings, and D. McVey. 1998. Using condom data to assess the impact of HIV/AIDS preventive interventions. *Health Education Research* 13(2): 267–74.

Görgen, Regina, Babette Pfander, Juma Bakari, and Akwillina Mlay. 2002. Youth involvement in IEC material production. In *Hands on! A manual for working with youth on sexual and reproductive health*, ed. Rollin and Gabriel, 137–46. Wiesbaden, Germany: Deutsche Gesellschaft für Technische Zusammenarbeit (GTZ).

Green, Edward C. 2011. *Broken promises: How the AIDS establishment has betrayed the developing world.* Sausalito, CA: PoliPointPress.

Green, Edward C., and Kim Witte. 2006. Can fear arousal in public health campaigns contribute to the decline of HIV prevalence? *Journal of Health Communication* 11(3): 245–59.

Greenberg, Judith, Laurence Magder, and Sevgi Aral. 1992. Age at first coitus: A marker for risky sexual behavior in women. *Sexually Transmitted Diseases* 19(6): 331–34.

Greenhalgh, T., E. Kristjansson, and V. Robinson. 2007. Realist review to understand the efficacy of school feeding programmes. *British Medical Journal* 335: 858–61.

Gregson, Simon, Constance A. Nyamukapa, Geoffrey P. Garnett, Peter R. Mason, Tom Zhuwau, Michel Caraël, Stephen K. Chandiwana, and Roy M. Anderson. 2002. Sexual mixing patterns and sex-differentials in teenage exposure to HIV infection in rural Zimbabwe. *Lancet* 359: 1896–1903.

Gregson, Simon, Jim Todd, and Basia Żaba. 2009. Sexual behaviour change in countries with generalised HIV epidemics? Evidence from population-based cohort studies in sub-Saharan Africa. *Sexually Transmitted Infections* 85(Supplement 1): i1–2.

Gregson, Simon, Nicola Terceira, Phyllis Mushati, Constance Nyamukapa, and Catherine Campbell. 2004. Community group participation: Can it help young women to avoid HIV? An exploratory study of social capital and school education in rural Zimbabwe. *Social Science and Medicine* 58(11): 2119–32.

Gregson, Simon, Tom Zhuwau, Roy M. Anderson, and Stephen K. Chandiwana. 1998. Is there evidence for behaviour change in response to AIDS in rural Zimbabwe? *Social Science and Medicine* 46(3): 321–30.

Grills, Nathan. 2006. Does a linear-received policy of condom promotion result in a myopic approach to HIV prevention? *African Journal of AIDS Research* 5(3): 289–93.

Groes-Green, Christian. 2009a. Health discourse, sexual slang and ideological contradictions among Mozambican youth: Implications for method. *Culture, Health and Sexuality* 11(6): 655–68.

Groes-Green, Christian. 2009b. Safe sex pioneers: Class identity, peer education and emerging masculinities among youth in Mozambique. *Sexual Health* 6(3): 233–40.

Grosskurth, Heiner, Frank Mosha, James Todd, Ezra Mwijarubi, Arnoud Klokke, Kesheni Senkoro, Phillipe Mayaud et al. 1995. Impact of improved treatment of sexually transmitted diseases on HIV infection in rural Tanzania: Randomised controlled trial. *Lancet* 346: 530–36.

Grunseit, Anne. 1997. *Impact of HIV and sexual health education on the sexual behaviour of young people: A review update.* Geneva: UNAIDS.

Gueye, Mouhamadou, Sarah Castle, and Mamadou Kani Konate. 2001. Timing of first intercourse among Malian adolescents: Implications for contraceptive use. *International Family Planning Perspectives* 27(2): 56–62 and 70.

Gumodoka, Balthazar, Isabelle Favot, and Wil Domans. 1997. Medical care-related transmission. In *HIV prevention and AIDS care in Africa: A district level approach,* ed. Japhet Ng'weshemi, Ties Boerma, John Bennett, and Dick Schapink, 280–91. Amsterdam: Royal Tropical Institute.

Gupta, Geeta Rao, Justin O. Parkhurst, Jessica A. Ogden, Peter Aggleton, and Ajay Mahal. 2008. Structural approaches to HIV prevention. *Lancet* 372: 764–75.

Guyon, A., A. Obasi, W. Lugoe, J. Wamoyi, G. Mshana, M. Plummer, D. Ross, and J. Ferguson. 2000. Evaluation of HIV/AIDS peer education in primary schools of Mwanza, Tanzania. 13th International AIDS Conference, Durban, South Africa. July 9–14, 2000. Abstract no. LbPeD7125.

Gysels, Marjolein, Robert Pool, and Betty Nnalusiba. 2002. Women who sell sex in a Ugandan trading town: Life histories, survival strategies and risk. *Social Science and Medicine* 54: 179–92.

Hageman, Kathy M., Hazel M. B. Dube, Owen Mugurungi, Loretta E. Gavin, Shannon L. Hader, and Michael E. St. Louis. 2010. Beyond monogamy: Opportunities to further reduce risk for HIV infection among married Zimbabwean women with only one lifetime partner. *AIDS and Behavior* 14: 113–24.

HALIRA. 2002. *HALIRA preliminary report on the* MEMA kwa Vijana *project intervention, June 2002.* Mwanza, Tanzania: Health and Lifestyles Research Project. Unpublished report.

Hallett, T. B., J. Aberle-Grasse, G. Bello, L.-M. Boulos, M. P. A. Cayemittes, B. Cheluget, J. Chipeta et al. 2006. Declines in HIV prevalence can be associated with changing sexual behaviour in Uganda, urban Kenya, Zimbabwe, and urban Haiti. *Sexually Transmitted Infections* 82(Supplement 1): i1–8.

Hallett, Timothy B., John Stover, Vinod Mishra, Peter D. Ghys, Simon Gregson, and Ties Boerma. 2010. Estimates of HIV incidence from household-based prevalence surveys. *AIDS* 24(1): 147–52.

Halperin, Daniel T., and Helen Epstein. 2004. Concurrent sexual partnerships help to explain Africa's high HIV prevalence: Implications for prevention. *Lancet* 364: 4–6.

Halperin, Daniel T., Owen Mugurungi, Timothy B. Hallett, Backson Muchini, Bruce Campbell, Tapuwa Magure, Clemens Benedikt, and Simon Gregson. 2011. A surprising prevention success: Why did the HIV epidemic decline in Zimbabwe? *PLoS Medicine* 8(2): e1000414.

Halperin. Daniel T. 2006. The controversy over fear arousal in AIDS prevention and lessons from Uganda. *Journal of Health Communication* 11(3): 266–67.

Han, Juliana, and Michael L. Bennish. 2009. Condom access in South African schools: Law, policy, and practice. *PLoS Medicine* 6(1): e1000006.

Hankins, Catherine A., and Barbara O. de Zalduondo. 2010. Combination prevention: A deeper understanding of effective HIV prevention. *AIDS* 24(Supplement 4): S70–80.

Harden, Angela, Ann Oakley, and Sandy Oliver. 2001. Peer-delivered health promotion for young people: A systematic review of different study designs. *Health Education Journal* 60: 339–53.

Hardon, Anita, and Hansjörg Dilger. 2011. Global AIDS medicines in East African health institutions. *Medical Anthropology* 30(2): 136–57.

Hardon, Anita. Emmy Kageha, John Kinsman, David Kyaddondo, Rhoda Wanyenze, and Carla Makhlouf Obermeyer. 2011. Dynamics of care, situations of choice: HIV tests in times of ART. *Medical Anthropology* 30(2): 183–201.

Hargreaves, J. R., and L. D. Howe. 2010. Changes in HIV prevalence among differently educated groups in Tanzania between 2003 and 2007. *AIDS* 24(5): 755–61.

Hargreaves, J. R., and T. Boler. 2006. *Girl power: The impact of girls' education on HIV and sexual health. Education and HIV Series 01.* Johannesburg, South Africa: ActionAid International.

Hargreaves, J. R., C. P. Bonell, T. Boler, D. Boccia, I. Birdthistle, A. Fletcher, P. M. Pronyk, and J. R. Glynn. 2008. Systematic review exploring time trends in the association between education attainment and risk of HIV infection in sub-Saharan Africa. *AIDS* 22: 403–14.

Harries, Anthony D., Rony Zachariah, Joep J. van Oosterhout, Steven D. Reid, Mina C. Hosseinipour, Vic Arendt, Zengani Chirwa, Andreas Jahn, Erik J. Schouten, and Kelita Kamoto. 2010. Diagnosis and management of antiretroviral-therapy failure in resource-limited settings in sub-Saharan Africa: Challenges and perspectives. *Lancet Infectious Diseases* 10: 60–65.

Harrison, Abigail, and Lucia F. O'Sullivan. 2010. In the absence of marriage: Long-term concurrent partnerships, pregnancy, and HIV risk dynamics among South African young adults. *AIDS and Behavior* 14(5): 991–1000.

Harrison, Abigail, Lucia F. O'Sullivan, Susie Hoffman, Curtis Dolezal, and Robert Morrell. 2006. Gender role and relationship norms among young adults in South Africa: Measuring the context of masculinity and HIV risk. *Journal of Urban Health* 83(4): 709–22.

Harrison, Abigail, Marie-Louise Newell, John Imrie, and Graeme Hoddinott. 2010. HIV prevention for South African youth: Which interventions work? A systematic review of current evidence. *BMC Public Health* 10: 102.

Hart, G. J., R. Pool, G. Green, S. Harrison, S. Nyanzi, and J. A. G. Whitworth. 1999. Women's attitudes to condoms and female-controlled means of protection against HIV and STDs in southwestern Uganda. *AIDS Care* 11(6): 687–98.

Harwood-Lejeune, Audrey. 2000. Rising age at marriage and fertility in southern and eastern Africa. *European Journal of Population* 17: 261–80.

Hastings, Gerard. 2007. *Social marketing: Why should the devil have the best tunes?* Oxford: Elsevier.

Hattori, Megan Klein, and F. Nii-Amoo Dodoo. 2010. Cohabitation, marriage, and 'sexual monogamy' in Nairobi's slums. *Social Science and Medicine* 64: 1067–78.

Hattori, Megan Klein, Kerry Richter, and Jessica L. Greene. 2008. Trust, caution and condom use with regular partners: An evaluation of the Trusted Partner Campaign targeting youth in four countries. *Social Marketing Quarterly* 16(2): 18–48.

Hayes, Richard J., John Changalucha, David A. Ross, Awene Gavyole, Jim Todd, Angela I. N. Obasi, Mary L. Plummer, Daniel Wight, David C. Mabey, and Heiner Grosskurth. 2005. The *MEMA kwa Vijana* Project: Design of a community-randomised trial of an innovative adolescent sexual health intervention in rural Tanzania. *Contemporary Clinical Trials* 26: 430–42.

Hayes, Richard, Saidi Kapiga, Nancy Padian, Sheena McCormack, and Judith Wasserheit. 2010. HIV prevention research: Taking stock and the way forward. *AIDS* 24(Supplement 4): S81–92.

Heald, Suzette. 1995. The power of sex: Some reflections on the Caldwells' "African sexuality" thesis. *Africa* 65(4): 489–505.

Hearst, Norman, and Sanny Chen. 2004. Condom promotion for AIDS prevention in the developing world: Is it working? *Studies in Family Planning* 35(1): 39–47.

Hecht, Robert. John Stover, Lori Bollinger, Farzana Muhib, Kelsey Case, and David de Ferranti. 2010. Financing of HIV/AIDS programme scale-up in low-income and middle-income countries, 2009–31. *Lancet* 376: 1254–60.

Heimer, Carol A. 2007. Old inequalities, new disease: HIV/AIDS in Sub-Saharan Africa. *Annual Review of Sociology* 33: 551–77.

Helleringer, Stéphane, and Hans-Peter Kohler. 2007. Sexual network structure and the spread of HIV in Africa: Evidence from Likoma Island, Malawi. *AIDS* 21(17): 2323–32.

Helle-Valle, Jo. 1999. Sexual mores, promiscuity and 'prostitution' in Botswana. *Ethnos* 64(3): 372–96.

Helle-Valle, Jo. 2004. Understanding sexuality in Africa: Diversity and contextualized dividuality. In *Re-thinking sexualities in Africa*, ed. Signe Arnfred, 195–210. Uppsala, Sweden: Nordiska Afrikainstitutet.

Helleve, Arnfinn, Alan J. Flisher, Hans Onya, Catherine Mathews, Leif Edvard Aarø, and Knut-Inge Klepp. 2011. The association between students' perceptions of a caring teacher and sexual initiation: A study among South African high school students. *Health Education Research* 26(5): 847–58.

Helleve, Arnfinn, Alan J. Flisher, Hans Onya, Wanjiru Mukoma, and Knut-Inge Klepp. 2009. South African teachers' reflections on the impact of culture on their teaching of sexuality and HIV/AIDS. *Culture, Health and Sexuality* 11(2): 189–204.

Helleve, Arnfinn, Alan J. Flisher, Hans Onya, Wanjiru Mūkoma, and Knut-Inge Klepp. 2011. Can any teacher teach sexuality and HIV/AIDS? Perspectives of South African Life Orientation teachers. *Sex Education* 11(1): 13–26.

Henderson, M., R. Ecob, D. Wight, and C. Abraham. 2008. What explains between-school differences in rates of smoking? *BMC Public Health* 8: 218.

Hendriksen, Ellen Setsuko, Audrey Pettifor, Sung-Jae Lee, Thomas J. Coates, and Helen V. Rees. 2007. Predictors of condom use among young adults in South Africa: The Reproductive Health and HIV Research Unit National Youth Survey. *American Journal of Public Health* 97(7): 1241–8.

Hewett, P. C., B. S. Mensch, and A. S. Erulkar. 2004. Consistency in the reporting of sexual behaviour by adolescent girls in Kenya: A comparison of interviewing methods. *Sexually Transmitted Infections* 80(Supplement 2): ii43–8.

Higbee, Kenneth L. 1969. Fifteen years of fear arousal: Research on threat appeals: 1953–1968. *Psychological Bulletin* 72(6): 426–44.

Hinde, Andrew, and Akim J. Mturi. 2000. Recent trends in Tanzanian fertility. *Population Studies* 54(2): 177–91.

Hirsch, Jennifer S., Holly Wardlow, Daniel Jordan Smith, Harriet M. Phinney, Shanti Parikh, and Constance A. Nathanson. 2009. *The secret: Love, marriage, and HIV.* Nashville: Vanderbilt University Press.

Hoffman, S., L. F. O'Sullivan, A. Harrison, C. Dolezal, and A. Monroe-Wise. 2006. HIV risk behaviors and the context of sexual coercion in young adults' sexual interactions: Results from a diary study in rural South Africa. *Sexually Transmitted Diseases* 33(1): 52–58.

Hoffmann, Oliver, Tania Boler, and Bruce Dick. 2006. Achieving the global goals on HIV among young people most at risk in developing countries: Young sex workers, injecting drug users and men who have sex with men. In *Preventing HIV/AIDS in young people: A systematic review of the evidence from developing countries,* ed. David A. Ross, Bruce Dick, and Jane Ferguson, 287–315. Geneva: WHO.

Holmes, King K., Ruth Levine, and Marcia Weaver. 2004. Effectiveness of condoms in preventing sexually transmitted infections. *Bulletin of the World Health Organization* 82: 454–61.

Hulton, Louise A., Rachel Cullen, and Symons Wamala Khalokho. 2000. Perceptions of the risks of sexual activity and their consequences among Ugandan adolescents. *Studies in Family Planning* 31: 35–46.

Hunter, M. 2002. The materiality of everyday sex: Thinking beyond prostitution. *African Studies* 61(1): 99–120.

Hunter, Mark. 2009. Providing love: Sex and exchange in twentieth-century South Africa. In *Love in Africa*, ed. Jennifer Cole and Lynn M. Thomas, 135–56. Chicago: University of Chicago Press.

Huygens, Pierre, Ellen Kajura, Janet Seeley, and Tom Barton. 1996. Rethinking methods for the study of sexual behavior. *Social Science and Medicine* 42(2): 221–31.

IFAD (International Fund for Agricultural Development). 2001. *Rural poverty report 2001: The challenge of ending rural poverty.* Oxford: Oxford University Press.

Inter-Agency Task Team on HIV and Young People. 2009. *Guidance brief: Overview of HIV interventions for young people.* New York: UNFPA.

International Group on Analysis of Trends in HIV Prevalence and Behaviours in Young People in Countries Most Affected by HIV. 2010. Trends in HIV prevalence and sexual behaviour among young people aged 15–24 years in countries most affected by HIV. *Sexually Transmitted Infections* 86(Supplement 2): ii72–83.

Isingo, Raphael, Basia Zaba, Milly Marston, Milalu Ndege, Julius Mngara, Wambura Mwita, Alison Wringe, David Beckles, John Changalucha, and Mark Urassa. 2007. Survival after HIV infection in the pre-antiretroviral therapy era in a rural Tanzanian cohort. *AIDS* 21(Supplement 6): S5–13.

Izugbara, Chimaraoke Otutubikey, and Felicia Nwabuawele Modo. 2007. Risks and benefits of multiple sexual partnerships: Beliefs of rural Nigerian adolescent males. *American Journal of Men's Health* 1(3): 197–207.

Izugbara, Chimaraoke Otutubikey. 2007. Representations of sexual abstinence among rural Nigerian adolescent males. *Sexuality Research and Social Policy* 4(2): 74–87.

Izugbara, Chimaraoke Otutubikey. 2008. Masculinity scripts and abstinence-related beliefs of rural Nigerian male youth. *Journal of Sex Research* 45(3): 262–76.

Jana, M., M. Nkambule, and D. Tumbo. 2008. *Onelove: Multiple and concurrent sexual partnerships. A ten country research report.* Soul City Institute Regional Program, Adelie Publishing.

Jankowiak, William R., and Edward F. Fischer. 1992. A cross-cultural perspective on romantic love. *Ethnology* 31(2): 149–55.

Jato, Miriam N., Calista Simbakalia, Joan M. Tarasevich, David N. Awasum, Clement N. B. Kihinga, and Edith Ngirwamungu. 1999. The impact of multimedia family planning promotion on the contraceptive behavior of women in Tanzania. *International Family Planning Perspectives* 25(2): 60–67.

Jewkes, R., M. Nduna, J. Levin, N. Jama, K. Dunkle, N. Khuzwayo, M. Koss, A. Puren, K. Wood, and N. Duvvury. 2006. A cluster randomized-controlled trial to determine the effectiveness of Stepping Stones in preventing HIV infections and promoting safer sexual behaviour amongst youth in the rural Eastern Cape, South Africa: Trial design, methods and baseline findings. *Tropical Medicine and International Health* 11(1): 3–16.

Jewkes, Rachel, Jonathan Levin, Nolwazi Mbananga, and Debbie Bradshaw. 2002. Rape of girls in South Africa. *Lancet* 359: 319–20.

Jewkes, Rachel, Katharine Wood, and Nata Duvvury. 2010. 'I woke up after I joined Stepping Stones': Meanings of an HIV behavioural intervention in rural South African young people's lives. *Health Education Research* 25(6): 1074–84.

Jewkes, Rachel, M. Nduna, J. Levin, N. Jama, K. Dunkle, A. Puren, and N. Duvvury. 2008. Impact of Stepping Stones on incidence of HIV and HSV-2 and sexual behaviour in rural South Africa: Cluster randomised controlled trial. *British Medical Journal* 337: a506.

Jewkes, Rachel, Mzikazi Nduna, and Nwabisa Jama. 2010. Stepping Stones: A training manual for sexual and reproductive health communication and relationship skills, edition III. South Africa: Medical Research Council.

Joel, M., A. Chukwuemeka, B. Amusa, and K. Klindera. 2004. Youth-friendly HIV voluntary counselling and testing services: From a youth perspective. 15th International AIDS Conference. Bangkok, Thailand. July 11–16, 2004. Abstract no. TuPeD5111.

Johns Hopkins University Center for Communication Programs. 2003. *Namibia research shows most youth don't understand the terms "abstinence" or "faithfulness" for HIV prevention.* Downloaded on December 20, 2011 from www.thefreelibrary.com/Johns+Hopkins%3A+Namibia+Research+Shows+Most+Youth+Don%27t+Understand+the...-a0102353813.

Johnson, Blair T., Michael P. Carey, Kerry L. Marsh, Kenneth D. Levin, and Lori A. J. Scott-Sheldon. 2003. Interventions to reduce sexual risk for the human immunodeficiency virus in adolescents, 1985–2000: A research synthesis. *Archives of Pediatrics and Adolescent Medicine* 157(4): 381–88.

Johnson, David. 2008. *The changing landscape of education in Africa: Quality, equality and democracy.* Oxford: Symposium Books.

Johnson, Leigh F., Rob E. Dorrington, Debbie Bradshaw, and David J. Coetzee. 2011. The effect of syndromic management interventions on the prevalence of sexually transmitted infections in South Africa. *Sexual and Reproductive Healthcare* 2: 13–20.

Joshi, Anil. 2010. Multiple sexual partners: Perceptions of young men in Uganda. *Journal of Health Organization and Management* 24(5): 520–27.

Jukes, Matthew, Stephanie Simmons, and Donald Bundy. 2008. Education and vulnerability: The role of schools in protecting young women and girls from HIV in southern Africa. *AIDS* 22(Supplement 4): S41–56.

Kaaya, Sylvia F., Alan J. Flisher, Jessie K. Mbwambo, Herman Schaalma, Leif Edvard Aarø, and Knut-Inge Klepp. 2002. A review of studies of sexual behaviour of school students in sub-Saharan Africa. *Scandinavian Journal of Public Health* 30: 148–60.

Kabiru, Caroline W., and Alex Ezeh. 2007. Factors associated with sexual abstinence among adolescents in four sub-Saharan African countries. *African Journal of Reproductive Health* 11(3): 111–32.

Kafewo, Samuel Ayedime. 2008. Using drama for school-based adolescent sexuality education in Zaria, Nigeria. *Reproductive Health Matters* 16(31): 202–10.

Kahn, Lauren. 2006. Narratives of sexual abstinence: A qualitative study of female adolescents in a Cape Town community. *Social Dynamics* 32(1): 75–101.

Kaluvya, S. E., T. J. Boerma, E. N. Mkumbo, and A. Klokke. 1998. The impact of HIV/AIDS on an urban hospital in Tanzania during 1994–1996. 12th International AIDS Conference. Geneva, Switzerland. 28 June–3 July, 1998. Abstract no. 12423.

Kamenga, Munkolenkole, Robert W. Ryder, Muana Jingu, Nkashama Mbuyi, Lubamba Mbu, Frieda Behets, Christopher Brown, and William L. Heyward. 1991. Evidence of marked sexual behavior change associated with low HIV-1 seroconversion in 149 married couples with discordant HIV-1 serostatus: Experience at an HIV counselling center in Zaire. *AIDS* 5: 61–67.

Kamo, Norifumi, Mary Carlson, Robert T. Brennan, and Felton Earls. 2008. Young citizens as health agents: Use of drama in promoting community efficacy for HIV/AIDS. *American Journal of Public Health* 98: 201–4.

Kaponda, Chrissie P. N., Kathleen F. Norr, Kathleen S. Crittenden, James L. Norr, Linda L. McCreary, Sitingawawo I. Kachingwe, Mary M. Mbeba, Diana L. N. Jere, and Barbara L. Dancy. 2011. Outcomes of an HIV prevention peer group intervention for rural adults in Malawi. *Health Education and Behavior* 38(2): 159–70.

Karau, P. B., M. S. Winnie, M. Geoffrey, and M. Mwenda. 2010. Responsiveness to HIV education and VCT services among Kenyan rural women: A community-based survey. *African Journal of Reproductive Health* 14(3): 165–69.

Karim, Quarraisha Abdool, Salim S. Abdool Karim, Janet A. Frohlich, Anneke C. Grobler, Cheryl Baxter, Leila E. Mansoor, Ayesha B. M. Kharsany et al. 2010. Effectiveness and safety of tenofovir gel, an antiretroviral microbicide, for the prevention of HIV infection in women. *Science* 329: 1168–74.

Karim, S. S. Abdool, Q. Abdool Karim, E. Preston-Whyte, and N. Sankar. 1992. Reasons for lack of condom use among high school students. *South African Medical Journal* 82(2): 107–10.

Karim, Salim S. Abdool , and Quarraisha Abdool Karim. 2011. Antiretroviral prophylaxis: A defining moment in HIV control. *Lancet* 378(9809): e23–25.

Katsidzira, Leolin, and James G. Hakim. 2011. HIV prevention in southern Africa: Why we must reassess our strategies? *Tropical Medicine and International Health* 16(9): 1120–30.

Katz, Itamar. 2006. Explaining the increase in condom use among South African young females. *Journal of Health Communication* 11: 737–53.

Kaufman, C. E., and S. E. Stavrou. 2004. "Bus fare, please": The economics of sex and gifts among young people in urban South Africa. *Culture, Health and Sexuality* 6(5): 377–91.

Kazaura, Method R., and Melkiory C. Masatu. 2009. Sexual practices among unmarried adolescents in Tanzania. *BMC Public Health* 9: 373.

Kenyon, Chris, Andrew Boulle, Motasim Badri, and Valerie Asselman. 2010. "I don't use a condom (with my regular partner) because I know that I'm faithful, but with everyone else I do": The cultural and socioeconomic determinants of sexual partner concurrency in young South Africans. *Journal of Social Aspects of HIV/AIDS* 7(3): 35–43.

Khan, Nazir. 2010. *Using football for HIV/AIDS prevention in Africa.* Coxswain: Social Investment Plus.

Kim, Caron R., and Caroline Free. 2008. Recent evaluations of the peer-led approach in adolescent sexual health education: A systematic review. *International Family Planning Perspectives* 34(2): 89–96.

Kim, Julia C., and Charlotte Watts. 2005. Gaining a foothold: Tackling poverty, gender equality, and HIV in Africa. *British Medical Journal* 331: 769–72.

Kim, Julia, Giulia Ferrari, Tanya Abramsky, Charlotte Watts, James Hargreaves, Linda Morison, Godfrey Phetla, John Porter, and Paul Pronyk. 2009. Assessing the incremental effects of combining economic and health interventions: The IMAGE study in South Africa. *Bulletin of the World Health Organization* 87(11): 824–32.

Kim, Young Mi, Adrienne Kols, Ronika Nyakauru, Caroline Marangwanda, and Peter Chibatamoto. 2001. Promoting sexual responsibility among young people in Zimbabwe. *International Family Planning Perspectives* 27(1): 11–19.

Kimuna, S., and Y. Djamba. 2005. Wealth and extramarital sex among men in Zambia. *International Family Planning Perspectives* 31(2): 83–89.

Kinfu, Yohannes, Mario R. Dal Poz, Hugo Mercer, and David B. Evans. 2009. The health worker shortage in Africa: Are enough physicians and nurses being trained? *Bulletin of the World Health Organization* 87: 225–30.

Kinsman, J., J. Nakiyingi, A. Kamali, L. Carpenter, M. Quigley, R. Pool, and J. Whitworth. 2001. Evaluation of a comprehensive school-based AIDS education programme in rural Masaka, Uganda. *Health Education Research* 16: 85–100.

Kinsman, J., S. Harrison, J. Kengeya-Kayondo, E. Kanyesigye, S. Musoke, and J. Whitworth. 1999. Implementation of a comprehensive AIDS education programme for schools in Masaka District, Uganda. *AIDS Care* 11(5): 591–601.

Kipp, Walter, Sunita Chacko, Lory Laing, and Geoffrey Kabagambe. 2007. Adolescent reproductive health in Uganda: Issues related to access and quality of care. *International Journal of Adolescent Medicine and Health* 19(4): 383–93.

Kippax, Susan, and Niamh Stephenson. 2005. Meaningful evaluation of sex and relationship education. *Sex Education* 5(4): 359–73.

Kippax, Susan. 2003. Sexual health interventions are unsuitable for experimental evaluation. In *Effective sexual health interventions: Issues in experimental evaluation*, ed. Judith M. Stephenson, John Imrie, and Chris Bonell, 17–34. Oxford: Oxford University Press.

Kirby, Doug. 2001. *The MEMA kwa Vijana curriculum: A review.* Unpublished report.

Kirby, Douglas B., B. A. Laris, M. P. H., and Lori A. Rolleri. 2007. Sex and HIV education programs: Their impact on sexual behaviors of young people throughout the world. *Journal of Adolescent Health* 40: 206–17.

Kirby, Douglas, Angela Obasi, and B. A. Laris. 2006. The effectiveness of sex education and HIV education interventions in schools in developing countries. In *Preventing HIV/AIDS in young people: A systematic review of the evidence from developing countries,* ed. David A. Ross, Bruce Dick, and Jane Ferguson, 103–50. Geneva: WHO.

Kirby, Douglas, Lynn Short, Janet Collins, Deborah Rugg, Lloyd Kolbe, Marion Howard, Brent Miller, Freya Sonenstein, and Laurie S. Zabin. 1994. School-based programs to reduce sexual risk behaviors: Review of effectiveness. *Public Health Reports* 109: 339–60.

Kirby, Douglas. 2006. Can fear arousal in public health campaigns contribute to the decline of HIV prevalence? *Journal of Health Communication* 11(3): 262–66.

Kirk, Dudley, and Bernard Pillet. 1998. Fertility levels, trends, and differentials in sub-Saharan Africa in the 1980s and 1990s. *Studies in Family Planning* 29(1): 1–22.

Kiš, Adam Daniel. 2010. ABC for AIDS prevention in Guinea: Migrant gold mining communities address their risks. *AIDS Care* 22(4): 520–25.

Kissling, Esther, Edward H. Allison, Janet A. Seeley, Steven Russell, Max Bachmann, Stanley D. Musgrave, and Simon Heck. 2005. Fisherfolk are among groups most at risk of HIV: Cross-country analysis of prevalence and numbers infected. *AIDS* 19: 1939–46.

Klepp, K. I., S. S. Ndeki, A. M. Seha, P. Hannan, B. A. Lyimo, M. H. Msuya, M. N. Irema, and A. Schreiner. 1994. AIDS education for primary school children in Tanzania: An evaluation study. *AIDS* 8: 1157–62.

Klepp, K.-I., S. Ndeki, M. T. Leshabari, P. J. Hannan, and B. A. Lyimo. 1997. AIDS education in Tanzania: Promoting risk reduction among primary school children. *American Journal of Public Health* 87(12): 1931–36.

Knerr, Wendy. 2011. Does condom social marketing improve health outcomes and increase usage and equitable access? *Reproductive Health Matters* 19(37): 166–73.

Koffi, Alain K., Visseho D. Adjiwanou, Stan Becker, Funmilola Olaolorun, and Amy O. Tsui. 2012. Correlates of and couples' concordance in reports of recent sexual behavior and contraceptive use. *Studies in Family Planning* 43(1): 33–42.

Konings, E., G. Bantebya, M. Caraël, D. Bagenda, and T. Mertens. 1995. Validating population surveys for the measurement of HIV/STD prevention indicators. *AIDS* 9: 375–82.

Kraut-Becher, Julie R., and Sevgi O. Aral. 2003. Gap length: An important factor in sexually transmitted disease transmission. *Sexually Transmitted Diseases* 30(3): 221–25.

Ku, Leighton, Freya L. Sonenstein, Charles F. Turner, Sevgi O. Aral, and Carolyn M. Black. 1997. The promise of integrated representative surveys about sexually transmitted diseases and behavior. *Sexually Transmitted Diseases* 24(5): 299–309.

Kuhn, L., M. Steinberg, and C. Mathews. 1994. Participation of the school community in AIDS education: An evaluation of a high school programme in South Africa. *AIDS Care* 6(2): 161–71.

Kumi-Kyereme, Akwasi, Kofi Awusabo-Asare, Ann Biddlecom, and Augustine Tanle. 2007. Influence of social connectedness, communication and monitoring on adolescent sexual activity in Ghana. *African Journal of Reproductive Health* 11(3): 133–47.

Kuran, T. 2004. Cultural obstacles to economic development. In *Culture and public action*, ed. V. Rao and M. Walton, 115–37. Palo Alto: Stanford University Press.

Kurowski, Christoph, Kaspar Wyss, Salim Abdulla, N'Diekhor Yémadji, and Anne Mills. 2003. *Human Resources for Health: Requirements and availability in the context of scaling-up priority interventions in low-income countries: Case studies from Tanzania and Chad.* Downloaded from info.worldbank.org/etools/docs/library/206875/HR%20DFID%20report%20final%20version.pdf on January 30, 2012.

Kurth, Ann E., Connie Celum, Jared M. Baeten, Sten H. Vermund, and Judith N. Wasserheit. 2011. Combination HIV prevention: Significance, challenges, and opportunities. *Current HIV/AIDS Reports* 8(1): 62–72.

Laga, Marie, Bernhard Schwärtlander, Elisabeth Pisani, Papa Salif Sow, and Michel Caraël. 2001. To stem HIV in Africa, prevent transmission to young women. *AIDS* 15(7): 931–34.

Laga, Marie, Deborah Rugg, Greet Peersman, and Martha Ainsworth. 2012. Evaluating HIV prevention effectiveness: The perfect as the enemy of the good. *AIDS* 26(7): 779–83.

Lagarde, E., B. Auvert, J. Chege, T. Sukwa, J. R. Glynn, H. A. Weiss, E. Akam, M. Laourou, M. Caraël, A. Buvé, and the Study Group on the Heterogeneity of HIV Epidemics in African Cities. 2001. Condom use and its association with HIV/ sexually transmitted diseases in four urban communities of sub-Saharan Africa. *AIDS* 15(Supplement 4): S71–78.

Lamptey, Peter, and Gail A. W. Goodridge. 1991. Condom issues in AIDS prevention in Africa. *AIDS* 5(Supplement 1): S183–91.

Landman, Keren Z., Jan Ostermann, John A. Crump, Anna Mgonja, Meghan K. Mayhood, Dafrosa K. Itemba, Alison C. Tribble et al. 2008. Gender differences in the risk of HIV infection among persons reporting abstinence, monogamy, and multiple sexual partners in northern Tanzania. *PLoS ONE* 3(8): e3075.

Langhaug. L. F., F. M. Cowan, T. Nyamurera, and R. Power. 2003. Improving young people's access to reproductive health care in rural Zimbabwe. *AIDS Care* 15(2): 147–57.

Larke, Natasha L., Bernadette Cleophas-Mazige, Mary L. Plummer, Angela I. Obasi, Merdard Rwakatare, Jim Todd, John Changalucha, Helen A. Weiss, Richard J. Hayes, and David A. Ross. 2010. Impact of the *MEMA kwa Vijana* adolescent sexual and reproductive health interventions on use of health services by young people in rural Mwanza, Tanzania: Results of a cluster randomised trial. *Journal of Adolescent Health* 47(5): 512–22.

Larsen, Ulla, and Marida Hollos. 2002. Women's empowerment and fertility decline among the Pare of Kilimanjaro region, Northern Tanzania. *Social Science and Medicine* 57: 1099–115.

Latkin, C. A., and A. R. Knowlton. 2005. Micro-social structural approaches to HIV prevention: A social ecological perspective. *AIDS Care* 17(Supplement 1): 102–13.

Le Blanc, Marie-Nathalie, Deidre Meintel, and Victor Piche. 1991. The African sexual system: Comment on Caldwell et al. *Population and Development Review* 17(3): 497–505.

Leclerc-Madlala, S. 2003 Transactional sex and the pursuit of modernity. *Social Dynamics* 29(2): 213–33.

LeClerc-Madlala, Suzanne. 2008. Age-disparate and intergenerational sex in southern Africa: The dynamics of hypervulnerability. *AIDS* 22(Supplement 4): S17–25.

Leclerc-Madlala, Suzanne. 2009. Cultural scripts for multiple and concurrent partnerships in southern Africa: Why HIV prevention needs anthropology. *Sexual Health* 6(2): 103–10.

Lees, Shelley, Nicola Desmond, Caroline Allen, Gilbert Bugeke, Andrew Vallely, and David Ross. 2009. Sexual risk behavior for women working in recreational venues in Mwanza, Tanzania: Considerations for the acceptability and use of vaginal microbicide gels. *Culture, Health and Sexuality* 11(6): 581–95.

Leiva, Anya, Matthew Shaw, Katie Paine, Kebba Manneh, Keith McAdam, and Philippe Mayaud. 2001. Management of sexually transmitted diseases in urban pharmacies in the Gambia. *International Journal of STD and AIDS* 12: 444–52.

Leshabari, Melkizedeck T., Sylvia F. Kaaya, and Anna Tengia-Kessy. 2008. Adolescent sexuality and the AIDS epidemic in Tanzania: What has gone wrong? In *Promoting adolescent sexual and reproductive health in east and southern Africa*, ed. Knut-Inge Klepp, Alan J. Flisher, and Sylvia F. Kaaya, 135–61. Capetown: HSRC Press.

Lewin, Simon, Claire Glenton, and Andrew D. Oxman. 2009. Use of qualitative methods alongside randomised controlled trials of complex healthcare interventions: Methodological study. *British Medical Journal* 339: b3496.

Lewinson, Anne. 2006. Love in the city: Navigating multiple relationships in Dar es Salaam, Tanzania. *City and Society* 18(1): 90–115.

Lillie, Tiffany, Julie Pulerwitz, and Barbara Curbow. 2009. Kenyan in-school youths' level of understanding of abstinence, being faithful, and consistent condom use terms: Implications for HIV prevention programs. *Journal of Health Communication* 14(3): 276–92.

Lloyd, Cynthia B., and Paul Hewett. 2009. Educational inequalities in the midst of persistent poverty: Diversity across Africa in educational outcomes. *Journal of International Development* 21: 1137–51.

Louie, Karly S., Silvia de Sanjose, and Philippe Mayaud. 2009. Epidemiology and prevention of human papillomavirus and cervical cancer in sub-Saharan Africa: A comprehensive review. *Tropical Medicine and International Health* 14(10): 1287–1302.

Lugoe, Wycliffe. 2001. *Evaluation of the teachers' training sessions for the MEMA kwa Vijana teacher-led component.* Unpublished report.

Luke, Nancy. 2003. Age and economic asymmetries in the sexual relationships of adolescent girls in sub-Saharan Africa. *Studies in Family Planning* 34(2): 67–86.

Lurie, Mark N., and Samantha Rosenthal. 2010. Concurrent partnerships as a driver of the HIV epidemic in Sub-Saharan Africa? The evidence is limited. *AIDS and Behavior* 14(1): 17–24.

Lutz, Brian. 2005. Marital status, sexual behavior and sexually transmitted infection in rural Tanzanian villages. Thesis for Master of Science in Epidemiology, London School of Hygiene and Tropical Medicine, UK.

Macdowall, Wendy, and Kirstin Mitchell. 2006. Sexual health communication: Letting young people have their say. In *Promoting young people's sexual health: International perspectives*, ed. Roger Ingham and Peter Aggleton, 174–91. Oxon, UK: Routledge.

Mack, Natasha, Cynthia Woodsong, Kathleen M. Macqueen, Greg Guest, and Emily Namey. 2005. *Qualitative research methods: A data collector's field guide.* Research Triangle Park, NC: Family Health International.

MacPhail, Catherine. 2003. Challenging dominant norms of masculinity for HIV prevention. *African Journal of AIDS Research* 2(2): 141–49.

MacPhail, Catherine, Audrey Pettifor, Sophie Pascoe, and Helen Rees. 2007. Predictors of dual method use for pregnancy and HIV prevention among adolescent South African women. *Contraception* 75: 383–89.

Madriz, Esther. 2000. Focus groups in feminist research. In *Handbook of qualitative research*, ed. Norman K. Denzin and Yvonna S. Lincoln, 835–50. Thousand Oaks, CA: Sage.

Mæstad, Ottar. 2006. *Human resources for health in Tanzania: Challenges, policy options and knowledge gaps.* Bergen, Norway: Chr. Michelsen Institute. Downloaded from www.cmi.no/publications/file/2175-human-resources-for-health-in-tanzania-challenges.pdf on January 30, 2012.

Maganja, R., S. Maman, A. Groves, and J. Mbwambo. 2007. Skinning the goat and pulling the load: Transactional sex among youth in Dar es Salaam, Tanzania. *AIDS Care* 19(8): 974–81.

Maharaj, Pranitha. 2006. Reasons for condom use among young people in KwaZulu-Natal: Prevention of HIV, pregnancy or both? *International Family Planning Perspectives* 32(1): 28–34.

Mahler, H., and N. Ndegwa. 2008. Championing the neglected "B": Tanzania's Sikia Kengele Initiative aims to promote faithfulness and partner reduction from a secular perspective. 17th International AIDS Conference, Mexico City, Mexico. 3–8 August, 2008. Abstract no. THPE0492.

Makokha, M., A. Obasi, K. Chima, B. Cleophas-Frisch, G. Mmassy, A. Guyon, W. Lugoe et al. 2002. Impact of environment on the effectiveness of peer education: Experiences from a teacher-led sexual and reproductive health programme in primary schools in rural Mwanza, Tanzania. 14th International AIDS Conference, Barcelona, Spain. 7–12 July, 2002. Abstract no. TuPeD5019.

Mamdani, Masuma, and Maggie Bangser. 2004. Poor people's experiences of health services in Tanzania: A literature review. *Reproductive Health Matters* 12(24): 138–53.

Manhart, Lisa E., Sevgi O. Aral, King K. Holmes, and Betsy Foxman. 2002. Sex partner concurrency: Measurement, prevalence, and correlates among urban 18–39-year-olds. *Sexually Transmitted Diseases* 29(3): 133–43.

Marindo, Ravai, Steve Pearson, and John B. Casterline. 2003. *Condom use and abstinence among unmarried young people in Zimbabwe: Which strategy, whose agenda? Policy Research Division Working Paper No. 170.* New York: Population Council.

Maro, C. N., G. C. Roberts, and M. Sørenson. 2009. Using sport to promote HIV/AIDS education for at-risk youths: An intervention using peer coaches in football. *Scandinavian Journal of Medicine and Science in Sports* 19(1): 129–41.

Mason-Jones, Amanda J., Catherine Mathews, and Alan J. Flisher. 2011. Can peer education make a difference? Evaluation of a South African adolescent peer education program to promote sexual and reproductive health. *AIDS and Behavior* 15: 1605–11.

Mathews, Catherine, Sally J. Guttmacher, Alan J. Flisher, Yolisa Y. Mtshizana, Tobey Nelson, Jean McCarthy, and Vanessa Daries. 2009. The quality of HIV testing services for adolescents in Cape Town, South Africa: Do adolescent-friendly services make a difference? *Journal of Adolescent Health* 44: 188–90.

Maticka-Tyndale, Eleanor, and Chris Brouillard-Coyle. 2006. The effectiveness of community interventions targeting HIV and AIDS prevention at young people in developing countries. In *Preventing HIV/AIDS in young people: A systematic review of the evidence from developing countries,* ed. David A. Ross, Bruce Dick, and Jane Ferguson, 243–86. Geneva: WHO.

Maticka-Tyndale, Eleanor, and Collins Kyeremeh. 2010. The trouble with condoms: Norms and meanings of sexuality and condom use among school-going youth in Kenya. *International Journal of Sexual Health* 22: 234–47.

Maticka-Tyndale, Eleanor, and Jessica Penwell Barnett. 2010. Peer-led interventions to reduce HIV risk of youth: A review. *Evaluation and Program Planning* 33: 98–112.

Matovu, Joseph K. B. 2011. HIV counselling and testing on the move. *Lancet Infectious Diseases* 11: 492–93.

Mattes, Dominik. 2011. "We are just supposed to be quiet": The production of adherence to antiretroviral treatment in urban Tanzania. *Medical Anthropology* 30(2): 158–82.

Mavedzenge, Sue M. Napierala, Aoife M. Doyle, and David A. Ross. 2011. HIV prevention in young people in sub-Saharan Africa: A systematic review. *Journal of Adolescent Health* 49(6): 568–86.

Mavedzenge, Sue Napierala, Rick Olson, Aoife M. Doyle, John Changalucha, and David A. Ross. 2011. The epidemiology of HIV among young people in sub-Saharan Africa: Know your local epidemic and its implications for prevention. *Journal of Adolescent Health* 49(6): 559–67.

Mbago, Maurice C. Y., and Francis J Sichona. 2010. Determinants of extramarital sex by men in Tanzania: A case study of Mbeya region. *Journal of Social Aspects of HIV/AIDS* 7(4): 33–38.

Mbonile, L., and E. J. Kayombo. 2008. Assessing acceptability of parents/guardians of adolescents towards introduction of sex and reproductive health education in schools at Kinondoni Municipal in Dar es Salaam city. *East African Journal of Public Health* 5(1): 26–31.

McCoy, Sandra I., Charlotte H. Watts, and Nancy S. Padian. 2010. Preventing HIV infection: Turning the tide for young women. *Lancet* 376: 1281–82.

McKinsey and Company. 2005. *Acting now to overcome Tanzania's greatest health challenge: Addressing the gap in Human Resources for Health: Report from field visit, Tanzania 2004.* Downloaded from www.touchfoundation.org/uploads/assets/documents/mckinsey_report_2004_CV7maemq.pdf on January 30, 2012.

Meekers, D., G. Ahmed, and M. T. Molathegi. 2001. Understanding constraints to adolescent condom procurement: The case of urban Botswana. *AIDS Care* 13(3): 297–302.

Meekers, Dominique, and Ronan Van Rossem. 2005. Explaining inconsistencies between data on condom use and condom sales. *BMC Health Services Research* 5: 5.

Meekers, Dominique, Sohail Agha, and Megan Klein. 2005. The impact on condom use of the "100 percent Jeune" social marketing program in Cameroon. *Journal of Adolescent Health* 36: 530.e1–530.e12.

Menon, Sonia. 2010. Early initiation of antiretroviral therapy and universal HIV testing in sub-Saharan Africa: Has WHO offered a milestone for HIV prevention? *Journal of Public Health Policy* 31(4): 385–400.

Mensch, Barbara S., Paul C. Hewett, and Annabel S. Erulkar. 2003. The reporting of sensitive behavior by adolescents: A methodological experiment in Kenya. *Demography* 40(2): 247–68.

Mensch, Barbara S., Wesley H. Clark, Cynthia B. Lloyd, and Annabel S. Erulkar. 2001. Premarital sex, schoolgirl pregnancy, and school quality in rural Kenya. *Studies in Family Planning* 32(4): 285–301.

Merson, Michael H., Jeffrey O'Malley, David Serwadda, and Chantawipa Apisuk. 2008. The history and challenge of HIV prevention. *Lancet* 372: 475–88.

Messersmith, Lisa J., Thomas T. Kane, Adetanwa I. Odebiyi, and Alfred A. Adewuyi. 2000. Who's at risk? Men's STD experience and condom use in southwest Nigeria. *Studies in Family Planning* 31(3): 203–16.

Michau, Lori. 2007. Approaching old problems in new ways: Community mobilisation as a primary prevention strategy to combat violence against women. *Gender and Development* 15(1): 95–109.

Michau, Lori, and Dipak Naker. 2003. *Mobilising communities to prevent domestic violence: A resource guide for organisations in East and Southern Africa.* Kampala, Uganda: Raising Voices.

Michie, S., M. Johnston, C. Abraham, R. Lawton, D. Parker, A. Walker, on behalf of the "Psychological Theory" Group. 2005. Making psychological theory useful for implementing evidence based practice: A consensus approach. *Quality and Safety in Health Care* 14: 26–33.

Michielsen, Kristien, Matthew F. Chersich, Stanley Luchters, Petra De Koker, Ronan Van Rossem, and Marleen Temmerman. 2010. Effectiveness of HIV prevention for youth in sub-Saharan Africa: Systematic review and meta-analysis of randomized and nonrandomized trials. *AIDS* 24: 1193–202.

Middelkoop, Keren, Landon Myer, Joalida Smit, Robin Wood, and Linda-Gail Bekker. 2006. Design and evaluation of a drama-based intervention to promote voluntary counseling and HIV testing in a South African community. *Sexually Transmitted Diseases* 33(8): 524–26.

Miller, Ann Neville, Lenette Golding, Kyalo wa Ngula, MaryAnne Wambua, Evans Mutua, Mary N. Kitizo, Caroline Teti, Nancy Booker, Kinya Mwithia, and Donald L. Rubin. 2009. Couples' communication on sexual and relational issues among the Akamba in Kenya. *African Journal of AIDS Research* 8(1): 51–60.

Mills, Edward J., Jean B. Nachega, David R. Bangsberg, Sonal Singh, Beth Rachlis, Ping Wu, Kumanan Wilson, Iain Buchan, Christopher J. Gill, and Curtis Cooper. 2006. Adherence to HAART: A systematic review of developed and developing nation patient-reported barriers and facilitators. *PLoS Medicine* 3(11): 2039–64.

Mindry, Deborah, Suzanne Maman, Admire Chirowodza, Tshifhiwa Muravha, Heidi van Rooyen, and Thomas Coates. 2011. Looking to the future: South African men and women negotiating HIV risk and relationship intimacy. *Culture, Health and Sexuality* 13(5): 589–602.

Mitchell, Kimberly J., Sheana Bull, Julius Kiwanuka, and Michele L. Ybarra. 2011. Cell phone usage among adolescents in Uganda: Acceptability for relaying health information. *Health Education Research* 26(5): 770–81.

Mkumbo, Kitila A. 2009. Content analysis of the status and place of sexuality education in the national school policy and curriculum in Tanzania. *Educational Research and Review* 4(12): 616–25.

Mkumbo, Kitila A. K. 2010. What Tanzanian young people want to know about sexual health; implications for school-based sex and relationships education. *Sex Education* 10(4): 405–12.

Mkumbo, Kitila A. K., and Roger Ingham. 2010. What Tanzanian parents want (and do not want) covered in school-based sex and relationships education. *Sex Education* 10(1): 67–78.

Mlemya, B., V. Justine, and Z. Mgalla. 1997. Country watch: Tanzania. *AIDS/STD Health Promotion Exchange* 1: 5–6.

Mmari, Kristin N., and Robert J. Magnani. 2003. Does making clinic-based reproductive health services more youth-friendly increase service use by adolescents? Evidence from Lusaka, Zambia. *Journal of Adolescent Health* 33: 259–70.

Mmbaga, Elia J., Germana H. Leyna, Kagoma S. Mnyika, Akthar Hussain, and Knut-Inge Klepp. 2007. Education attainment and the risk of HIV-1 infections in rural Kilimanjaro Region of Tanzania, 1991–2005: A reversed association. *Sexually Transmitted Diseases* 34(12): 947–53.

Modjarrad, Kayvon, and Sten H. Vermund. 2010. Effect of treating co-infections on HIV-1 viral load: A systematic review. *Lancet Infectious Diseases* 10: 455–63.

Mojola, Sanyu A. 2011. Fishing in dangerous waters: Ecology, gender and economy in HIV risk. *Social Science and Medicine* 72: 149–56.

Molassiotis, Alexander, Irene Saralis-Avis, Wilson Nyirenda, and Nina Atkins. 2004. The Simalelo Peer Education Programme for HIV prevention: A qualitative process evaluation of a project in Zambia. *African Journal of AIDS Research* 3(2): 183–90.

Molla, Mitike, Yemane Berhane, and Bernt Lindtjørn. 2008. Traditional values of virginity and sexual behavior in rural Ethiopian youth: Results from a cross-sectional study. *BMC Public Health* 8: 9.

Montgomery, C. M., S. Lees, J. Stadler, N. S. Morar, A. Ssali, B. Mwanza, M. Mntambo, J. Phillip, C. Watts, and R. Pool. 2008. The role of partnership dynamics in determining the acceptability of condoms and microbicides. *AIDS Care* 20(6): 733–40.

Montgomery, Catherine M., Victoria Hosegood, Joanna Busza, and Ian M. Timæus. 2006. Men's involvement in the South African family: Engendering change in the AIDS era. *Social Science and Medicine* 62: 2411–19.

Moody, James. 2002. The importance of relationship timing for diffusion. *Social Forces* 81(1): 25–56.

Morgan, Dilys, Cedric Mahe, Billy Mayanja, J. Martin Okongo, Rosemary Lubega, and James A. G Whitworth. 2002. HIV-1 infection in rural Africa: Is there a difference in median time to AIDS and survival compared with that in industrialized countries? *AIDS* 16: 597–603.

Morris, Martina, and Mirjam Kretzschmar. 1997. Concurrent partnerships and the spread of HIV. *AIDS* 11: 641–48.

Morris, Martina. 2010. Barking up the wrong evidence tree. Comment on Lurie and Rosenthal, "Concurrent partnerships as a driver of the HIV epidemic in sub-Saharan Africa? The evidence is limited". *AIDS and Behavior* 14: 31–33.

Moyo, W., B. A. Levandowski, C. MacPhail, H. Rees, and A. Pettifor. 2008. Consistent condom use in South African youths most recent sexual relationships. *AIDS and Behavior* 12: 431–40.

Mpofu, Elias, Alan J. Flisher, Khalipha Bility, Hans Onya, and Carl Lombard. 2006. Sexual partners in a rural south African setting. *AIDS and Behavior* 10(4): 399–404.

Mukoma, Wanjiru, Alan J. Flisher, Nazeema Ahmed, Shahieda Jansen, Catherine Mathews, Knut-Inge Klepp, and Herman Schaalma. 2009. Process evaluation of a school-based HIV/AIDS intervention in South Africa. *Scandinavian Journal of Public Health* 37(Supplement 2): 37–47.

Munguti, Katua, Heiner Grosskurth, James Newell, Kesheni Senkoro, Frank Mosha, James Todd, Philippe Mayaud, Awena Gavyole, Maria Quigley, and Richard Hayes. 1997. Patterns of sexual behaviour in a rural population in north-western Tanzania. *Social Science and Medicine* 44(10): 1553–61.

Murphy, Elaine M., Margaret E. Greene, Alexandra Mihailovic, and Peter Olupot-Olupot. 2006. Was the "ABC" approach (Abstinence, Being Faithful, Using Condoms) responsible for Uganda's decline in HIV? *PLoS Medicine* 3(9): 1443–47.

Muyinda, H., J. Nakuya, R. Pool, and J. Whitworth. 2003. Harnessing the senga institution of adolescent sex education for the control of HIV and STDs in rural Uganda. *AIDS Care* 15(2): 159–67.

Muyinda, Herbert, Jane Kengeya, Robert Pool, and James Whitworth. 2001. Traditional sex counselling and STI/HIV prevention among young women in rural Uganda. *Culture, Health and Sexuality* 3(3): 353–61.

Mwaanga, Oscar. 2010. Sport for addressing HIV/AIDS: Explaining our convictions. *LSA Newsletter* No. 85: 61–67.

Mwaluko, Gabriel, Mark Urassa, Raphael Isingo, Basia Zaba, and J. Ties Boerma. 2003. Trends in HIV and sexual behaviour in a longitudinal study in a rural population in Tanzania, 1994–2000. *AIDS* 17: 2645–51.

Myer, L., C. Mathews, and F. Little. 2002. Improving the accessibility of condoms in South Africa: The role of informal distribution. *AIDS Care* 14(6): 773–78.

Naker, Dipak, and Lori Michau. 2004. *Rethinking domestic violence: A training process for community activists.* Kampala, Uganda: Raising Voices.

National Bureau of Statistics, and ICF Macro. 2011. *Tanzania Demographic and Health Survey 2010.* Dar es Salaam, Tanzania: National Bureau of Statistics and ICF Macro.

National Bureau of Statistics, and Macro International Inc. 2000. *Tanzania Reproductive and Child Health Survey 1999.* Calverton, MD: National Bureau of Statistics and Macro International Inc.

National Bureau of Statistics, and ORC Macro. 2004. *2002 Population and Housing Census: The regional and district census data in brief (Volume IV).* Dar es Salaam, Tanzania: National Bureau of Statistics and ORC Macro.

National Bureau of Statistics, and ORC Macro. 2005. *Tanzania Demographic and Health Survey 2004–05.* Dar es Salaam, Tanzania: National Bureau of Statistics and ORC Macro.

National Research Council. 2002. *Geographic information for sustainable development in Africa.* Washington, DC: National Academies Press.

Nelson, Sara J., Lisa E. Manhart, Pamina M. Gorbach, David H. Martin, Bradley P. Stoner, Sevgi O. Aral, and King K. Holmes. 2007. Measuring sex partner concurrency: It's what's missing that counts. *Sexually Transmitted Diseases* 34(10): 801–7.

Neukom, Josselyn and Lori Ashford. 2003. *Changing youth behavior through social marketing: Program experiences and research findings from Cameroon, Madagascar, and Rwanda.* Washington, DC: Population Services International.

Ngom, Pierre, Monica A. Magadi, and Tom Owuor. 2003. Parental presence and adolescent reproductive health among Nairobi urban poor. *Journal of Adolescent Health* 33: 369–77.

Nilsson, Paula. 2003. *Education for all: Teacher demand and supply in Africa. Education International Working Paper No. 12.* Brussels: Education International.

Nixon, Stephanie A., Clara Rubincam, Marisa Casale, and Sarah Flicker. 2011. Is 80 percent a passing grade? Meanings attached to condom use in an abstinence-plus HIV prevention programme in South Africa. *AIDS Care* 23(2): 213–20.

Njau, B., M. H. Watt, J. Ostermann, R. Manongi, and K. J. Sikkema. 2011. Perceived acceptability of home-based couples voluntary HIV counseling and testing in Northern Tanzania. *AIDS Care* 24(4): 413–19.

Njau, Bernard, Sabina Mtweve, Rachel Manongi, and Hector Jalipa. 2010. Gender differences in intention to remain a virgin until marriage among school pupils in rural northern Tanzania. *African Journal of AIDS Research* 8(2): 157–66.

Njue, Carolyne, Charles Nzioka, Beth-Maina Ahlberg, Anne M. Pertet, and Helene A. C. M. Voeten. 2009. "If you don't abstain, you will die of AIDS": AIDS education in Kenyan public schools. *AIDS Education and Prevention* 21(2): 169–79.

Nnko, Soori, J. Ties Boerma, Mark Urassa, Gabriel Mwaluko, and Basia Zaba. 2004. Secretive females or swaggering males? An assessment of the quality of sexual partnership reporting in rural Tanzania. *Social Science and Medicine* 59: 299–310.

Ntabaye, M., and J. McMahan. 2008. Increasing the people who know their status: Scaling up provider-initiated testing and counseling in Tanzania. 17th International AIDS Conference, Mexico City, Mexico. 3–8 August 2008. Abstract no. WEPE0045.

Nzioka, C. 2001. Perspectives of adolescent boys on the risks of unwanted pregnancy and sexually transmitted infections: Kenya. *Reproductive Health Matters* 9(17): 108–17.

Nzioka, Charles. 2004. Unwanted pregnancy and sexually transmitted infection among young women in rural Kenya. *Culture, Health and Sexuality* 6(1): 31–44.

O'Farrell, Nigel. 1999. Increasing prevalence of genital herpes in developing countries: Implications for heterosexual HIV transmission and STI control programs. *Sexually Transmitted Infections* 75(6): 377–84.

O'Grady, Mary. 2006. Just inducing fear of HIV/AIDS is not just. *Journal of Health Communication* 11(3): 261–62.

O'Hara, H. B., H. A. C. M. Voeten, A. G. Kuperus, J. M. Otido, J. Kusimba, J. D. F. Habbema, J. J. Bwayo, and J. O. Ndinya-Achola. 2001. Quality of health education during STD case management in Nairobi, Kenya. *International Journal of STD and AIDS* 12: 315–22.

O'Reilly, K. R., A. Medley, J. Dennison, G. P. Schmid, and M. D. Sweat. 2004. Systematic review of the impact of abstinence-only programmes on risk behavior in developing countries. 15th International AIDS Conference. Bangkok, Thailand. 11–16 July 2004. Abstract no. TuPeC4899.

Oakley, Ann, Vicki Strange, Chris Bonell, Elizabeth Allen, Judith Stephenson, and RIPPLE Study Team. 2006. Process evaluation in randomised controlled trials of complex interventions. *British Medical Journal* 332: 413–16.

Obasi, A. I. N., K. Chima, B. Cleophas-Frisch, G. Mmassy, M. Makokha, M. L. Plummer, M. Kudrati, and D. A. Ross. 2002a. *Good things for young people: Reproductive health education for primary schools: Teacher's guide for Standard 5.* Mwanza, Tanzania: *MEMA kwa Vijana.* Downloaded from www.memakwavijana .org on October 4, 2011.

Obasi, A. I. N., K. Chima, B. Cleophas-Frisch, G. Mmassy, M. Makokha, M. L. Plummer, M. Kudrati, and D. A. Ross. 2002b. *MEMA kwa Vijana: Elimu ya afya ya uzazi kwa shule za msingi: Kiongozi cha mwalimu: Darasa la 5.* Mwanza, Tanzania: *MEMA kwa Vijana.* Downloaded from www.memakwavijana.org on October 4, 2011.

Obasi, A. I. N., K. Chima, B. Cleophas-Frisch, G. Mmassy, M. Makokha, M. L. Plummer, M. Kudrati, and D. A. Ross. 2002c. *Good things for young people: Reproductive health education for primary schools: Teacher's guide for Standard 6.* Mwanza, Tanzania: *MEMA kwa Vijana.* Downloaded from www.memakwavijana .org on October 4, 2011.

Obasi, A. I. N., K. Chima, B. Cleophas-Frisch, G. Mmassy, M. Makokha, M. L. Plummer, M. Kudrati, and D. A. Ross. 2002d. *MEMA kwa Vijana: Elimu ya afya ya uzazi kwa shule za msingi: Kiongozi cha mwalimu: Darasa la 6.* Mwanza, Tanzania: *MEMA kwa Vijana.* Downloaded from www.memakwavijana.org on October 4, 2011.

Obasi, A. I. N., K. Chima, B. Cleophas-Frisch, G. Mmassy, M. Makokha, M. L. Plummer, M. Kudrati, and D. A. Ross. 2002e. *Good things for young people: Reproductive health education for primary schools: Teacher's guide for Standard 7.* Mwanza, Tanzania: *MEMA kwa Vijana.* Downloaded from www.memakwavijana .org on October 4, 2011.

Obasi, A. I. N., K. Chima, B. Cleophas-Frisch, G. Mmassy, M. Makokha, M. L. Plummer, M. Kudrati, and D. A. Ross. 2002f. *MEMA kwa Vijana: Elimu ya afya ya uzazi kwa shule za msingi: Kiongozi cha mwalimu: Darasa la 7.* Mwanza, Tanzania: *MEMA kwa Vijana.* Downloaded from www.memakwavijana.org on October 4, 2011.

Obasi, A. I. N., K. Chima, B. Cleophas-Frisch, G. Mmassy, M. Makokha, M. L. Plummer, M. Kudrati, and D. A. Ross. 2002g. *Good things for young people: Reproductive health education for primary schools: Teacher's resource book.*

Mwanza, Tanzania: *MEMA kwa Vijana.* Downloaded from www.memakwavijana .org on October 4, 2011.

Obasi, A. I. N., K. Chima, B. Cleophas-Frisch, G. Mmassy, M. Makokha, M. L. Plummer, M. Kudrati, and D. A. Ross. 2002h. *MEMA kwa Vijana: Elimu ya afya ya uzazi kwa shule za msingi: Kiongozi cha mwalimu: Vielelezo vya ziada kwa ajili ya walimu.* Mwanza, Tanzania: *MEMA kwa Vijana.* Downloaded from www .memakwavijana.org on October 4, 2011.

Obasi, A. I., B. Cleophas, D. A. Ross, K. L. Chima, G. Mmassy, A. Gavyole et al. 2006. Rationale and design of the *MEMA kwa Vijana* adolescent sexual and reproductive health intervention in Mwanza Region, Tanzania. *AIDS Care* 18(4): 311–22.

Obasi, A. I., K. L. Chima, G. Mmassy, B. Cleophas-Frisch, B. Mujaya, D. Ross, and R. Hayes. 2002. Impact of a training programme on teacher knowledge and attitudes to reproductive health education in primary schools in Mwanza, Tanzania. 14th International AIDS Conference, Barcelona, Spain. 7–12 July, 2002. Abstract no. MoPeD3626.

Obasi, A., B. Cleophas-Frisch, K. L. Chima, S. Mataba, G. Mmassy, R. Balira, J. Todd, D. Ross, and B. Mujaya. 2000. Health worker and head teacher attitudes to the provision of reproductive health education and services to adolescents in rural Mwanza region, Tanzania. 13th International AIDS Conference, Durban, South Africa. 9–14 July, 2000. Abstract no. WePpD1334.

Obasi, Angela I., Rebecca Balira, Jim Todd, David A. Ross, John Changalucha, Frank Mosha, Heiner Grosskurth, Rosanna Peeling, David C. W. Mabey, and Richard J. Hayes. 2001. Prevalence of HIV and *Chlamydia trachomatis* infection in 15–19–year olds in rural Tanzania. *Tropical Medicine and International Health* 6(7): 517–25.

Obasi, Angela. 2001. *Report of the development, pre-testing and pilot testing of the Year 1 Teacher's Guide.* Mwanza, Tanzania: *MEMA kwa Vijana.* Unpublished report.

Okonofua, Friday E., Paul Coplan, Susan Collins, Frank Oronsaye, Dapo Ogunsakin, James T. Ogonor, Joan A. Kaufman, and Kris Heggenhougen. 2003. Impact of an intervention to improve treatment-seeking behavior and prevent sexually transmitted diseases among Nigerian youths. *International Journal of infectious Diseases* 7: 61–73.

Okware, S., J. Kinsman, S. Onyango, A. Opio, and P. Kaggwa. 2005. Revisiting the ABC strategy: HIV prevention in Uganda in the era of antiretroviral therapy. *Postgraduate Medical Journal* 81: 625–28.

Oladepo, Oladimeji, and Mojisola M. Fayemi. 2011. Perceptions about sexual abstinence and knowledge of HIV/AIDS prevention among in-school adolescents in a western Nigerian city. *BMC Public Health* 11: 304.

Omorodion, Francisca Isi. 1993. Sexual networking among market women in Benin City, Bendel State, Nigeria. *Health Transition Review* 3(Supplement): 1–11.

Onya, Hans, Leif Edvard Aarø, and Sylvester N. Madu. 2009. Social outcome expectations regarding delayed sexual debut among adolescents in Mankweng, South Africa. *Scandinavian Journal of Public Health* 37(Supplement 2): 92–100.

Onyango-Ouma, W., J. Aagaard-Hansen, and B. B. Jensen. 2005. The potential of schoolchildren as health change agents in rural western Kenya. *Social Science and Medicine* 61: 1711–22.

Oraby, Doaa, Cherif Soliman, Sherif Elkamhawi, and Rawya Hassan. 2008. *Assessment of youth friendly clinics in teaching hospitals in Egypt. Family Health International Assessment Report.* Downloaded on August 21, 2010 from www.fhi .org/NR/rdonlyres/esvin7blgv2r3bq6dqhpiwbyzthu3wvu7oa7gzqaunnsctfnohdiad wcy4bjqep66xubgutujbhykm/Assessmentreportmay28final2.pdf.

O-saki, Kalafunja Mlang'a, and Augustine Obeleagu Agu. 2002. A study of classroom interaction in primary schools in the United Republic of Tanzania. *Prospects* 32: 103–16.

Ostermann, Jan, Elizabeth A. Reddy, Meghan M. Shorter, Charles Muiruri, Antipas Mtalo, Dafrosa K. Itemba, Bernard Njau, John A. Bartlett, John A. Crump, and Nathan M. Thielman. 2011. Who tests, who doesn't, and why? Uptake of mobile HIV counseling and testing in the Kilimanjaro Region of Tanzania. *PLoS ONE* 6(1): e16488.

Oyugi, Jessica H., Jayne Byakika-Tusiime, Kathleen Ragland, Oliver Laeyendecker, Roy Mugerwa, Cissy Kityo, Peter Mugyenyi, Thomas C. Quinn, and David R. Bangsberg. 2007. Treatment interruptions predict resistance in HIV-positive individuals purchasing fixed-dose combination antiretroviral therapy in Kampala, Uganda. *AIDS* 21: 965–71.

Padian, Nancy S., Ariane van der Straten, Gita Ramjee, Tsungai Chipato, Guy de Bruyn, Kelly Blanchard, Stephen Shiboski et al. 2007. Diaphragm and lubricant gel for prevention of HIV acquisition in southern African women: A randomized controlled trial. *Lancet* 370: 251–61.

Padian, Nancy S., Sandra I. McCoy, Salim S. Abdool Karim, Nina Hasen, Julia Kim, Michael Bartos, Elly Katabira, Stefano M. Bertozzi, Bernhard Schwartländer, and Myron S. Cohen. 2011. HIV prevention transformed: The new prevention research agenda. *Lancet* 378: 269–78.

Painter, Thomas M. 2001. Voluntary counseling and testing for couples: A high-leverage intervention for HIV/AIDS prevention in sub-Saharan Africa. *Social Science and Medicine* 53: 1397–1411.

Painter, Thomas M., Kassamba L. Diaby, Danielle M. Matia, Lillian S. Lin, Toussaint S. Sibailly, Moïse K. Kouassi, Ehounou R. Ekpini, Thierry H. Roels, and Stefan Z. Wiktor. 2007. Faithfulness to partners: A means to prevent HIV infection, a source of HIV infection risks, or both? A qualitative study of women's experiences in Abidjan, Côte d'Ivoire *African Journal of AIDS Research* 6(1): 25–31.

Palen, Lori-Ann, Edward A. Smith, Linda L. Caldwell, Alan J. Flisher, Lisa Wegner, and Tania Vergnani. 2008. Inconsistent reports of sexual intercourse among South African high school students. *Journal of Adolescent Health* 42(3): 221–27.

Palmer, Robert, Ruth Wedgwood, and Rachel Hayman, with Kenneth King and Neil Thin. 2007. *Educating out of poverty? A synthesis report on Ghana, India, Kenya, Rwanda, Tanzania and South Africa. Department for International Development: Educational Paper no. 70.* Edinburgh, UK: Centre of African Studies, University of Edinburgh.

Panos Institute. 2003. *Beyond victims and villains: Addressing sexual violence in the education sector. PANOS Report No. 47.* London: Panos.

Papa, Michael J., Arvind Singhal, Sweety Law, Saumya Pant, Suruchi Sood, Everett M. Rogers, and Corrine L. Shefner-Rogers. 2000. Entertainment-education and social change: An analysis of parasocial interaction, social learning, collective efficacy, and paradoxical communication. *Journal of Communication* 50(4): 31–55.

Papo, Jacqueline K., Evasius K. Bauni, Eduard J. Sanders, Peter Brocklehurst, and Harold W. Jaffe. 2011. Exploring the condom gap: Is supply or demand the limiting factor—condom access and use in an urban and a rural setting in Kilifi district, Kenya. *AIDS* 25(2): 247–55.

Parikh, Shanti A. 2007. The political economy of marriage and HIV: The ABC approach, safe infidelity, and managing moral risk in Uganda. *American Journal of Public Health* 97(7): 1198–208.

Parker, R. G., G. Herdt, and M. Carballo. 1991. Sexual culture, HIV transmission, and AIDS research. *The Journal of Sex Research* 28(1): 77–98.

Parker, Richard G., Delia Easton, and Charles H. Klein. 2000. Structural factors and facilitators in HIV prevention: A review of international research. *AIDS* 14(Supplement 1): S22–32.

Partnership for Child Development. 1998. Implications for school-based health programmes of age and gender patterns in the Tanzanian primary school. *Tropical Medicine and International Health* 3: 850–53.

Paruk, Zubeda, Inge Petersen, and Arvin Bhana. 2009. Facilitating health-enabling social contexts for youth: Qualitative evaluation of a family-based HIV-prevention pilot programme. *African Journal of AIDS Research* 8(1): 61–68.

Paruk, Zubeda, Inge Petersen, Arvin Bhana, Carl Bell, and Mary McKay. 2005. Containment and contagion: How to strengthen families to support youth HIV prevention in South Africa. *African Journal of AIDS Research* 4(1): 57–63.

Pattman, Rob, and Fatuma Chege. 2003. 'Dear diary I saw an angel, she looked like heaven on earth': Sex talk and sex education. *African Journal of AIDS Research* 2(2): 103–12.

Paul-Ebhohimhen, Virginia A., Amudha Poobalan, and Edwin R. van Teijlingen. 2008. A systematic review of school-based sexual health interventions to prevent STI/HIV in sub-Saharan Africa. *BMC Public Health* 8: 4.

Pawson, R., and N. Tilley. 1997. *Realistic evaluation.* London: Sage.

Peacock, Dean, Jean Redpath, Mark Weston, Kieran Evans, Andrew Daub, and Alan Greig for Sonke Gender Justice Network. 2008. *Literature review on men, gender, health and HIV and AIDS in South Africa.* Johannesburg, South Africa: Sonke Gender Justice Network.

Pechmann, C. 1997. Does antismoking advertising combat underage smoking? A review of past practices and research. In *Social marketing: Theoretical and practical perspectives,* ed. Marvin E. Goldberg, Martin Fishbein, and Susan E. Middlestadt, 189–216. Mahwah, New Jersey: Lawrence Erlbaum Associates.

Pellati, Donatella, Ioannis Mylonakis, Giulio Bertoloni, Cristina Fiore, Alessandra Andrisani, Guido Ambrosini, and Decio Armanini. 2008. Genital tract infections and infertility. *European Journal of Obstetrics and Gynecology and Reproductive Biology* 140: 3–11.

Peltzer, K. 2009. Health behavior and protective factors among school children in four African countries. *The International Journal of Behavioral Medicine* 16(2): 172–80.

Peltzer, Karl, and Phillip Seoka. 2004. Evaluation of HIV/AIDS prevention intervention messages on a rural sample of South African youth's knowledge, attitudes, beliefs and behaviours over a period of 15 months. *Journal of Child and Adolescent Mental Health* 16(2): 93–102.

Pettifor, Audrey E., Ariane van der Straten, Megan S. Dunbar, Stephen C. Shiboski, and Nancy S. Padian. 2004. Early age of first sex: A risk factor for HIV infection among women in Zimbabwe. *AIDS* 18: 1435–42.

Pettifor, Audrey E., Brooke A. Levandowski, Catherine MacPhail, Nancy S. Padian, Myron S. Cohen, and Helen V. Rees. 2008. Keep them in school: The importance of education as a protective factor against HIV infection among young South African women. *International Journal of Epidemiology* 37: 1266–73.

Pettifor, Audrey E., Catherine MacPhail, Stefano Bertozzi, and Helen V. Rees. 2007. Challenge of evaluating a national HIV prevention programme: The case of loveLife, South Africa. *Sexually Transmitted Infections* 83(Supplement 1): i70–74.

Pettifor, Audrey E., Helen V. Rees. Immo Kleinschmidt, Annie E. Steffenson, Catherine MacPhail, Lindiwe Hlongwa-Madikizela, Kerry Vermaak, and Nancy S. Padian. 2005. Young people's sexual health in South Africa: HIV prevalence and sexual behaviors from a nationally representative household survey. *AIDS* 19: 1525–34.

Pfeiffer, James. 2004. Condom social marketing, Pentecostalism, and structural adjustment in Mozambique: A clash of AIDS prevention messages. *Medical Anthropology Quarterly* 18(1): 77–103.

Phetla, G., J. Busza, J. R. Hargreaves, P. M. Pronyk, J. C. Kim, L. A. Morison, C. Watts, and J. D. H. Porter. 2008. They have opened our mouths: Increasing women's skills and motivation for sexual communication with young people in rural South Africa. *AIDS Education and Prevention* 20(6): 504–18.

Philpott, Anne, Wendy Knerr, and Vicky Boydell. 2006. Pleasure and prevention: When good sex is safer sex. *Reproductive Health Matters* 14(28): 23–31.

Pilcher, Christopher D., Hsiao Chuan Tien, Joseph J. Eron Jr., Pietro L. Vernazza, Szu-Yun Leu, Paul W. Stewart, Li-Ean Goh, and Myron S. Cohen, for the Quest Study and the Duke-UNC-Emory Acute HIV Consortium. 2004. Brief but efficient: Acute HIV infection and the sexual transmission of HIV. *Journal of Infectious Diseases* 189: 1785–92.

Piot, Peter, Michael Bartos, Heidi Larson, Debrework Zewdie, and Purnima Mane. 2008. Coming to terms with complexity: A call to action for HIV prevention. *Lancet* 372: 845–59.

Plautz, Andrea, and Dominique Meekers. 2007. Evaluation of the reach and impact of the 100% Jeune youth social marketing program in Cameroon: Findings from three cross-sectional surveys. *Reproductive Health* 4: 1.

Plummer, M. L., D. A. Ross, D. Wight, J. Changalucha, G. Mshana, J. Wamoyi, J. Todd et al. 2004. 'A bit more truthful': The validity of adolescent sexual behavior data collected in rural northern Tanzania using five methods. *Sexually Transmitted Infections* 80(Supplement 2): ii49–56.

Plummer, Mary L. 1994. Development, implementation and evaluation of a secondary school AIDS education programme. In *Consultancy report for Kuleana Centres for Children's Rights and AIDS Action, June 1994*, 6–83. Mwanza, Tanzania: Kuleana. Unpublished report.

Plummer, Mary L., D. Wight, A. I. N. Obasi, J. Wamoyi, G. Mshana, J. Todd, B. C. Mazige, M. Makokha, R. J. Hayes, and D. A. Ross. 2007. A process evaluation of a school-based adolescent sexual health intervention in rural Tanzania: The *MEMA kwa Vijana* programme. *Health Education Research* 22(4): 500–12.

Plummer, Mary L., Daniel Wight, David A. Ross, Rebecca Balira, Alessandra Anemona, Jim Todd, Zachayo Salamba et al. 2004. Asking semi-literate adolescents about sexual behavior: The validity of assisted self-completion questionnaire (ASCQ) data in rural Tanzania. *Tropical Medicine and International Health* 9: 737–54.

Plummer, Mary Louisa, and Daniel Wight. 2011. *Young people's lives and sexual relationships in rural Africa: Findings from a large qualitative study in Tanzania*. Lanham, MD: Lexington Books.

Plummer, Mary, and Mary Maswe. 1998. *Evaluation report for the TANESA primary school health education program, February 1998*. Mwanza, Tanzania: Tanzania Netherlands Project to Support HIV/AIDS Control in Mwanza Region, Tanzania (TANESA). Unpublished report.

Pool, R., A. Kamali, and J. A. G. Whitworth. 2006. Understanding sexual behavior change in rural southwest Uganda: A multi-method study. *AIDS Care* 18(5): 479–88.

Pool, R., and W. Geissler. 2005. *Medical anthropology*. Berkshire, England: Open University Press.

Porco, Travis C., Jeffrey N. Martin, Kimberly A. Page-Shafer, Amber Cheng, Edwin Charlebois, Robert M. Grant, and Dennis H. Osmond. 2004. Decline in HIV infectivity following the introduction of highly active antiretroviral therapy. *AIDS* 18: 81–88.

Potterat, John J., Helen Zimmerman-Rogers, Stephen Q. Muth, Richard B. Rothenberg, David L. Green, Jerry E. Taylor, Mandy S. Bonney, and Helen A. White. 1999. *Chlamydia* transmission: Concurrency, reproduction number, and the epidemic trajectory. *American Journal of Epidemiology* 150(12): 1331–9.

Poulsen, Melissa N., Hilde Vandenhoudt, Sarah C. Wyckoff, Christopher O. Obong'o, Juliet Ochura, Gillian Njika, Nelson Juma Otwoma, and Kim S. Miller. 2010. Cultural adaptation of a U.S. evidence-based parenting intervention for rural western Kenya: From parents matter! To families matter! *AIDS Education and Prevention* 22(4): 273–85.

Prata, Ndola, Leo Morris, Elizio Mazive, Farnaz Vahidnia, and Mark Stehr. 2006. Relationship between HIV risk perception and condom use: Evidence from a population-based survey in Mozambique. *International Family Planning Perspectives* 32(4): 192–200.

Price, Neil, and Kirstan Hawkins. 2002. Researching sexual and reproductive behavior: A peer ethnographic approach. *Social Science and Medicine* 55(8): 1325–36.

Price, Neil. 2001. The performance of social marketing in reaching the poor and vulnerable in AIDS control programmes. *Health Policy and Planning* 16(3): 231–39.

Pronyk, Paul M., James R. Hargreaves, Julia C. Kim, Linda A. Morison, Godfrey Phetla, Charlotte Watts, Joanna Busza, and John D. H. Porter. 2006. Effect of a structural intervention for the prevention of intimate-partner violence and HIV in rural South Africa: A cluster randomised trial. *Lancet* 368: 1973–83.

Pronyk, Paul M., Julia C. Kim, Tanya Abramsky, Godfrey Phetla, James R. Hargreaves, Linda A. Morison, Charlotte Watts, Joanna Busza, and John D. H. Porter. 2008. A combined microfinance and training intervention can reduce HIV risk behaviour in young female participants. *AIDS* 22: 1659–65.

Puffer, Eve S., Christina S. Meade, Anya S. Drabkin, Sherryl A. Broverman, Rose A. Ogwang-Odhiambo, and Kathleen J. Sikkema. 2011. Individual- and family-level psychosocial correlates of HIV risk behavior among youth in rural Kenya. *AIDS and Behavior* 15: 1264–74.

Pulerwitz, Julie, Annie Michaelis, Ravi Verma, and Ellen Weiss. 2010. Addressing gender dynamics and engaging men in HIV programs: Lessons learned from Horizons research. *Public Health Reports* 125(2): 282–92.

Quinn, Thomas C., and David Serwadda. 2011. The future of HIV/AIDS in Africa: A shared responsibility. *Lancet* 377: 1133–34.

Radcliffe-Brown, Alfred Reginald. 1950. Introduction. In *African systems of kinship and marriage*, ed. Alfred Reginald Radcliffe-Brown and Cyril Daryll Forde, 1–85. Oxford: Oxford University Press.

Ramjee, Gita, Anatoli Kamali, and Sheena McCormack. 2010. The last decade of microbicide clinical trials in Africa: From hypothesis to facts. *AIDS* 24(Supplement 4): S40–9.

Reed, Jenny, and Jean Baxen. 2010. Understanding HIV/AIDS prevention programmes through the use of process evaluation. *Journal of Education* 50: 115–38.

Remes, Pieter, Jenny Renju, Kija Nyalali, Lemmy Medard, Michael Kimaryo, John Changalucha, Angela Obasi, and Daniel Wight. 2010. Dusty discos and dangerous desires: Community perceptions of adolescent sexual and reproductive health risks and vulnerability and the potential role of parents in rural Mwanza, Tanzania. *Culture, Health and Sexuality* 12(3): 279–92.

Reniers, Georges. 2008. Marital strategies for regulating exposure to HIV. *Demography* 45(2): 417–38.

Reniers, Georges, and Rania Tfaily. 2008. Polygyny and HIV in Malawi. *Demographic Research* 19: 1781–1800.

Reniers, Georges, and Susan Watkins. 2010. Polygyny and the spread of HIV in sub-Saharan Africa: A case of benign concurrency. *AIDS* 24: 299–307.

Renju, Jenny R., Bahati Andrew, Lemmy Medard, Coleman Kishamawe, Michael Kimaryo, John Changalucha, and Angela Obasi. 2010. Scaling up adolescent sexual and reproductive health interventions through existing government systems? A detailed process evaluation of a school-based intervention in Mwanza Region in the northwest of Tanzania. *Journal of Adolescent Health* 48(1): 79–86.

Renju, Jenny, Bahati Andrew, Kija Nyalali, Coleman Kishamawe, Charles Kato, John Changalucha, and Angela Obasi. 2010. A process evaluation of the scale up of a youth-friendly health services initiative in northern Tanzania. *Journal of the International AIDS Society* 13: 32.

Renju, Jenny, Maende Makokha, Charles Kato, Lemmy Medard, Bahati Andrew, Pieter Remes, John Changalucha, and Angela Obasi. 2010. Partnering to proceed: Scaling up adolescent sexual reproductive health programmes in Tanzania. Operational research into the factors that influenced local government uptake and implementation. *Health Research Policy and Systems* 8: 12.

Research to Prevention. 2009. *Concurrent partnerships and HIV/AIDS in Tanzania: Evidence from the literature, June 2009*. Baltimore, Maryland: Johns Hopkins University Center for Communication Programs.

Robins, Steven. 2009. Foot soldiers of global health: Teaching and preaching AIDS science and modern medicine on the frontline. *Medical Anthropology* 28(1): 81–107.

Roehr, Bob. 2005. Abstinence programmes do not reduce HIV prevalence in Uganda. *British Medical Journal* 330: 496.

Rogers, Everett M., Peter W. Vaughan, Ramadhan M. A. Swalehe, Nagesh Rao, Peer Svenkerud, and Suruchi Sood. 1999. Effects of an entertainment-education radio soap opera on family planning behavior in Tanzania. *Studies in Family Planning* 30(3): 193–211.

Rosen, Sydney, Matthew P. Fox, and Christopher J. Gill. 2007. Patient retention in antiretroviral therapy programs in sub-Saharan Africa: A systematic review. *PLoS Medicine* 4(10): e298.

Ross, David A. 2010. Behavioural interventions to reduce HIV risk: What works? *AIDS* 24(Supplement 4): S4–14.

Ross, David A., John Changalucha, Angela I. Obasi, Jim Todd, Mary L. Plummer, Bernadette Cleophas-Mazige, Alessandra Anemona et al. 2007. Biological and behavioral impact of an adolescent sexual health intervention in Tanzania: A community-randomized trial. *AIDS* 21(14): 1943–55.

Rutenberg, Naomi, and Susan Cotts Watkins. 1997. The buzz outside of clinics: Conversations and contraception in Nyanza Province, Kenya. *Studies in Family Planning* 28(4): 290–307.

Rutherford, George W. 2008. Condoms in concentrated and generalised HIV epidemics. *Lancet* 372: 275–76.

Rutter, Michael, Barbara Maughan, Peter Mortimore, and Janet Ouston. 1979. *Fifteen thousand hours: Secondary schools and their effects on children*. Boston: Harvard University Press.

Sahin-Hodoglugil, Nuriye Nalan, Ariane van der Straten, Helen Cheng, Elizabeth T. Montgomery, Deborah Kacanek, Sibongile Mtetwa, Neetha Morar, Jane Munyoro, Nancy Padian, and the MIRA Team. 2009. Degrees of disclosure: A study of women's covert use of the diaphragm in an HIV prevention trial in sub-Saharan Africa. *Social Science and Medicine* 69: 1547–55.

Saïd Business School, Oxford University. 2010. *New study shows sanitary protection for girls in developing countries may provide a route to raising their educational standards.* Downloaded from www.modernghana.com/news/262658/1/new-study -shows-sanitary-protection-for-girls-in-d.html on February 27, 2012.

Sambisa, William, and C. Shannon Stokes. 2006. Rural/urban residence, migration, HIV/AIDS, and safe sex practices among men in Zimbabwe. *Rural Sociology* 71(2): 183–211.

Sambisa, William, Sian L. Curtis, and C. Shannon Stokes. 2010. Ethnic differences in sexual behaviour among unmarried adolescents and young adults in Zimbabwe. *Journal of Biosocial Science* 42: 1–26.

Samuelsen, Helle. 2006. Love, lifestyles and the risk of AIDS: The moral worlds of young people in Bobo-Dioulasso, Burkina Faso. *Culture, Health and Sexuality* 8(3): 211–24.

Sandøy, Ingvild F., Charles Michelo, Seter Siziya, and Knut Fylkesnes. 2007. Associations between sexual behaviour change in young people and decline in HIV prevalence in Zambia. *BMC Public Health* 7: 60.

Sandøy, Ingvild F., Kumbutso Dzekedzeke, and Knut Fylkesnes. 2010. Prevalence and correlates of concurrent sexual partnerships in Zambia. *AIDS and Behavior* 14: 59–71.

Saunders, Ruth P., Martin H. Evans, and Praphul Joshi. 2005. Developing a process evaluation plan for assessing health promotion program implementation: A how-to guide. *Health Promotion Practice* 6(2): 134–47.

Sauvain-Dugerdil, Claudine, Bassoutoura Gakou, Fatou Berthé, Abdoul Wahab Dieng, Gilbert Ritschard, and Mathias Lerch. 2008. The start of the sexual transition in Mali: Risks and opportunities. *Studies in Family Planning* 39(4): 263–80.

Sawers, Larry, and Eileen Stillwaggon. 2010a. Understanding the southern African 'anomaly': Poverty, endemic disease and HIV. *Development and Change* 41(2): 195–224.

Sawers, Larry, and Eileen Stillwaggon. 2010b. Concurrent sexual partnerships do not explain the HIV epidemics in Africa: A systematic review. *Journal of the International AIDS Society* 13: 34.

Sayles, Jennifer N., Audrey Pettifor, Mitchell D. Wong, Catherine MacPhail, Sung-Jae Lee, Ellen Hendriksen, Helen V. Rees, and Thomas Coates. 2006. Factors associated with self-efficacy for condom use and sexual negotiation among South African youth. *Journal of Acquired Immune Deficiency Syndromes* 43: 226–33.

Schachter, J., and J. M. Chow. 1995. The fallibility of diagnostic tests for sexually transmitted diseases: The impact on behavioral and epidemiologic studies. *Sexually Transmitted Diseases* 22: 191–96.

Schapink, Dick, Jumanne Hema, and Bartimayo Mujaya. 1997. Youth and HIV/AIDS programmes. In *HIV prevention and AIDS care in Africa: A district level approach,* ed. Japhet Ng'weshemi, Ties Boerma, John Bennett, and Dick Schapink, 163–84. Amsterdam: Royal Tropical Institute.

Schomogyi, Mark, Anna Wald, and Lawrence Corey. 1998. Herpes Simplex Virus-2: An emerging disease? *Infectious Disease Clinics of North America* 12(1): 47-61.

Sedere, Upali M., Helima Mengele, and Teferi Kajela. 2008. *Evaluation of the Education Quality Improvement Through Pedagogy (EQUIP) Project in Shinyanga, Tanzania. Full report, Oxfam GB Programme Evaluation December 2008.* Downloaded from www.oxfam.org.uk/resources/evaluations/downloads/1208_p00048_tanzania_pedagogy_education_exec.pdf on August 6, 2010.

Seeley, Janet, Jessica Nakiyingi-Miiro, Anatoli Kamali, Juliet Mpendo, Gershim Asiki, Andrew Abaasa, Jan De Bont, Leslie Nielsen, and Pontiano Kaleebu, on behalf of the CHIVTUM Study Team. 2012. High HIV incidence and socio-behavioral risk patterns in fishing communities on the shores of Lake Victoria, Uganda. *Sexually Transmitted Diseases* 39(6): 433–39.

Seidenfeld, David. 2010. Obstacles to access: An evaluation of a condom distribution program in rural Zambia. A Dissertation in Education presented to the Faculties of the University of Pennsylvania in Partial Fulfillment for the Requirements for the Degree of Doctor of Philosphy, 2010.

Selikow, Terry-Ann, Nazeema Ahmed, Alan J. Flisher, Catherine Mathews, and Wanjiru Mukoma. 2009. I am not "umqwayito": A qualitative study of peer pressure and sexual risk behavior among young adolescents in Cape Town, South Africa. *Scandinavian Journal of Public Health* 37: 107–12.

Setel, Philip W. 1999a. Comparative histories of sexually transmitted diseases and HIV/AIDS in Africa: An introduction. In *Histories of sexually transmitted diseases and HIV/AIDS in sub-Saharan Africa*, ed. Philip W. Setel, Milton Lewis, and Maryinez Lyons, 1–15. Westport, Connecticut: Greenwood Press.

Setel, Philip W. 1999b. *A plague of paradoxes: AIDS, culture and demography in northern Tanzania*. Chicago: University of Chicago Press.

Shai, Nwabisa Jama, R. Jewkes, Jonathan Levin, K. Dunkle, and Mzikazi Nduna. 2010. Factors associated with consistent condom use among rural young women in South Africa. *AIDS Care* 22(11): 1379–85.

Sheeran, Paschal, and Charles Abraham. 1994. Measurement of condom use in 72 studies of HIV-preventive behaviour: A critical review. *Patient Education and Counseling* 24: 199–216.

Shelton, James D., and Beverly Johnston. 2001. Condom gap in Africa: Evidence from donor agencies and key informants. *British Medical Journal* 323: 139.

Shelton, James D., Daniel T. Halperin, Vinand Nantulya, Malcolm Potts, Helene D. Gayle, and King K. Holmes. 2004. Partner reduction is crucial for balanced ABC approach to HIV prevention. *British Medical Journal* 328: 891–94.

Sherr, L. 1990. Fear arousal and AIDS: Do shock tactics work? *AIDS* 4(4): 361–64.

Shuey, Dean A., Bernadette B. Babishangire, Samuel Omiat, and Henry Bagarukayo. 1999. Increased sexual abstinence among in-school adolescents as a result of school health education in Soroti district, Uganda. *Health Education Research* 14: 411–19.

Silberschmidt, Margrethe, and Vibeke Rasch. 2001. Adolescent girls, illegal abortions and "sugar daddies" in Dar es Salaam: Vulnerable victims and active social agents. *Social Science and Medicine* 52: 1815–26.

Singh, Kavita, William Sambisa, Shungu Munyati, Brian Chandiwana, Alfred Chingono, Roeland Monash, and Sharon Weir. 2010. Targeting HIV interventions for adolescent girls and young women in southern Africa: Use of the place methodology in Hwange District, Zimbabwe. *AIDS and Behavior* 14: 200–208.

Singh, Susheela, Akinrinola Bankole, and Vanessa Woog. 2005. Evaluating the need for sex education in developing countries: Sexual behaviour, knowledge of preventing sexually transmitted infections/HIV and unplanned pregnancy. *Sex Education* 5(4): 307–31.

Singh, Susheela, Deirdre Wulf, Renee Samara, and Yvette P. Cuca. 2000. Gender differences in the timing of first intercourse: Data from 14 countries. *International Family Planning Perspectives* 26(1): 21–28 and 43.

Singh, Susheela, Jacqueline E. Darroch, and Akinrinola Bankole. 2003. *A, B and C in Uganda: The roles of abstinence, monogamy and condom use in HIV decline. Occasional Report No. 9.* New York: The Alan Guttmacher Institute.

Singhal, Arvind, Michael J. Cody, Everett M. Rogers, and Miguel Sabido. 2004. *Entertainment-education and social change: History, research, and practice.* New Jersey: Erlbaum Associates, Inc.

Slavin, S., C. Batrouney, and D. Murphy. 2007. Fear appeals and treatment side-effects: An effective combination for HIV prevention? *AIDS Care* 19(1): 130–37.

Slaymaker, E. 2004. A critique of international indicators of sexual risk behaviour. *Sexually Transmitted Infections* 80(Supplement 2): ii13–21.

Smith, Daniel Jordan. 2009. Managing men, marriage, and modern love: Women's perspectives on intimacy and male infidelity in southeastern Nigeria. In *Love in Africa*, ed. Jennifer Cole and Lynn M. Thomas, 157–80. Chicago: University of Chicago Press.

Smith, Jennifer S., Stephen Moses, Michael G. Hudgens, Corette B. Parker, Kawango Agot, Ian Maclean, Jeckoniah O. Ndinya-Achola, Peter J. F. Snijders, Chris J. L. M. Meijer, and Robert C. Bailey. 2010. Increased risk of HIV acquisition among Kenyan men with Human Papillomavirus infection. *Journal of Infectious Diseases* 201(11): 1677–85.

Smith, Peter G., and Richard H. Morrow. 1996. *Field trials of health interventions: A Toolbox.* Oxford: Macmillan.

Somi, G., S. C. Keogh, J. Todd, B. Kilama, A. Wringe, J. van den Hombergh, K. Malima et al. 2012. Low mortality risk but high loss to follow-up among patients in the Tanzanian national HIV care and treatment programme. *Tropical Medicine and International Health* 17(4): 497–506.

Sommer, Marni. 2009. Ideologies of sexuality, menstruation and risk: Girls' experiences of puberty and schooling in northern Tanzania. *Culture, Health and Sexuality* 11(4): 383–98.

Sommer, Marni. 2010. Where the education system and women's bodies collide: The social and health impact of girls' experiences of menstruation and schooling in Tanzania. *Journal of Adolescence* 33: 521–29.

Speizer, Ilene S., and Justin S. White. 2008. The unintended consequences of intended pregnancies: Youth, condom use, and HIV transmission in Mozambique. *AIDS Education and Prevention* 20(6): 531–46.

Speizer, Ilene S., B. Oleko Tambashe, and Simon-Pierre Tegang. 2001. An evaluation of the "Entre Nous Jeunes" peer-educator program for adolescents in Cameroon. *Studies in Family Planning* 32(4): 339–51.

Stadler, Jonathan, and Eirik Saethre. 2011. Blockage and flow: Intimate experiences of condoms and microbicides in a South African clinical trial. *Culture, Health and Sexuality* 13(1): 31–44.

Steele, Matthew S., Elizabeth Bukusi, Craig R. Cohen, Bettina A. Shell-Duncan, and King K. Holmes. 2006. The ABCs of HIV prevention in men: Associations with HIV risk and protective behaviors. *Journal of Acquired Immune Deficiency Syndromes* 43: 571–76.

Sterne, J. A. C., A. C. Turner, J. A. Connell, J. V. Parry, P. E. M. Fine, J. M. Ponnighaus, S. Nyasulu, and P. K. Mkandwire. 1993. Human immunodeficiency virus: GACPAT and GACELISA as diagnostic tests for antibodies in urine. *Transactions of the Royal Society of Tropical Medicine and Hygiene* 87: 181–83.

Stone, Nicole, and Roger Ingham. 2006. Young people and sex and relationships education. In *Promoting young people's sexual health: International perspectives*, ed. Roger Ingham and Peter Aggleton, 192–208. Oxon, UK: Routledge.

Stoneburner, Rand L., and Daniel Low-Beer. 2004. Population-level HIV declines and behavioral risk avoidance in Uganda. *Science* 304(5671): 714–18.

Stroeken, Koen, Pieter Remes, Petra De Koker, Kristien Michielsen, Anke Van Vossole, and Marleen Temmerman. 2012. HIV among out-of-school youth in Eastern and Southern Africa: A review. *AIDS Care* 24(2): 186–94.

Stycos, J. Mayone. 2000. Sample surveys for social science in underdeveloped areas. In *Social research in developing countries: Surveys and censuses in the Third World*, ed. Martin Bulmer and Donald P. Warwick, 53–64. London: University College London.

Sunmola, A. M., Dada O. Adebayo, and Kayode O. Ogungbemi. 2008. Patterns of condom acquisition and its association with consistent use among young men in Nigeria. *AIDS Care* 20(7): 791–95.

Swart, Dehran, and Priscilla Reddy. 1999. Establishing networks for health promoting schools in South Africa. *Journal of School Health* 69(2): 47–50.

Swidler, Ann, and Susan C. Watkins. 2007. Ties of dependence: AIDS and transactional sex in rural Malawi. *Studies in Family Planning* 38(3): 147–62.

TACAIDS, ZAC, NBS, OCGS, and Macro International Inc. 2008. *HIV/AIDS and Malaria Indicator Survey 2007–08*. Dar es Salaam, Tanzania: Tanzania Commission for AIDS (TACAIDS), Zanzibar AIDS Commission (ZAC), National Bureau of Statistics (NBS), Office of Chief Government Statistician (OCGS), and Macro International Inc.

TACAIDS. 2007. *National Multi-Sectoral Framework on HIV and AIDS, 2008–2012*. Dar es Salaam: Tanzania Commission for AIDS (TACAIDS).

TACAIDS. 2008. *UNGASS country progress report: Tanzania Mainland: Reporting period: January 2006–December 2007*. Dar es Salaam: Tanzania Commission for AIDS (TACAIDS).

Tamale, Sylvia. 2006. Eroticism, sensuality and women's secrets among the Baganda. *IDS Bulletin* 37(5): 89–97.

Tanner, R. E. S. 1955a. Maturity and marriage among the northern Basukuma of Tanganyika. *African Studies* 14(3): 123–33.

Tanner, R. E. S. 1955b. The sexual mores of the Basukuma, Tanganyika. *International Journal of Sexology* 8(4): 238–41.

Tanser, Frank, Till Bärnighausen, Lauren Hund, Geoffrey P. Garnett, Nuala McGrath, and Marie-Louise Newell. 2011. Effect of concurrent sexual partnerships on rate of new HIV infections in a high-prevalence, rural South African population: A cohort study. *Lancet* 378: 247–55.

Tassiopoulos, Katherine K., George R. Seage, Noel E. Sam, Trong T. H. Ao, Elisante J. Masenga, Michael D. Hughes, and Saidi H. Kapiga. 2006. Sexual behavior, psychosocial and knowledge differences between consistent, inconsistent and non-users of condoms: A study of female bar and hotel workers in Moshi, Tanzania. *AIDS and Behavior* 10: 405–13.

Tavory, Iddo, and Ann Swidler. 2009. Condom semiotics: Meaning and condom use in rural Malawi. *American Sociological Review* 74: 171–89.

Tawfik, L., and S. C. Watkins. 2007. Sex in Geneva, sex in Lilongwe, and sex in Balaka. *Social Science and Medicine* 64: 1090–101.

Taylor, Christopher C. 1990. Condoms and cosmology: The 'fractal' person and sexual risk in Rwanda. *Social Science and Medicine* 31(9): 1023–28.

Taylor, Myra, Siyabonga B. Dlamini, Anna Meyer-Weitz, Reshma Sathiparsad, Champak C. Jinabhai, and Tonya Esterhuizen. 2010. Changing sexual behaviour to reduce HIV transmission: A multi-faceted approach to HIV prevention and treatment in a rural South African setting. *AIDS Care* 22(11): 1395–1402.

Tenkorang, Eric Y., Fernando Rajulton, and Eleanor Maticka-Tyndale. 2009. Perceived risks of HIV/AIDS and first sexual intercourse among youth in Cape Town, South Africa. *AIDS and Behavior* 13: 234–45.

Tenkorang, Eric Yeboah, and Eleanor Maticka-Tyndale. 2008. Factors influencing the timing of first sexual intercourse among young people in Nyanza, Kenya. *International Family Planning Perspectives* 34(4): 177–88.

Terceira, Nicola, Simon Gregson, Basia Zaba, and Peter R. Mason. 2003. The contribution of HIV to fertility decline in rural Zimbabwe, 1985–2000. *Population Studies* 57(2): 149–64.

Terris-Prestholt, Fern, Lilani Kumaranayake, Angela I. N. Obasi, Bernadette Cleophas-Mazige, Maende Makokha, Jim Todd, David A. Ross, and Richard J. Hayes. 2006. From trial intervention to scale-up: Costs of an adolescent sexual health program in Mwanza, Tanzania. *Sexually Transmitted Diseases* 33(10 Supplement): S133–39.

Thaler, Richard H., and Cass R. Sunstein. 2009. *Nudge: Improving decisions about health, wealth and happiness.* London: Penguin Books.

Thomsen, S., M. Stalker, and C. Toroitich-Ruto. 2004. Fifty ways to leave your rubber: How men in Mombasa rationalise unsafe sex. *Sexually Transmitted Infections* 80(6): 430–34.

Thornton, Robert J. 2008. *Unimagined community: Sex, networks, and AIDS in Uganda and South Africa.* Berkeley, California: University of California Press.

Todd, J., I. Cremin, N. McGrath, J. Bwanika, A. Wringe, M. Marston, I. Kasamba et al. 2009. Reported number of sexual partners: Comparison of data from four African longitudinal studies. *Sexually Transmitted Infections* 85(Supplement 1): i72–80.

Todd, J., J. Changalucha, D. A. Ross, F. Mosha, A. I. N. Obasi, M. Plummer, R. Balira, H. Grosskurth, D. C. W. Mabey, and R. Hayes. 2004. The sexual health of pupils in years 4 to 6 of primary schools in rural Tanzania. *Sexually Transmitted Infections* 80: 35–42.

Topan, Farouk. 2008. Tanzania: The development of Swahili as a national and official language. In *Language and national identity in Africa*, ed. Andrew Simpson, 252–66. New York: Oxford University Press.

Towse, Peter, David Kent, Funja Osaki, and Noah Kirua. 2002. Non-graduate teacher recruitment and retention: Some factors affecting teacher effectiveness in Tanzania. *Teaching and Teacher Education* 18: 637–52.

Turner, Abigail Norris, Alana E. De Kock, Amy Meehan-Ritter, Kelly Blanchard, Mohlatlego H. Sebola, Anwar A. Hoosen, Nicol Coetzee, and Charlotte Ellertson. 2009. Many vaginal microbicide trial participants acknowledged they had misreported sensitive sexual behavior in face-to-face interviews. *Journal of Clinical Epidemiology* 62(7): 759–65.

Turner, Charles F., and Heather G. Miller. 1997. Zenilman's anomaly reconsidered: Fallible reports, ceteris paribus, and other hypotheses. *Sexually Transmitted Diseases* 24: 522–27.

Turner, G., and J. Shepherd. 1999. A method in search of a theory: Peer education and health promotion. *Health Education Research* 14(2): 235–47.

Tylee, Andre, Dagmar M. Haller, Tanya Graham, Rachel Churchill, and Lena A Sanci. 2007. Youth-friendly primary-care services: How are we doing and what more needs to be done? *Lancet* 369: 1565–73.

Uiso, F. C., E. J. Kayombo, Z. H. Mbwambo, Y. Mgonda, R. L. A. Mahunnah, and M. J. Moshi. 2006. Traditional healer's knowledge and implications to the management and control of HIV/AIDS in Arusha, Tanzania. *Tanzania Health Research Bulletin* 8(2): 95–100.

UNAIDS and WHO. 2003. *AIDS epidemic update December 2003.* Geneva: UNAIDS and WHO.

UNAIDS and WHO. 2009. *AIDS epidemic update December 2009.* Geneva: UNAIDS and WHO.

UNAIDS. 1999a. *Sexual behavioural change for HIV: Where have theories taken us?* Geneva: UNAIDS.

UNAIDS. 1999b. *Peer education and HIV/AIDS: Concepts, uses and challenges.* Geneva: UNAIDS.

UNAIDS. 2004. *2004 report on the global HIV/AIDS epidemic: 4th global report.* Geneva: UNAIDS.

UNAIDS. 2005. *Evidence for HIV decline in Zimbabwe: A comprehensive review of the epidemiological data.* Geneva: UNAIDS.

UNAIDS. 2007. *UNAIDS expert consultation on behaviour change in the prevention of sexual transmission of HIV: Highlights and recommendations.* Geneva: UNAIDS.

UNAIDS. 2010. *Global report: UNAIDS report on the global AIDS epidemic 2010.* Geneva: UNAIDS.

Underhill, Kristen, Don Operario, and Paul Montgomery. 2007. Systematic review of abstinence-plus HIV prevention programs in high-income countries. *PLoS Medicine* 4(9): 1471–85.

Underhill, Kristen, Paul Montgomery, and Don Operario. 2007. Sexual abstinence only programmes to prevent HIV infection in high income countries: Systematic review. *British Medical Journal* 335: 248.

Underwood, Carol, Holo Hachonda, Elizabeth Serlemitsos, and Uttara Bharath-Kumar. 2006. Reducing the risk of HIV transmission among adolescents in Zambia: Psychosocial and behavioral correlates of viewing a risk-reduction media campaign. *Journal of Adolescent Health* 38: 55.e1–13.

Underwood, Carol, Joanna Skinner, Nadia Osman, and Hilary Schwandt. 2011. Structural determinants of adolescent girls' vulnerability to HIV: Views from community members in Botswana, Malawi, and Mozambique. *Social Science and Medicine* 73: 343–50.

Undie, Chi-Chi, and Kabwe Benaya. 2006. The state of knowledge on sexuality in sub-Saharan Africa: A synthesis of literature. *Jenda: A Journal of Culture and African Women Studies* (8): 1–33.

Undie, Chi-Chi, Joanna Crichton, and Eliya Zulu. 2007. Metaphors we love by: Conceptualizations of sex among young people in Malawi. *African Journal of Reproductive Health* 11(3): 221–35.

UNESCO. 2008. *Review of sex, relationships and HIV education in schools: Prepared for the first meeting of UNESCO's Global Advisory Group, 13–14 December 2007.* Paris: UNESCO.

UNESCO. 2009a. *International technical guidance on sexuality education: An evidence-informed approach for schools, teachers and health educators: Volume I: The rationale for sexuality education.* Paris: UNESCO.

UNESCO. 2009b. *International technical guidance on sexuality education: An evidence-informed approach for schools, teachers and health educators: Volume II: Topics and learning objectives.* Paris: UNESCO.

United Nations. 2004. *World population to 2300.* New York: United Nations.

United Nations. 2007. *World urbanization prospects: The 2006 revision: Executive Summary.* New York: United Nations.

United Republic of Tanzania (Ministry of Education and Culture). 1996. *Guidelines for HIV/AIDS/STDs preventive education for schools.* Dar es Salaam: United Republic of Tanzania.

United Republic of Tanzania (Ministry of Education and Culture). 2004. *Guidelines for implementing HIV/AIDS and life-skills education programmes in schools.* Dar es Salaam: United Republic of Tanzania.

United Republic of Tanzania (Ministry of Education and Culture). 2000. *Policy guidelines of school health promotion in Tanzania.* Dar es Salaam: United Republic of Tanzania.

United Republic of Tanzania. 1997. *Mwanza Region socio-economic profile.* Dar es Salaam: United Republic of Tanzania.

United Republic of Tanzania. 1999. *Education for all: The 2000 assessment. National report, second draft.* Dar es Salaam: United Republic of Tanzania.

United Republic of Tanzania. 2003. *Basic statistics in education 2003: Regional data.* Dar es Salaam: United Republic of Tanzania.

Van den Bergh, Graziella. 2008. To risk or not to risk? Is it a question? Sexual debut, poverty and vulnerability in times of HIV: A case from Kigoma Region, Tanzania. In *Promoting adolescent sexual and reproductive health in east and southern Africa*, ed. Knut-Inge Klepp, Alan J. Flisher, and Sylvia F. Kaaya, 162–82. Capetown: HSRC Press.

van der Velde, Frank W., and Joop van der Pligt. 1991. AIDS-related health behavior: Coping, protection motivation, and previous behavior. *Journal of Behavioral Medicine* 14(5): 429–51.

Van Dyk, Alta C. 2008. Perspectives of South African school children on HIV/AIDS, and the implications for education programmes. *African Journal of AIDS Research* 7(1): 79–93.

Van Rossem, Ronan, and Dominique Meekers. 2007. The reach and impact of social marketing and reproductive health communication campaigns in Zambia. *BMC Public Health* 7: 352.

Vandenhoudt, Hilde, Kim S. Miller, Juliet Ochura, Sarah C. Wyckoff, Christopher O. Obong'o, Nelson J. Otwoma, Melissa N. Poulsen, Joris Menten, Elizabeth Marum, and Anne Buve. 2010. Evaluation of a U.S. evidence-based parenting intervention for rural western Kenya: From parents matter! To families matter! *AIDS Education and Prevention* 22(4): 328–43.

Varkevisser, Corlien M. 1973. *Socialization in a changing society: Sukuma childhood in rural and urban Mwanza, Tanzania.* The Hague: Centre for the Study of Education in Changing Societies.

Vaughan, Meghan. 2009. *The history of romantic love in sub-Saharan Africa.* Presented as part of the Raleigh Lecture on History series at the British Academy, 26 February, 2009. Podcast downloaded on February 5, 2010 from www.britac.ac.uk/events/archive/raleigh-podcast.cfm.

Vaughan, Peter W., Everett M. Rogers, Arvind Singhal, and Ramadhan M. Swalehe. 2000. Entertainment-education and HIV/AIDS prevention: A field experiment in Tanzania. *Journal of Health Communication* 5(Supplement 1): 81–100.

Venkatesh, Kartik K., Guy de Bruyn, Mark N. Lurie, Tebogo Modisenyane, Elizabeth W. Triche, Glenda E. Gray, Alex Welte, and Neil A. Martinson. 2012. Sexual risk behaviors among HIV-infected South African men and women with their partners in a primary care program: Implications for couples-based prevention. *AIDS and Behavior* 16: 139–50.

Vijayakumar, G., Z. Mabude, J. Smit, M. Beksinska, and M. Lurie. 2006. A review of female-condom effectiveness: Patterns of use and impact on protected sex acts and STI incidence. *International Journal of STD and AIDS* 17(10): 652–59.

Visser, M. 1996. Evaluation of the first AIDS kit, the AIDS and lifestyle education programme for teenagers. *South African Journal of Psychology* 26(2): 103–13.

Visser, Maretha J., Johan B. Schoeman, and Jan J. Perold. 2004. Evaluation of HIV/AIDS prevention in South African schools. *Journal of Health Psychology* 9: 263–80.

Vissers, Debby C. J., Helene A. C. M. Voeten, Mark Urassa, Raphael Isingo, Milalu Ndege, Yusufu Kumogola, Gabriel Mwaluko, Basia Zaba, Sake J. De Vlas, and J.

Dik F. Habbema. 2008. Separation of spouses due to travel and living apart raises HIV risk in Tanzanian couples. *Sexually Transmitted Diseases* 35(8): 714–20.

Voétèn, Helene A. C. M., Omar B. Egesah, and J. Dik F. Habbema. 2004. Sexual behavior is more risky in rural than in urban areas among young women in Nyanza Province, Kenya. *Sexually Transmitted Diseases* 31(8): 481–87.

Vos, J., B. Gumodoka, Z. A. Berege, W. M. Dolmans, and M. W. Borgdorff. 1992. Patient demand for injections, a contributing factor to HIV transmission? 8th International AIDS Conference. Amsterdam, the Netherlands. 19–24 July 1992. Abstract no. PuC 8240.

Wall, Kristin, Etienne Karita, Azhar Nizam, Brigitte Bekan, Gurkiran Sardar, Deborah Casanova, Davora Joseph Davey et al. 2012. Influence network effectiveness in promoting couples' HIV voluntary counseling and testing in Kigali, Rwanda. *AIDS* 26: 217–27.

Wamoyi, Joyce, and Gerry Mshana. 2010. *Qualitative research sub-study on the MEMA kwa Vijana cohort long term follow-up: Final report, January 2010.* Unpublished report.

Wamoyi, Joyce, Angela Fenwick, Mark Urassa, Basia Zaba, and William Stones. 2011a. "Women's bodies are shops": Beliefs about transactional sex and implications for understanding gender power and HIV prevention in Tanzania. *Archives of Sexual Behavior* 40(1): 5–15.

Wamoyi, Joyce, Angela Fenwick, Mark Urassa, Basia Zaba, and William Stones. 2011b. Parental control and monitoring of young people's sexual behaviour in rural North-Western Tanzania: Implications for sexual and reproductive health interventions. *BMC Public Health* 11: 106.

Wamoyi, Joyce, Angela Fenwick, Mark Urassa, Basia Zaba, and William Stones. 2011c. Parent-child communication about sexual and reproductive health in rural Tanzania: Implications for young people's sexual health interventions. *Reproductive Health* 7: 6.

Warenius, Linnéa U., Elisabeth A. Faxelid, Petronella N. Chishimba, Joyce O. Musandu, Antony A. Ong'any, and Eva B-M. Nissen. 2006. Nurse-midwives' attitudes towards adolescent sexual and reproductive health needs in Kenya and Zambia. *Reproductive Health Matters* 14(27): 119–28.

Warenius, Linnéa, Karen O. Pettersson, Eva Nissen, Bengt Höjer, Petronella Chishimba, and Elisabeth Faxelid. 2007. Vulnerability and sexual and reproductive health among Zambian secondary school students. *Culture, Health and Sexuality* 9(5): 533–44.

Warrington, Molly, and Susan Kiragu. 2011. "It makes more sense to educate a boy": Girls 'against the odds' in Kajiado, Kenya. *International Journal of Educational Development* 32(2): 301–9.

Watkins, Susan Cotts. 2004. Navigating the AIDS epidemic in rural Malawi. *Population and Development Review* 30(4): 673–705.

Wawer, Maria J., Ronald H. Gray, Nelson K. Sewankambo, David Serwadda, Xianbin Li, Oliver Laeyendecker, Noah Kiwanuka et al. 2005. Rates of HIV-1 transmission per coital act, by stage of HIV-1 infection, in Rakai, Uganda. *Journal of Infectious Diseases* 191: 1403–9.

Weber, Jonathan, Roger Tatoud, and Sarah Fidler. 2010. Postexposure prophylaxis, preexposure prophylaxis or universal test and treat: The strategic use of antiretroviral drugs to prevent HIV acquisition and transmission. *AIDS* 24 (Supplement 4): S27–39.

Wechsberg, Wendee M., Winnie K. Luseno, Tracy L. Kline, Felicia A. Browne, and William A. Zule. 2010. Preliminary findings of an adapted evidence-based woman-focused HIV intervention on condom use and negotiation among at-risk women in Pretoria, South Africa. *Journal of Prevention and Intervention in the Community* 38(2): 132–46.

Wegbreit, Jeny, Stefano Bertozzi, Lisa M. DeMaria, and Nancy S. Padian. 2006. Effectiveness of HIV prevention strategies in resource-poor countries: Tailoring the intervention to the context. *AIDS* 20: 1217–35.

Weir, S. S., and P. J. Feldblum. 1996. Condom use to prevent incident STDs. *Sexually Transmitted Diseases* 23(1): 76–77.

Weiss, Helen A., Kim E. Dickson, Kawango Agot, and Catherine A. Hankins. 2010. Male circumcision for HIV prevention: Current research and programmatic issues. *AIDS* 24 (Supplement 4): S61–69.

Wellings, Kaye, Martine Collumbien, Emma Slaymaker, Susheela Singh, Zoé Hodges, Dhaval Patel, and Nathalie Bajos. 2006. Sexual behaviour in context: A global perspective. *Lancet* 368(9548): 1706–28.

West, P., H. Sweeting, and A. Leyland. 2004. School effects of pupils' health behaviors: Evidence in support of the health promoting school. *Research Papers in Education* 19(3): 261–91.

WHO and UNESCO. 1994a. *School health education to prevent AIDS and STD: A resource package for curriculum planners: Handbook for curriculum planners.* Geneva: WHO.

WHO and UNESCO. 1994b. *School health education to prevent AIDS and STD: A resource package for curriculum planners: Students activities.* Geneva: WHO.

WHO and UNESCO. 1994c. *School health education to prevent AIDS and STD: A resource package for curriculum planners: Teachers' guide.* Geneva: WHO.

WHO. 1993. *The European Network of Health Promoting Schools.* Copenhagen: WHO.

WHO. 1997. *Promoting health through schools: Report of a WHO Expert Committee on Comprehensive School Health Education and Promotion.* Geneva: WHO.

WHO. 2001. *Global prevalence and incidence of selected curable sexually transmitted infections: Overview and estimates.* Geneva: WHO.

WHO. 2002. *Adolescent friendly health services: An agenda for change.* Geneva: WHO.

WHO. 2003a. *Skills for health: Skills-based health education including life skills: An important component of a Child-Friendly/Health-Promoting School.* Geneva: WHO.

WHO. 2003b. *Creating an environment for emotional and social well-being: An important responsibility of a Health-Promoting and Child Friendly School.* Geneva: WHO.

WHO. 2006. *Working together for health: The World Health Report 2006.* Geneva: WHO.

WHO. 2007a. *Helping parents in developing countries improve adolescents' health.* Geneva: WHO.

WHO. 2007b. *Summaries of projects in developing countries assisting the parents of adolescents.* Geneva: WHO.

Wight, Daniel, and Angela Obasi. 2003. Unpacking the black box: The importance of process data to explain outcomes. In *Effective sexual health interventions: Issues in experimental evaluation,* ed. Judith M. Stephenson, John Imrie, and Chris Bonell, 151–66. Oxford: Oxford University Press.

Wight, Daniel, and M. Barnard. 1993. The limits of participant observation in HIV/AIDS research. *Practicing Anthropology* 15(4): 66–69.

Wijsen, Frans, and Ralph Tanner. 2002. *"I am just a Sukuma": Globalization and identity construction in northwest Tanzania.* Amsterdam: Rodopi.

Williamson, Lisa M., Alison Parkes, Daniel Wight, Mark Petticrew, and Graham J. Hart. 2009. Limits to modern contraceptive use among women in developing countries: A systematic review of qualitative research. *Reproductive Health* 6: 3.

Williamson, Nancy E., Jennifer Liku, Kerry McLoughlin, Isaac K. Nyamongo, and Flavia Nakayima. 2006. A qualitative study of condom use among married couples in Kampala, Uganda. *Reproductive Health Matters* 14(28): 89–98.

Wilson, Craig M., Peter F. Wright, Jeffrey T. Safrit, and Bret Rudy. 2010. Epidemiology of HIV infection and risk in adolescents and youth. *Journal of Acquired Immune Deficiency Syndromes* 54(Supplement 1): S5–6.

Wilson, D. 2004. Partner reduction and the prevention of HIV/AIDS. *British Medical Journal* 328: 848–49.

Wilson, David, and Daniel T. Halperin. 2008. "Know your epidemic, know your response": A useful approach, if we get it right. *Lancet* 372: 423–26.

Winskell, Kate, Laura K. Beres, Elizabeth Hill, Benjamin Chigozie Mbakwem, and Oby Obyerodhyambo. 2011. Making sense of abstinence: Social representations in young Africans' HIV-related narratives from six countries. *Culture, Health and Sexuality* 13(8): 945–59.

Witte, Kim, and Mike Allen. 2000. A meta-analysis of fear appeals: Implications for effective public health campaigns. *Health Education and Behavior* 27: 591–615.

Wolf, R. Cameron, Linda A. Tawfik, and Katherine C. Bond. 2000. Peer promotion programs and social networks in Ghana: Methods for monitoring and evaluating AIDS prevention and reproductive health programs among adolescents and young adults. *Journal of Health Communication* 5(Supplement): 61–80.

Wolff, Brent, Barbara Nyanzi, George Katongole, Deo Ssesanga, Anthony Ruberantwari, and Jimmy Whitworth. 2005. Evaluation of a home-based voluntary counselling and testing intervention in rural Uganda. *Health Policy and Planning* 20(2): 109–16.

Wood, Kate, and Rachel Jewkes. 2006. Blood blockages and scolding nurses: Barriers to adolescent contraceptive use in South Africa. *Reproductive Health Matters* 14(27): 109–18.

World Bank. 2004. *User fees in primary education.* Washington, DC: The World Bank.

World Bank. 2005a. *World development report 2006: Equity and development.* Washington, DC: World Bank.

World Bank. 2005b. *Improving educational quality through interactive radio instruction: A toolkit for policy makers and planners. Africa Region Human Development Working Papers Series no. 52.* Washington, DC: World Bank.

World Bank. 2006. *World development report 2007: Development and the next generation.* Washington, DC: World Bank.

Wright, Susan. 1998. The politicization of 'culture'. *Anthropology Today* 14(1): 7–15.

Yamanis, Thespina J., Suzanne Maman, Jessie K. Mbwambo, Jo Anne E. Earp, and Lusajo J. Kajula. 2010. Social venues that protect against and promote HIV risk for young men in Dar es Salaam, Tanzania. *Social Science and Medicine* 71: 1601–9.

Żaba, B., R. Isingo, A. Wringe, M. Marston, E. Slaymaker, and M. Urassa. 2009. Influence of timing of sexual debut and first marriage on sexual behavior in later life: Findings from four survey rounds in the Kisesa cohort in northern Tanzania. *Sexually Transmitted Infections* 85(Supplement 1): i20–26.

Zabin, Laurie Schwab, and Karungari Kiragu. 1998. The health consequences of adolescent sexual and fertility behavior in sub-Saharan Africa. *Studies in Family Planning* 29(2): 210–32.

Zenilman, J. M., C. S. Weisman, A. M. Rompalo, N. Ellish, D. M. Upchurch, E. W. Hook, and D. Celentano. 1995. Condom use to prevent incident STDs: The validity of self-reported condom use. *Sexually Transmitted Diseases* 22(1): 15–21.

Zulu, Eliya Msiyaphazi, and Gloria Chepngeno. 2003. Spousal communication about the risk of contracting HIV/AIDS in rural Malawi. *Demographic Research* 1: 247–78.

Index

abstinence, 17–18, *224*, 257–86; factors associated with, 257, 270, 272–74, 282–83, 362–66; primary, 17, *224*, 257–64, 274–79, 287–93; promotion, 17–18, 125, 138–41, 163–64, 221, 231–35, 272–73, 282–86, 355, *370–71*, 374–77, 389, 396, 404; secondary, 17, 264–70, 279–82, 290–93, 330–36; social ideals, 6–7, 17–18, 83–85, 111–12, 235, 271–72, 274–75, 305–6, 318, 363, 383; theoretical determinants of, 231–35. *See also* data validity; HIV prevention interventions; sexual behavior of unmarried youth

being faithful (including limiting partner number and/or being monogamous), 18–21, *224–25*, 287–320; before marriage, 183, 307–10, 378, 392–95; factors associated with, 287, 296–97, 302, 304–5, 307, 362–66; in marriage, 310–13, 395–96; promotion, 20–21, 139–40, 183, 221–22, 236–41, 299, 313–20, *370–71*, 373–78, 389–98, 402; social ideals, 6–7, 83–84, 11–12, 237–38, 240, 304–7, 313–14, 318, 363, 395; theoretical determinants of, 236–41; variable interpretation of,

18–19, 297, 300–301, 306, 375. *See also* data validity; HIV prevention interventions; sexual behavior of unmarried youth; sexual partner selectivity; sexual relationships of married youth

case study series, 38–39, 67; series 1 (youth who abstained), 257–70; series 2 (youth who limited partner number and/or were monogamous), 3, 287–97; series 3 (youth who used condoms), 3–4, 321–36

community-based programs, 23–24, *370–72*, 378–81, 384–402; couples, 285, 316, 319–20, *370–74*, 390–96; health worker, 23, 191–92, *370*, *372*, 399–400; mass media, 23, 27, 251, 314, 316–17, 351–52, *370*, 400–402; men, *370–72*, 388–91; microfinance and cash transfers, 15, 254, *370*, 383, 386–88, 397; out-of-school youth, *370*, 379–80, 384–86; parents, 317–19, *370–74*, 383–84, 396–98; peer education, 154, 356, *370*, 384–85, 389; people living with HIV/AIDS, *370*, 400; sport, 283, *370*, 385–86, 390–91; women, 15, 254, *370–72*, 386–88, 397. *See*

About the Author

Mary Louisa Plummer has worked in HIV/AIDS education, curriculum development, and program evaluation since 1988. Her academic background is in social sciences, biology, and languages (Swahili, Mandarin Chinese, and German). Her HIV-related work in Tanzania began with the development and testing of a secondary school curriculum in urban Mwanza in 1994. This was followed by process evaluations of two rural Mwanza primary school programs in 1997–1998. From 1999 to 2009, Mary was employed by the London School of Hygiene and Tropical Medicine, UK, first as a research fellow and then as a lecturer. From 1999 to 2002, she was also the social science coordinator for the *MEMA kwa Vijana* adolescent sexual health trial in Mwanza. In that capacity she co-led several of the trial impact and process evaluation surveys, and she coordinated the HALIRA qualitative study that is the basis for this book and its companion volume, *Young People's Lives and Sexual Relationships in Rural Africa* (2011). Mary has a PhD in comparative social and natural science methods (2004) and she is a British Academy Post-Doctoral Fellow (2005–2008). Currently she is an independent consultant based in Dar es Salaam, Tanzania, where she lives with her husband and three children. She can be contacted at mary.louisa.plummer@gmail.com.

Edwards Brothers Malloy
Thorofare, NJ USA
March 22, 2013